Behavioral concepts & nursing intervention

contributing authors

Margaret Baumgartner, R.N., M.S.
    Professor of Nursing, Fresno State College, Fresno, California

Betty Blackwell, R.N., M.S.
    Professor, Psychiatric Nursing, California State College, Los Angeles

Dorothy W. Bloch, R.N., M.S.
    Formerly Coordinator and Associate Professor of Psychiatric Nursing, University of Colorado School of Nursing, Denver

Perquilla Callaghan, R.N., M.N.
    Clinical Nursing Specialist, San Francisco General Hospital; Formerly Assistant Professor of Nursing, San Francisco State College, California

Carolyn E. Carlson, R.N., M.S.
    Formerly Assistant Professor of Nursing, University of California, Los Angeles

Rose Kemp, R.N., M.S.
    Formerly Assistant Professor of Psychiatric Nursing, Loretto Heights College, Denver, Colorado

Sister Mary Martha Kiening, R.N., M.S.
    Associate Professor of Nursing; Director Psychiatric and Mental Health Nursing Integration Project, University of San Francisco, California

Silvia Lange, R.N., M.N.
    Psychiatric Nurse, Community Mental Health Services, Day Center, San Diego, California; Formerly Assistant Professor and Director, Mental Health Program, Seattle University, Washington

Mary R. Lawrence, R.N., M.S.
    Associate Professor of Nursing, San Jose State College, California

Lucile L. Love, R.N., M.S.N.
    Assistant Professor of Nursing, University of Hawaii

Florence M. McDonald, R.N., M.A.
    Assistant Professor, School of Nursing, Stanford University, California

Dorothy V. Moses, R.N., M.S.
    Professor of Psychiatric and Geriatric Nursing, San Diego State College, California

Catherine M. Norris, R.N., Ed.D.
    Associate Professor of Nursing, University of Kansas, Kansas City

Vera M. Robinson, R.N., M.Litt.
    Associate Professor of Psychiatric Nursing, Indiana University, Indianapolis; Formerly Associate Professor of Mental Health Nursing, Colorado State College, Greeley

Mary Durand Thomas, R.N., M.S.N.
    Assistant Professor, Psychiatric Nursing Program, University of Washington, Seattle

Lucille M. Wilson, R.N., M.S.
    Associate Professor, School of Nursing, Montana State University, Bozeman

Behavioral concepts & nursing intervention

Coordinated by
CAROLYN E. CARLSON
*Formerly Assistant Professor of Nursing,
University of California, Los Angeles*

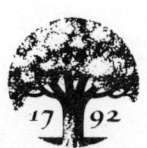

J. B. LIPPINCOTT COMPANY
Philadelphia   Toronto

This work was supported in large part by Grant Number 5 T 31 MH-9509 from the National Institute of Mental Health.

Copyright © 1970, by J. B. Lippincott Company

> This book is fully protected by copyright and, with the exception of brief excerpts for review, no part of it may be reproduced in any form, by print, photoprint, microfilm, or any other means, without the written permission of the publishers.

Distributed in Great Britain by
Blackwell Scientific Publications, Oxford and Edinburgh

Library of Congress Catalog Card Number 73-109948

Printed in the United States of America

foreword

By Esther A. Garrison, R.N., D. Sc., L.L.D.

Lecturer, School of Nursing, University of California, San Francisco; formerly Chief, Psychiatric Nursing Training Branch, Division of Manpower and Training Programs, National Institute of Mental Health, Public Health Service, U. S. Department of Health Education and Welfare.

Those persons responsible for the integration of social-behavioral and mental health content in nursing curricula will find this book particularly useful. Likewise, practitioners in all fields of nursing will welcome it as an invaluable source as they seek to increase their understanding and render more effective care to patients.

Behavioral Concepts and Nursing Intervention adds a new dimension and considerable expansion to a similar project undertaken and completed by the Southern Regional Education Board. It reflects a particular approach which allows for considerable variation not only in individual approach but in form and focus. The 18 concepts included herein are developed and presented with clarity worthy of note.

Obviously nurse educators and students in all types of programs will find this book an excellent teaching and learning tool. It is equally appropriate for use in formal academic courses and in continuing education.

acknowledgments

The coordinator, in behalf of the contributors, wishes to gratefully acknowledge some of the many persons and organizations who have contributed to the publication of this book. First, I would like to thank Lulu Wolf Hassenplug for her constant support and for making it possible for me to administer the project with complete freedom. I am greatly indebted to the deans and directors of the nursing programs where project participants were employed, for their support of the project and for their generous consent and administrative efforts in enabling participants to be away for two weeks during each academic year. Marguerite Cobb, Colette Kerlin, Alice Robinson and Shirley Yee gave meaningful critiques of the work midway in the project, and Elizabeth Cunningham, Cynthia H. Kelly, Edith P. Lewis and Thelma M. Schorr added the essential editorial consultation during the project's final stages. The efforts of all of these consultants are greatly appreciated.

Thanks also go to the Western Council on Higher Education in Nursing, which provided the impetus for the works herein, and to Esther Garrison and the National Institute of Mental Health, who gave their continuous consultation and support.

contents

Introduction 1
    Carolyn E. Carlson and Betty Blackwell

1. Denial of Illness 9
    Sister Mary Martha Kiening

2. Empathy 29
    Margaret Baumgartner

3. The Professional Nurse and Body Image 39
    Catherine M. Norris

4. Shame 67
    Silvia Lange

5. Grief and Mourning 95
    Carolyn E. Carlson

6. Trust in the Nurse-Patient Relationship 117
    Mary Durand Thomas

7. Humor in Nursing 129
    Vera M. Robinson

8. Listening 153
    Lucille M. Wilson

9. Reality Orientation in the Aging Person 171
    Dorothy V. Moses

10. Hostility 187
    Sister Mary Martha Kiening

11. Ambivalence 207
    Rose Kemp

12. Transactional Analysis and Nursing 227
    Silvia Lange

13. Privacy 251
    Dorothy Bloch

14. Inquiry 269
    Florence McDonald

15. Development of Awareness of Self for the Professional Nursing Student 283
    Perquilla Callaghan
16. The Process of Role Change 303
    Lucile L. Love
17. Stigma 317
    Betty Blackwell
18. Relationship Control 331
    Mary R. Lawrence

Introduction

Carolyn E. Carlson and Betty Blackwell

The focus of this book is on a vitally important but underdeveloped area of nursing knowledge. Popular phrases such as "meeting patient's emotional needs", "giving emotional support" and "preventing emotional stress" have been with us for years; sprinkling them throughout the literature has become ritual. However, the meaning of such statements, and methods of accomplishing the goals associated with them, have not been adequately defined. In the development of the content of this book, the authors have attempted to create a prototype wherein relevant behavioral-mental health concepts are identified, examined, and demonstrated in a nursing context.

In recent years the Federal Government and nursing organizations have supported many projects designed to strengthen and to integrate social-behavioral and mental health content in nursing curricula. Several publications have focused on the integration of these concepts in nursing, yet the emphases have largely been on process and problems involved in integrating the concepts rather than on their content. For example, the proceedings of the 1958 Regional Conferences on Psychiatric Nursing Education[1] exemplify the focus on process and problems; however, psychiatric or mental health concepts were not delineated or operationalized. At another conference in 1959 an attempt was made to identify some mental health concepts that should be integrated in the nursing curricula.[2] One criticism of the description of these concepts was that they were stated much too broadly and generally to be meaningful. The report of a work conference in 1962[3] also demonstrates the need for clearly defined and operationalized mental health concepts. Some concepts were listed, but criteria for selection of the concepts and the scope and depth of the concepts were not included. Pesznecker and Hewitt[4] sum up the problem in stating the "progress toward identifying the appropriate concepts and content to be included throughout the basic program has really just begun." These early projects paved the way for present and future efforts to add to nursing knowledge and improve the quality of patient care. They provided the necessary foundation for continued pursuit of these goals.

Concern over lack of definition and operationalization of behavioral and mental health concepts is based on the assumption that the nurse practitioner needs an understanding of these concepts in order to promote emotional health of patients beyond that which she could do by chance or intuition. Anyone who has cared for others can recall situations in which she wished she could understand and comfort, or in which she said or did something that helped but did not know why or how. Both circumstances find the care giver without the knowledge or ability to understand what the receiver of care is experiencing. She doesn't know what in her own behavior has helped the patient, and is not able to analyze the nurse-patient interaction. Such lack of knowledge or understanding makes it difficult to transfer learning from one situation to another.

Understanding of concepts that help to explain behavior is considered essential for promoting emotional health; however, understanding alone will not necessarily lead to the desired outcome. Each individual must learn to put this understanding into action. In part, this requires the study of how the nurse's behavior is perceived by the patient and vice versa.

At least two recent projects provide evidence that concern over the development of content to explain patient behavior is being complemented by action. In 1968 the Southern Regional Education Board published the results of a project that focused on *Developing Behavioral Concepts in Nursing*[5]. Five concepts for nursing intervention that were developed are included in its report.

The chapters in this book represent the work of a second project group consisting of nurse educators in the Western Region.[6] A detailed report of the project was published by the Western Interstate Commission for Higher Education[7] in 1970. The purpose of this project was to identify, define and develop behavioral and mental health content that nurses need to acquire in order to meet the emotional needs of patients. Since there was no tried and true method previously established for identifying and defining this content, only general guidelines were adopted for participants to follow in selecting and developing their respective areas of content. Absence of a rigid format led to considerable variation in the way the authors approached the task, as well as in the form and focus of the work produced. Thus, the chapters that follow represent various philosophies of nursing and, consequently, different conceptual and theoretical frames of reference.

There are, perhaps, advantages in not requiring a common frame of reference. At present, members of the nursing profession are attempting to define the role of nursing in the health care system which has become extremely complex owing to the increasing numbers of types of health workers and the changing needs of society. Stands on this issue vary, and it is difficult at this point in time to accept or reject any of them unconditionally. Until the issue is clarified or resolved, it seems that much can be gained from individuals' developing content according to their own individual views of nursing. The increasing popularity of the use of compilations of readings in courses in nursing can be viewed as an indication that nurse practitioners and educators desire exposure to many points of view, or wish to select articles which support or extend their individual conceptions of nursing.

The following discussion utilizes one theoretical frame of reference in which the content of the articles might be applied in nursing practice and nursing education.

THE EVOLUTION OF NURSING CONTENT AND ONE FRAME OF REFERENCE IN WHICH TO VIEW THE CONTENT

Man makes his world understandable, and hence manageable, by reliance on a system of beliefs which tend to explain the phenomena he encounters in his everyday life. In the Western world, these explanatory concepts are derived increasingly from the body of scientific knowledge. For the nurse, knowledge and theory derive from those truths discovered or postulated by the natural and behavioral scientists. The selection by nurses of certain of these truths as ones which will best explain the interactional phenomena of their professional everyday life not only makes everyday situations manageable but also contributes to the ongoing development of the interaction itself.

In the past when nursing education and practice derived the bulk of their operational principles from the natural and medical sciences, the value that every patient was entitled to equal care meant such things as: he would be kept clean; his medications and treatments would be given on time and in the proper dosages; his eliminative needs would be provided for; and he would receive humane treatment regardless of his socioeconomic status, race or religion. Contextual factors such as severity of illness and availability of personnel were used to delimit the definition of equal treatment.

This combination of natural and medical science principles and the value of equal treatment may be seen as one causative factor in the ritualization of certain nursing practices. Included among these practices are strict adherence to the time scheduling of the patient's activities of daily living, functional assignment of nursing personnel, increased bureaucratization of the health agencies and isolation of the patient from his family and community.

More recently, psychiatric principles have been added to those of the natural and medical sciences to be used as explanatory tools in defining the tasks and functions of the nurse's role. The value of equal treatment has been joined by one stressing the uniqueness of each individual, as well as his sharing of mental-emotional processes with other human beings. Acceptance of this value meant not only the substitution of jargon such as "anxiety" for "nervousness", but also adding the nursing task of "talking to" (psychotherapeutic interviewing) to the previously defined one of "doing for." Variables such as severity of illness, availability of personnel, the ambivalence of physicians toward psychiatry, and the nurse's definition of proper utilization of time were used to delimit the definition of mental-emotional uniqueness or similarity of the individual patient.

This combination of psychiatric, medical and natural science concepts with the values of equal treatment and the individual's mental-emotional uniqueness or similarity, has resulted in the deritualization of some nursing and health agency practices. Examples of "personalization of care" include consideration for patient preference in the timing of his activities of daily living, liberalization of policies concerning family participation in patient care and emotional support, assignment to nurses of total patient care, and alteration of the role expectation for the nursing supervisor from that of disciplinarian to human relations expert.

Most recently, findings from psychology, anthropology and sociology have been added to those mentioned previously. The values of equal treatment and individual uniqueness and emotional-mental similarity have been expanded by selected concepts from the behavioral sciences such as ethnic-socioeconomic differences, small-group influences on behavior, and health organizations as social systems. Acceptance of this expanded definition of the values of equal treatment and individual uniqueness had led to the expectation that the nurse will consciously consider the patient's ethnicity and socioeconomic status as variables influencing his response to illness and to treatment. Consideration of the influences of the small group and the organization as a social system have led to changes in nursing practice such as utilization of the team approach, of the therapeutic community, of group teaching to patients and their families, of in-outpatient care continuity and, incidentally, of power politics in the redefinition of the nurse's status within the organization hierarchy. To delimit the definition of equal care and individual uniqueness, contextual factors such as those previously mentioned have been joined by society's assessment of the worth of particular ethnic and socio-economic groups and inter- and intra- profession disagreements on the proper use of the nurse's time.

The articles in this volume illustrate the applications of concepts from single or from several academic disciplines. For example, Blackwell's article on *Stigma* is almost completely dependent upon a sociological frame of reference; Lange's on *Shame* and Bloch's on *Privacy* combine sociological, psychological and psychiatric frames; Norris's on *Body Image* adds to these three disciplines concepts from medicine and natural science.

Utilizing these four typical articles to demonstrate one possible method of application of the content reveals the following features:

1. The concepts are universally applicable. They are not restricted by type or severity of illness or by specific social contexts.

2. Definitions of each concept involve discussion of what it is not. For instance, Lange must define guilt in order to clearly delineate the features of shame.

3. Individually, the concepts do not explain fully any everyday occurrence. Despite the universal applicability of certain individual concepts, each of the authors in suggesting application to nursing

practice brings in the influence of additional concepts to explain the phenomena occurring in the actual situation.

4. The elaboration of the concept does not spell out under what circumstances that particular concept would best explain the phenomena under observation. Nor does it predict specific behavior as a consequence of application of the concept.

A careful reading of these four articles will demonstrate the first two features mentioned above. The interrelatedness of the selected concepts is demonstrated by the inability of any one of them to be fully persuasive without consideration of each of the other three. One cannot imagine an everyday situation in which shame is recognized without equal recourse to the ideas of stigma, privacy, and body image—although, as Lange points out, these three concepts do not compose the totality of explanatory conceptualizations presently available to the practitioner.

The fourth feature mentioned above perhaps is most demonstrative of the state of tested knowledge in both nursing and the behavioral sciences. Norris in the introduction to her paper on body image suggests that adequate conceptualization is one of the first steps in developing nursing knowledge. The authors of this volume have endeavored to achieve such adequate conceptualizations.

USE OF THE BOOK

Since the articles have not been written from a common philosophical or conceptual base and were not written expressly for a specific course or curriculum, it is not necessary that they be read in sequence. Sections can be used individually or in combination with others. The interrelatedness of some of the concepts has been discussed. The content is sufficiently broad to be applicable in any setting in which nursing is practiced, and in a wide variety of courses in nursing curricula. Examples might be fundamentals and the clinical areas, plus more specialized courses such as interpersonal processes in nursing, introduction to nursing problems, and nursing seminars.

These topics are relevant for students at any point in their education. The content can be used to introduce the student to the world of the patient and the process of identifying patient problems, or to suggest methods of intervention in situations involving particular nursing or patient problems. It can also be helpful as background for developing research problems. In many cases it will be meaningful to re-read certain articles at various stages in the curriculum to accomplish different objectives or to become resensitized to the phenomena that patients experience. Thus, the book can be used as a text in many courses in nursing, for inservice educational programs, and as a resource book for the nurse practitioner to use on her own.

The reader will find that the topics covered here are neither exhaustive nor disjointed. The understanding of any nurse-patient interaction or specific patient problems requires the synthesis of knowledge from numerous sources. No doubt, the unknown by far outweighs the known with regard to understanding behavior. The various authors have attempted to draw upon pertinent knowledge to answer some questions and to raise questions for future study.

REFERENCES

1. National League for Nursing: Concepts of the Behavioral Sciences in Basic Nursing Education. Proceedings of the 1958 Regional Conferences in Psychiatric Nursing Education sponsored by the National League for Nursing, 1958.
2. National League for Nursing: Psychiatric Nursing Concepts and Basic Nursing Education. Proceedings of the Conference at Boulder, Colorado, June 15-18, 1959. pp. 121-149. New York, National League for Nursing, 1960.
3. National League for Nursing: Integration of Psychiatric Nursing Concepts in Baccalaureate Basic Programs. Report of Work Conference held at Chicago, April, 1962. New York, National League for Nursing, 1963.
4. Pesznecker, B. L., and Hewitt, H. E.: Psychiatric Content in the Nursing Curriculum. p. 102. Seattle, University of Washington Press, 1963.
5. Zderad, L. T., and Belcher, H. C.: Developing Behavioral Concepts in Nursing. Atlanta, Southern Regional Education Board, 1968.
6. Four year project supported by Grant Number 5 T 31 MH-9509 from the National Institute of Mental Health, Public Health Service, U.S. Department of Health, Education and Welfare, awarded to the Department of Continuing Education in Medicine and Health Sciences, University of California, Los Angeles.
7. Carlson, C. E., Norris, C. M., Lange, S., Blackwell, B., and Moses, D.: Identification of Basic Mental Health Content in Nursing. Boulder, Western Interstate Commission for Higher Education, 1970.

1
Denial of Illness

Sister Mary Martha Kiening

The impact of illness, and its many implications concerning the sick person's ability to deal with a changed life situation, has important connotations for the effectiveness of nursing care. The threat to the self-system depends not only upon the actual degree of physical disequilibrium brought about by the illness itself but, more importantly, upon the alteration of the self-concept that takes place as a result of impaired physical functioning. One of the ways in which an individual may deal with the stress produced by the threat to his integrity is to deny the threat. Denial operates to allay anxiety by reducing the perception of the threat.

The concept of denial has been treated extensively in psychiatric literature; more recently, there has been increasing focus on denial as an adaptive maneuver used to reduce anxiety generated by crippling, disabling or socially unacceptable diseases. That the nursing profession is beginning to recognize the importance of denial as a nursing problem that sometimes seriously interferes with the patient's plan of care is attested to by the still more recent articles written by nurses.[1,2]

The tendency to deny the seriousness of an illness and its possible outcome for the individual has long been noted by health workers. Perhaps one of the earliest comments on this tendency is by Benjamin Rush in his account of the yellow fever epidemic in Philadelphia in the year 1793. With something akin to wonder, he remarks that these patients, even in the advanced stages of the disease:

> did not acknowledge that they had any other indisposition than a common cold. I was particularly struck with the self-deception in many persons who had nursed relatives who had died with yellow fever and who had

been exposed to it in neighborhoods where it had prevailed for days and even weeks with great mortality...Perhaps it would be proper to rank that self-deception with respect to the nature and danger of the disease which was so universal among the instances of derangement of mind.[3]

It may be said that all defenses operate to deny reality in one way or another. Such terms as dissociation, repression, selective inattention and suppression all have to do with unconsciously denying entry of material into consciousness. Freud distinguishes between repression and denial when he says:

> If we wish to differentiate between what happens to the idea distinct from the affect we can restrict 'repression' to relate to the affect; the correct word for what happens to the idea is then 'denial'.[4]

Denial is a defense mechanism operating outside of and beyond conscious awareness in the endeavor to resolve emotional conflict and to allay anxiety. It achieves its purpose by disowning, rejecting or ignoring one or more of the elements of the conflict. Obvious reality factors that the person finds painful or unpleasant are perceived as a threat to the self-structure and treated as if they did not exist. If the threat cannot be escaped or attacked, anxiety may be reduced and comfort re-established by denying its existence. Reality is rejected or distorted and replaced by wish-fulfilling or "as-if" behavior. The person may explicitly deny verbally what is perceived, or he may act as if the painful situation did not exist. Unpleasant and intolerable facts, wishes, thoughts and actions are disowned by an unconscious process of elimination.

For purposes of this discussion, denial is defined as the kind of behavior that indicates a failure to accept either an obvious fact or its significance to the individual involved in the situation. Operationally, we may say that denying behavior includes the following steps:

1. A reality situation exists.
2. The individual perceives or anticipates some element in the situation as threatening.
3. Anxiety occurs in response to the perceived threat.
4. Either the facts, or their significance in the threat-producing situation, are completely or partially disclaimed.
5. Psychological equilibrium is temporarily regained and maintained by ignoring or rejecting objective evidence connected with the threatening situation.

The denial, however, serves only to cover or minimize the anxiety-provoking aspects of the reality that constitutes the threat. So long as the person can maintain his denial in the face of objective evidence, it serves as an effective protection against overwhelming anxiety. Its inconsistency with reality makes it a very brittle defense, however, and when it finally must come face to face with reality it crumbles, leaving the person defenseless. As reality begins to storm the bastion of denial, depression may result, possibly leading to personality disorganization or even suicide.

Denial is one of the earliest and most primitive of the defense mechanisms and is thought to precede even the mechanism of repression in the developing infantile ego. Its earliest and most rudimentary manifestations may be seen in the very young infant who deals with disturbing external stimuli by closing his eyes, then by turning his head away. In this early stage, it consists, perhaps, simply of a separation of that which is unpleasant or anxiety-producing from the rest of the emerging personality organization. By the time the infant begins to experience the early forms of anxiety, the mechanism of denial has been established and soon begins to operate automatically in the service of the ego. Miller classes denial with the "first family" of defenses, all of which have four common features: (a) they seem applicable to every type of conflict, (b) their use requires no previous learning, (c) they distort reality markedly and (d) they are of little help in solving real social difficulties.[5]

Denial as a part of the normal developmental process is readily observed in the play of children in which the child uses fantasy to live in a world of his own creation and in which unpleasant reality can be reversed or blotted out. The normal child, however, can readily abandon his play and return to the everyday world upon demand. Although vestiges of this mechanism linger even into mature adulthood, frank denial in the face of obvious reality in an adult is usually an indication of serious mental illness, particularly if it persists for any length of time.

Interruptions to health always pose some threat to the individual's life situation. Although the fear of death or disability looms as an important factor in the patient's response to the impact of illness, there are many other needs the fulfillment of which is jeopardized by an alteration in physical or psychological well-being. Even a minor health problem calls for some readjustment in the self-concept of the person who has previously seen himself as "whole" or "well" and is

12   Denial of Illness

now faced with a change in body image, be it ever so slight. Pride, self-esteem, sense of achievement and power, self-identity, and sexual identification are only a few of the self-attributes which undergo change as the individual finds himself thrust away from wellness and mastery into illness and loss of control over his life situation.

Denial of illness can, at times, seriously interfere with the treatment program. It may defeat the nurse's best efforts to establish a helping relationship with her patient. On the other hand it may, and often does, serve as a protection for the ego, preventing the person from becoming overwhelmed by anxiety and averting extensive emotional disorganization. If this defense is too forcibly undermined in an attempt to make the patient "deal with reality," he may become increasingly disorganized, and a severe depression may be the result. It is important, then, that the nurse learn to: (1) recognize the manifestations of denial, (2) be able to assess the degree to which it is impeding the patient's progress toward regained health, (3) understand the dynamics of the behavior, (4) try to determine the need which the denial is serving and then, (5) make a nursing decision that best serves the needs of the patient at this time. This decision must take into account the fact that ego support must be given high priority in the treatment goal. If the behavior by which the patient communicates his distortions or rejection of reality is not understood, it is more likely to trigger anxiety, resentment and anger on the nurse's part, thus making it even more difficult for the patient to obtain the help which he needs at this time.

The range of behavior along the continuum of denial is wide. There are differences, both in the level of awareness at which denial operates, and in the degree to which reality is excluded. Explicit verbal denial can be a symptom of severe emotional disturbance; the blind person who denies that he cannot see, the paraplegic who insists that he can move the paralyzed arm or leg. This complete denial can only occur as a result of serious psychological disequilibrium; yet the vestiges of this primitive, automatic response to sudden threat remain even in the mature, normal adult. The shocked, "Oh, no," "It can't be," "I can't believe it!" with which tragic news is often met is denial operating on a higher level of awareness and in a much shorter time-span, but completely shutting out the unwelcome fact. It is as if the ego needs to stand back in order to gain time to absorb a shattering emotional impact. Full realization and acceptance are never accomplished all at once.

A more common way of denying illness is by disowning or ignoring only certain aspects of it. This is typified by the coronary patient who experiences substernal pain, but attributes it to something he ate; or by the injured athlete who makes plans to play in the next big game in spite of rather extensive incapacitation. The ideals of health, beauty and eternal youth fostered in our society exploit the tendency to deny the realities of a changing body image concomitant with maturity and aging. Tenure, prestige and social advancement that come with increasing years are goals for which to strive, but the physical marks of aging, grey hair, wrinkles and decreasing physical vitality, are aspects of aging that are ignored, disowned—in short, denied—a denial actively encouraged in our contemporary culture.

Some patients, while not denying explicitly, tend to minimize the illness or certain aspects of it. Expressions such as "It's not so bad," "It could be worse," "It will all turn out all right" may be used to minimize the entire unpleasant experience of the illness. Or certain symptoms and syndromes may be minimized, as in the case of Benjamin Rush's yellow fever patients who acknowledged the symptoms, but attributed them to a cold.

Where denial is explicitly verbalized, the evidence is clear and the nurse can validate her hypothesis that the patient is denying, simply by listening to what he says and then consulting obvious reality as she sees it and as it has been consensually validated by others.

Behavioral clues to implicit denial may pose more of a problem for the nurse. Because they are often acted out, these clues may not be so easily recognized. Here again, the range of the behavior is wide—from the quiet, reticent, model patient whose understatement of his needs may be so great that the medical staff and his family overlook his real feelings and requirements to the hostile, "uncooperative" patient who flagrantly violates his medical orders. Clues to denial may be picked up all along the continuum by the observant, knowledgeable nurse. How the nurse validates these clues and follows through on them will depend first of all, upon her astuteness, and then upon the need they serve for the patient, the patient's tolerance for stress and, of course, upon the nurse's own feelings and degree of self-awareness and her ability to cope with her feelings.

Fisher, in speaking of patients with severe, long-term physical disability such as amputation, says that if the basic emotions of anxiety, depression and anger are not exhibited, one should suspect the presence of defenses such as denial, for "such feelings are a normal and realistic reaction to a genuine threat."[6] Other manifestations of implicit denial may include missed clinic appointments, failure to carry out a prescribed treatment regimen, refusal of medication, selective inattention to the symptoms of the illness, or a cheerfulness that seems inappropriate in the face of the reality factors. Changes relating to attitudes about food, bowel and urinary function, physical contacts and sexual behavior were reported by Weinstein in his group of patients with neurological damage.[7] Humor is frequently employed as a denial mechanism. Some patients may use the second or third person in referring to the illness. A common form of implicit denial is the displacement of concern about the illness to another person or describing the illness in terms of what other people said or did: "The doctor said I had a stroke." Many people tend to reassure themselves by plunging into over-activity as if to convince themselves that the symptoms are an illusion or at least trivial. Some men see their masculinity threatened by illness and so may engage in a dangerous denial of symptoms through over-activity.

Basic to any discussion of behavioral dynamics is the question: "What need is the behavior serving?" Denial has been classed as one of the major defense mechanisms and, as such, came to have a somewhat negative connotation. Recent literature, however, reflects a more positive view. Although most authorities agree that support or reinforcement of the denial are highly questionable therapeutically, there is a growing respect for the protection which this mechanism affords the ego in times of overwhelming emotional onslaught. All authorities seem to agree that the defense should certainly not be attacked directly, and most seem to think that as the stress of the anxiety-producing situation is ameliorated, the person's need will likewise decrease.

An area receiving increasing attention is that of the psychological needs of the dying patient. In a review of the literature, only one author favored support of the denial, Whal.[8] He states that the physician's task is to strengthen and buttress the natural and ever-present defenses of denial, and adds that no patient should ever be told he is going to die, even if he assures the physician that he wants the "naked truth." This is an extreme position with which most authorities do not agree. Among those who have reported extensive work with dying patients, Glaser and Strauss state emphatically, "on the whole, there is much to recommend giving the patient an opportunity actively to manage his own dying . . . staff members could soften the disclosure, handle the depression so as to encourage acceptance and guide the patient into active preparation for death."[9] This latter position seems more in accord with a philosophy that acknowledges the right of the individual to know whatever facts will enable him to make judgments and decisions based on reality and his dignity as a human person.

Chodoff and Hamburg make some interesting observations on denial as a "normal" way of dealing with anxiety, and they remind the reader that so much of the knowledge of the defense mechanisms has been derived from the study of neurotic persons that there is danger of considering these mechanisms as pathogenic in themselves. Viewed from the standpoint of normality, denial may be thought of as coping behavior, that is, one of the "psychic activities by which the adaptive process is brought about. It (coping behavior) can be seen as consisting of two aspects, an externally directed one judged for its effectiveness in social terms and an internally directed or defensive aspect which serves to protect the individual from disruptive degrees of anxiety and which is judged for adequacy by the degree of comfort resulting."[10] In fact, denial is so closely related to hope that it may be difficult for the nurse to make a distinction in terms of observable behavior on which to validate her assumption that denial is really operating.

Speaking of the anxiety generated in the patient by the knowledge that he has cancer, Brauer makes the point that the patient usually has available counterbalancing, reconstructive forces within himself which can be encouraged and supported by the therapist. He goes on to say that the average patient is susceptible to a healthy reorientation and adjustment and can balance the reality of his disease with the proper amount of denial.[11]

The process by which adaptation takes place, beginning with denial and progressing through various stages of coping behavior, has been delineated by Visotsky and his associates. These authors noted much individual variation, but were able to perceive a broad sequence which characterized the stages most of these patients went through over the months and years.[12] Although the transition from one phase to another is a gradual process with no clearly perceptible line of demarcation, it can be described as occurring in a more or less sequential fashion. Garrard and Richmond, in working with the parents of children with a chronic illness or handicap, have identified three phases in the sequence:

1. *A period of disorganization*
    a. Great anxiety is usually present. There are efforts to deny or minimize the impact in one way or another, but the defensive mechanisms are almost completely ineffective in coping with the stress.
2. *A period of reintegration*
    a. During this period, which usually coincides with the acute period of the illness, there is extensive use of defenses—in this case, extensive denial of the nature of the illness, its seriousness and its probable outcome.
    b. Denial is rarely effective in completely relieving distress. There is gradual acknowledgement of some of the more obvious aspects of reality about the illness.
3. *A period of mature adaptation*
    a. Most of the realities of the situation can be faced.
    b. There is an appropriate response to this confrontation with reality, such as seeking information about the factors relevant to the illness and assessments of the probable long-term limitations.
    c. This phase is usually characterized by periods of depression which may be looked upon as normal grief and mourning.
    d. Resolution of the conflict by the slow transition from a self-concept of physical vigor to one of physical limitations.[13]

Although phases 1 and 2 have been most extensively dealt with in the literature, the series of approximations and adaptive behavior that follows the initial phase may have been given less recognition than it deserves, and may have more significant implications for the nurse. Phase 3 is, of course, the desirable goal in psychological management, and it is one that some persons never reach or attain only incompletely. It is while the patient is gradually coming to a realization of his changed life situation that the nurse's understanding, acceptance and support become increasingly important. An accurate assessment of his anxiety level, and appropriate nursing intervention (or non-intervention), may be crucial in helping him to regain emotional equilibrium and to focus on the problem to be mastered.

Denial of illness, either explicit or implicit, is not confined to the person who is ill. It is a behavioral pattern commonly encountered in the family threatened by the illness of a member. In speaking of the coping ability of patients with cancer, Brauer says that it is not the patient as much as the family who needs our help.[14]

Extensive studies of family denial in relation to children have been carried out by a number of investigators. Woodfall, in working with the families of mentally retarded children, reports a range of behavior in parents from complete denial to denial of certain aspects of the problem.[15] The sense of failure generated by the production of a defective child, whom the parent sees as a projection of himself, may lead to attempts to minimize or disown the obvious signals of arrested development in the child's behavior. When there is complete denial, the parents are prevented from using available community services and thus providing the child with the professional help needed. In cases of minimal denial, the parents may not accept certain aspects of the illness. They may have a more constructive approach toward treatment goals, but their goals tend to be limited because of the inability to acknowledge the full reality of the illness.

Garrard and Richmond, who observed the use of denial by parents of children with chronic disease, report that this denial occurred to some extent in all such parents until a more mature adaptation was achieved.[16] This was revealed in such behavior as misunderstanding the physician's explanation, repetitious questions and "shopping around" for medical advice or treatment. Davidman and his associates cited resentment, avoidance, seclusion and over-protection as manifestations of denial in the parents of deaf, blind and mute children.[17] Such reactions cause the parents to avoid teaching the child and to prevent him from learning such special skills as he would need to foster the ability to communicate.

Bozeman, in working with mothers of leukemic children, found that all mothers in the series attempted to deny, in one way or another, the implications of the diagnosis, either by screening out the reality of the situation or engaging in compulsive efforts to reverse it. In some instances, the denial could not be relinquished for several months; however, none of the mothers attempted to deny the illness itself.[18]

Chodoff reports a series of observations of parents who seemed to be projecting their denial onto their chronically ill children. The parents could not acknowledge that their children were aware of what was happening, although there seemed to be ample evidence that the latter were not being fooled by the elaborate stratagems employed to keep them in ignorance of the real facts.[19]

Denial may be employed by members of the helping professions as well as by patients and their families, and it is here, perhaps, that it has its greatest effect on the quality of care. Bernstein, in a pithy article on the unmarried mother, has this to say:

> the unmarried mother's use of denial is a source of some concern to social workers. . . . in assessing the meaning of denial we may do well to take cognizance of our own role in fostering it. As agents of the community we offer the unmarried pregnant girl anonymity in a protected shelter; we provide out-of-town mailing addresses; we encourage her to deny her maternity by plans for the early placement of her baby so she can resume her place in the community as though nothing had happened.[20]

Medical and nursing staff may actively foster and encourage denial in patients and families as a result of their own reactions of helplessness, frustration, or anger in an emotionally charged situation. References in the literature to the use of denial by the staff are somewhat scanty, particularly when one considers the rather extensive treatment of this mechanism in relation to patients and families.

However, a recent study by Glaser and Strauss explores in some detail the many ways in which both the physician and the nursing staff attempt to deny or avoid the issue when it is known that a patient's illness is terminal. Observed behavior ranged from elaborate rituals for keeping patient and family unaware, to elaborate games of mutual pretension in which both staff member and patient were aware, but neither wished to admit this openly to the other.[21]

In dealing with denial of illness as a nursing problem, the nurse needs to to able to assess, first of all, the extent to which the denial is harmful, and, then, the extent to which it is therapeutic for the patient. For example, the psychiatric patient who completely and actively denies his illness cannot benefit from a therapeutic program until this problem is recognized and at least partially resolved. In other circumstances, denial may be recognized as operating, but not as presenting a particular nursing problem at the time—in fact, it may be the emergency "brake" that prevents complete disorganization in the face of a crisis with which the person has not yet been able to cope. What is sometimes interpreted as pathology may be the valid use of a healthy protecting mechanism, or it may not even be denial at all, since many patients are very well aware of their illness and its implications, but choose consciously to face this alone rather than add to the stress and anxiety of other family members.

The nurse is perhaps more intimately involved than any other person on the health team with patients' behavior and its effect on the success or failure of medical treatment. She is in a unique position, not only to observe denial of illness, but also to make the necessary nursing judgments, and to intervene therapeutically in reducing anxiety in assisting the patient and family to accept and to deal with the painful reality factors that are being denied. However, before she can begin to be effective on any level with the person who is denying illness, the nurse must first be able to look at herself and her own reactions. How she sees the situation and what she does about it will both depend upon: (1) her own awareness of her feelings regarding the patient and his illness; (2) the coping patterns which she has developed as part of her behavior for meeting stress situations; (3) her perception of herself in the professional role as a member of the treatment team; and (4) her relationships with the rest of the nursing staff and other members of the health team.

In a series of observations made by a group of faculty members in various clinical settings to which students were assigned for learning experiences, denial was found to be employed frequently by patients, family members and staff. In some of the following examples, nursing intervention was effective in reducing anxiety and reducing the need for denial; in others, it was only partially effective or not effective at all. The manifestations of denial ranged from a sudden reaction, to increased anxiety, or a well-entrenched pattern of behavior of pathological proportions.

In a sudden reaction, intervention may be effective or ineffective.

A newly admitted patient was scheduled for a complete diagnostic study on the following morning. The evening of his admission, the nursing aide approached the patient, saying: "Mr. A, you have been scheduled for an arteriogram in the morning. Has anyone told you what to expect?"

Patient (angrily): "No, and I don't want to know. Why is everyone so anxious to give me all the information? I'm better off if I don't know what's going to happen."

The aide excused herself and left the room.

A more sensitive appraisal of the patient's anxiety level might have elicited a less dramatic response on the part of the patient. The failure to recognize the high anxiety level resulted in a nursing action which increased rather than reduced the anxiety so that the nurse aide's attempt to be helpful precipitated the need to deny. A more therapeutic approach might have resulted in the patient's being helped to deal with the anxiety in a more constructive way.

A middle-aged woman patient, scheduled for minor surgery in the morning, approached the nurse. Anxiety was obvious: the pallor, dry lips, the worried look on her face and the wringing of her hands as she spoke:
Patient: "I'm so afraid I'll hemorrhage again. It's crazy to be so frightened, just crazy."
Nurse: "You're afraid you will hemorrhage?"
Patient: "Oh, now you do frighten me . . . you think I can hemorrhage?"
Nurse: "But you said that at the beginning . . ."
Patient: "No. I didn't say that. Do you think I might have a cardiac arrest?"

The nurse at this point decided to remain and listen. For half an hour she sat with the patient, permitting her to talk freely of her fears about the coming surgery. At the end of this time she appeared much calmer and mentioned a television show which she had planned to watch that evening. The nurse helped her select the channel and remained long enough to assure herself that the patient was involved in the program.

The nurse's intervention was based on accurate assessment of the patient's anxiety—the quick denial seemed to indicate the patient's extreme need for help in dealing with her anxiety at this time. It was neither necessary nor desirable to deal directly with the denial since the real issue was not the fact that the patient was using the mechanism but the fact that anxiety had to be dealt with and reduced to manageable proportions if this patient was to successfully weather this particular crisis situation.

Denial is also used as an attempt to adjust to the threat of loss or change.

A former nursing supervisor, nearing 75 years of age, was retired when certain positions were restructured in her hospital. After retirement, she suffered what appeared to be a "little stroke." However, she was not incapacitated and she decided that she could do volunteer work regularly at the hospital. It soon became evident that this schedule was too strenuous for her, but she insisted that she could continue. When her relatives insisted that she discontinue this work she said: "I don't know why I am not allowed to do this. There is nothing wrong with me." When she was reminded that she had been ill: "I didn't have a stroke, and there is nothing wrong with me. The doctor said that he wanted me to keep busy." She engaged in many activities and went to many community affairs and events.

One of the nurses at the hospital, recognizing this behavior as part of the crisis of aging, found opportunities to engage in conversation with her. She attempted to emphasize the things the patient could still do well and to help her find less demanding activities in which she could still feel useful and productive.

Here again, a frontal attack on the denial might have resulted in even greater efforts on the part of the patient to retain the one mechanism which allayed the anxiety and restored at least a measure of comfort and security. The nurse correctly assessed the behavior as indicating a need to feel wanted and productive and geared her efforts toward an attempt to work with the patient's strengths in a positive way. It is quite probable that the denial will reoccur if the patient again finds herself in a position where her self-concept is threatened; or she may go on further to depression if the situation continues and her denial begins to lose its effectiveness over the long haul of adjusting to loss of self-esteem and usefulness.

The following situation illustrates how the nurse assisted a family member to begin to adjust to the loss of a loved one. It is important to note that the nurse's role was two-fold: first, in assisting the mother to face reality and, perhaps more importantly, supporting her in the difficult period which immediately followed this realization.

The mother of an eight-year-old child who lay dying of a fatal illness, repeatedly turned to the nurse with such comments as: "She is going to get well, isn't she?" The nurse met each question with a simple statement of fact: "She is very, very sick." Since the mother spoke English very poorly, a Spanish-speaking aide was found to explain to the mother in her own language that the little girl did not have much longer to live. After the aide left, the nurse remained in the room with the mother, offering support by her physical presence and empathic attitude. She permitted the mother to give as much physical care and comfort to the little girl as she wished.

Nursing intervention here was directed, first, toward relief of the mother's anxiety. The nurse's supportive attitude was one factor; establishing a more familiar psychological climate for the mother by providing someone who spoke her language was another. When denial was recognized the need for it was accepted, but it was not reinforced; the nurse pointed out reality by a simple statement of fact. Anxiety was then again anticipated and reduced by the helping relationship of the nurse and her co-worker and by permitting the mother to become actively involved in a specific task directed toward the comfort and relief of her child.

22 Denial of Illness

An attractive woman in her late thirties was admitted for investigation of a lump in her breast. She denied concern by talking incessantly, joking and laughing with everyone who came into her room. The nurse, observing this behavior, tried first of all to adopt a quiet, accepting, listening attitude. She walked up and down the corridor with the patient as a means of helping reduce anxiety and making herself available. No attempt was made to comment on the patient's behavior or to explore her feelings about the forthcoming surgery. Although the nurse recognized the need for this, the patient was apparently not yet ready for such intervention.

In this case, further nursing intervention would have been for the nurse to plan frequent short contacts with the patient. During these periods the nurse would attempt to gain the patient's trust by establishing herself as an interested, helpful person, and would listen for cues that might indicate the patient's readiness to talk about herself, the forthcoming surgery, and what it meant to her. This should be done before the operation, because a secondary reaction later might result in a depression and a more serious problem for the patient and for her subsequent nursing care.

In working with the patient who seems to be using denial as a coping mechanism, the nurse must first determine:

1. How well defined the reality factors are.

2. What aspects of the patient's behavior are open to direct observation and can therefore be checked.

3. What protective function denial is serving at this time and how strong the patient's need for it is.

4. What other means are available to him for the reduction of his anxiety at this time.

Particularly in making this last judgment, the nurse needs all her skill in carefully and continually assessing the patient's anxiety level and his ability to tolerate the stress precipitating the denying behavior.

She also needs to know and to be able to recognize the phases through which the individual passes as he gradually works through the denial and again begins to be able to deal with reality. This sensitivity to verbal clues from the patient that he is beginning to accept reality may be seen in the following example:

A patient on the psychiatric service had been informed that plans had been concluded for his transfer to another hospital nearer his own home. He had steadfastly refused to accept this in spite of specific information regarding these plans. During one interview with the nurse he stated:

"I'm glad you're taking notes about me. They might be valuable some time. Maybe you should send them to my doctor in L----."

Nurse: Then you will be seeing your doctor in L----?"

Patient: "Well, just in case he ever needs them. I'm going to stay here for a year and then I'll transfer to L----."

Although the patient evaded the issue as soon as he was confronted with it, denial was not as complete as it had been; he had been willing to admit one small aspect of reality, if only for a moment. The task of the nurse then became to focus more on this breakthrough and to aid him through the anxiety-laden period by her understanding, support, and assistance in further exploring the reality of the situation and what it meant for him.

There are many unanswered questions concerning the background and preparation of the nurse who is to intervene actively in so complex a situation as denial often presents. Because denial operates almost universally to some degree in all patients, and because it can so often block the goals of nursing therapy, it would seem reasonable to expect that the professional nurse should be able to:

1. Recognize her own feelings regarding the patient and his illness, and the coping patterns she herself has developed as part of her own behavior in meeting stress situations.

2. Perceive her professional role and her relationship with staff and other members of the treatment team.

3. Recognize denying behavior in herself, her patients and other members of the team.

4. Avoid reinforcing patterns of denial as observed in others.

5. Continually assess the level of anxiety as she maintains her role as the representative of reality.

6. Seek additional information and collaboration from other members of the health team.

7. Maintain a supportive, helping relationship as the patient begins to move toward a more reality-based orientation in working through his problem.

As a professional, the nurse needs continually to assess and to evaluate her own learning needs and to plan purposefully for her own professional growth. As she adds to her knowledge and experience, the young graduate should, with further preparation, be able to work at ever deeper and more therapeutic levels with patients and families.

REFERENCES

1. American Nurses' Association: Nursing Approaches to Denial of Illness. Monograph No. 12. Report of the A.N.A. Clinical Session, Detroit, 1962.
2. King, J. M.: Denial. Am. J. Nurs., 66:1010-1013, 1966.
3. Schneck, J. S.: Benjamin Rush on denial of illness. Am. J. Psychiat., 120:1129, 1964.
4. Freud, S.: Collected Papers. Vol. 5, Strachey, J. (ed.). pp. 199-200. New York, Basic Books, 1959.
5. Miller, D., and Swanson, B.: The study of conflict. In Jones, M. R. (ed.): Nebraska Symposium on Motivation. p. 163. Lincoln, University of Nebraska Press, 1965.
6. Fisher, S.: Psychological aspects of rehabilitation. In Lief, H. I., Lief, V., and Lief, N. (eds.): The Psychological Basis of Medical Practice. p. 525. New York, Harper & Row, 1963.
7. Weinstein, E. A., and Kahn, R. L.: Denial of Illness. Springfield, Ill., Charles C Thomas, 1956.
8. Wahl, C.: The physician's management of the dying patient. In Masserman, J. H. (ed.): Current Psychiatric Therapies. Vol. 2, p. 127. New York, Grune & Stratton, 1962.
9. Glaser, B. G., and Strauss, A. L.: Awareness of Dying. p. 135. Chicago, Aldine, 1965.
10. Chodoff, P., Friedman, S., and Hamburg, D.: Stress, defenses and coping behavior: Observations in parents of children with malignant diseases. Am. J. Psychiat., 120:745, February, 1964.
11. Brauer, P. H.: Should the patient be told the truth? In Skipper, J. K., and Leonard, R. C. (eds.): Social Interaction and Patient Care. p. 177. Philadelphia, J. B. Lippincott, 1965.
12. Visotsky, H., Hamburg, D., and Goss, M.: Coping behavior under extreme stress. Arch. Gen. Psychiat., 5:445, November, 1961.
13. Garrard, S., and Richmond, J.: Psychological aspects of the management of chronic diseases and handicapping conditions of childhood. In Lief, H. I., Lief, V., and Lief, N. (eds.): The Psychological Basis of Medical Practice. p. 391. New York, Harper & Row, 1963.
14. Brauer, P. H.: loc. cit.
15. Woodfall, R.: The nurse, the mentally retarded child and his family. In Nursing Approaches to Denial of Illness. p. 5, loc. cit.
16. Ibid.

17. Davidman, H.: Psychological problems of deafness, blindness and muteness in children. *In* The Psychological Basis of Medical Practice. p. 405, *loc. cit.*
18. Bozeman, M., Orbach, C., and Sutherland, A.: Psychological impact of cancer and its treatment. Part I. Cancer, *8*:4, 1955.
19. Chodoff, P., Friedman, S., and Hamburg, D.: Stress, denial and coping behavior. p. 744, *loc. cit.*
20. Bernstein, R.: Are we still stereotyping the unmarried mother? *In* Parad, H. J. (ed.): Crisis Intervention. p. 108. New York, Family Service Association of America, 1966.
21. Glaser, B. G., and Strauss, A. L.: Awareness of Dying. p. 137. Chicago, Aldine, 1964.

BIBLIOGRAPHY

American Nurses' Association: Nursing Approaches to Denial of Illness. Monograph 12, Report of the A.N.A. Clinical Sessions. Detroit, 1962.

Bernstein, R.: Are we still stereotyping the unmarried mother? *In* Parad, H. J. (ed.): Crisis Intervention. New York, Family Service Association of America, 1966.

Bozeman, M., Orbach, C., and Sutherland, A.: Psychological impact of cancer and its treatment. Part I. Cancer, *8*:1-19, 1955.

Brauer, P. H.: Should the patient be told the truth? *In* Skipper, J. K., and Leonard, R. C. (eds.): Social Interaction and Patient Care. Philadelphia, J. B. Lippincott, 1965.

Cameron, N. A.: Personality Development and Psychopathology. Boston, Houghton Mifflin, 1963.

Chodoff, P.: Adjustment to disability. J. Chronic Dis., *9*:653-659, 1959.

Chodoff, P., Friedman, S., and Hamburg, D.: Stress, defenses and coping behavior: Observations in parents of children with malignant diseases. Am. J. Psychiat., *120*:744-749, 1964.

Davidman, H.: Psychological problems of deafness, blindness and muteness in children. *In* Lief, H. I., Lief, V., and Lief, N. (eds.): The Psychological Basis of Medical Practice. p. 404. New York, Harper & Row, 1963.

Dunbar, H. F.: Emotions and Bodily Changes: A Survey of Literature on Psychosomatic Interrelationships, 1910-1953. New York, Columbia University Press, 1954.

Fenichel, O.: Psychoanalytic Theory of Neurosis. New York, W. W. Norton & Co., 1945.

Fisher, S.: Psychological aspects of rehabilitation. *In* Lief, H. I., Lief, V., and Lief, N. (eds.): The Psychological Basis of Medical Practice. p. 525. New York, Harper & Row, 1963.

Freud, A.: The Ego and the Mechanisms of Defense. New York, International Universities Press, 1964.

Freud, S.: Collected Papers. Strachey, J. (ed.). New York, Basic Books, 1959.

Garrard, S., and Richmond, J.: Psychological aspects of the management of chronic disease and handicapping conditions of childhood. *In* Lief, H. I., Lief, V., and Lief, N. (eds.): The Psychologi-

cal Basis of Medical Practice. p. 391. New York, Harper & Row, 1963.
Grinker, R.: Mentally healthy young males. Arch. Gen. Psychiat., 6:405-453, 1962.
Hackett, T., and Weisman, A.: The treatment of the dying. *In* Masserman, J. H. (ed.): Current Psychiatric Therapies. New York, Grune & Stratton, 1962.
Hankoff, L., *et al.*: Denial of illness in schizophrenic outpatients: Effects of psychopharmacological treatment. Arch. Gen. Psychiat., 3:657-664, 1960.
Horney, K.: Neurotic Personality of Our Time. New York, W. W. Norton & Co., 1937.
Jacobson, E.: Denial and repression. J. Am. Psychoanal. Assn., 5:61-62.
Kassebaum, G., and Baumann, B.: Dimensions of the sick role in chronic illness. J. Health Hum. Behav., 6:1, 1965.
King, J. M.: Denial. Am. J. Nurs., 66:1010-1013, 1966.
Lederer, H. D.: How the sick view their world. *In* Skipper, J. K., and Leonard, R. C. (eds.): Social Interaction and Patient Care. Philadelphia, J. B. Lippincott, 1965.
Marmor, J.: The cancer patient and his family. *In* Lief, H. I., Lief, V., and Lief, N. (eds.): The Psychological Basis of Medical Practice. p. 312. New York, Harper & Row, 1963.
Miller, D., and Swanson, G.: The study of conflict. *In* Jones, M. R. (ed.): Nebraska Symposium on Motivation. p. 163. Lincoln, University of Nebraska Press, 1956.
Murphy, L. B.: Coping devices and defense mechanisms in relation to autonomous ego function. *In* Palmer, J. O., and Goldstein, M. J. (eds.): Perspectives of Psychopathology. New York, Oxford University Press, 1966.
Noyes, A. P., and Kolb, L. C.: Modern Clinical Psychiatry. ed. 6. Philadelphia, W. B. Saunders, 1963.
Orbach, C., Sutherland, A., and Bozeman, M.: Adaptation of mothers to the threatened loss of their children through leukemia. Part 2. Cancer, 8:20-33, 1955.
Rogers, C. R.: Client-Centered Therapy. Boston, Houghton Mifflin, 1956.
Rothenberg, A.: Psychological problems in terminal cancer management. Cancer, 14:1063-1073, 1961.

Schneck, J. S.: Benjamin Rush on denial of illness. Am. J. Psychiat., *120*:1129-1130, 1964.

Schwartz, D. A.: Psychotic reactions, a result of the breakdown of defense by denial. Arch. Gen. Psychiat., *4*:119-123, 1961.

Seidenberg, R.: Omnipotence, denial and psychosomatic medicine. Psychosom. Med., *25*:31-36, 1963.

Singer, H. L.: The indefinite you, a common defense mechanism. Compr. Psychiat., *5*:358-363, 1963.

Visotsky, H., Hamburg, D., and Goss, M.: Coping behavior under extreme stress. Arch. Gen. Psychiat., *5*:423-448, 1961.

Wahl, C. W.: The physician's management of the dying patient. *In* Masserman, J. H. (ed.): Current Psychiatric Therapies. Vol. 2, p. 127. New York, Grune & Stratton, 1962.

Weinstein, E. A., and Kahn, R. L.: Denial of Illness. Springfield, Ill., Charles C Thomas, 1955.

Woodfall, R.: The nurse, the mentally retarded child and his family. *In* Nursing Approaches to Denial of Illness. Report of the A.N.A. Clinical Sessions. Detroit, 1962.

2
Empathy

Margaret Baumgartner

The ability to empathize, according to Sister Madeleine Clemence,[1] is the distinguishing characteristic of the committed nurse. Through empathy she meets the patient in an I-thou relationship. In contrast the uncommitted nurse functions on the I-it plane. She bestows her services on the patient without engaging in any interpersonal relationship at all. Similarly, Katz notes that ". . . anyone who takes the role of a helper . . . is confronted with the complexities of empathic involvement no matter what level or depth the relationship takes."[2]

Empathy involves both the intellectual and emotional nature of man. To understand its complexities it is necessary to comprehend how it is developed. Some of the processes involved are imagination, the power of the will, identification, insight, compassion and sympathy.

Those who enter nursing seek self-fulfillment through altruism—helping others, attempting to alleviate their suffering, expressing concern for their welfare. To achieve such self-fulfillment in the art of nursing, the nurse must be able to put herself "in another's place." Empathy, as the term is used in this paper, is the ability to use imagination and will to project oneself into the emotions of another in the pursuit of altruistic purposes.

Modern nursing and medicine have both been criticized for the loss of the qualities of compassion and sympathy.[3,4] Perhaps nurses, in their struggle for professionalism, have focused too much on the science rather than on the art of nursing, with the result that humanitarianism in patient care has been neglected. To many of the public even the term "professional nurse" has a connotation of cold and machine-like efficiency, objectivity, lack of feeling, or even hostility.

Nurses who express hostility toward patients through use of such labels as "uncooperative" have forgotten the art of nursing. Self-concern prevents them from putting themselves "in the patient's place"—i.e., from achieving empathy. This inability produces an unfavorable and unwanted public image and is probably the reason for the public's longing for the old-fashioned nurse.

No one would advocate weakening the much emphasized science content in nursing curricula. However, unless equal attention is given to courses that nourish the humanitarian emotions, stimulate the imagination, and deepen human understanding, it is doubtful that modern nurses will be prepared to practice the altruistic art of nursing.

To acquire the quality of empathy is in itself an art. It implies self-knowledge, including a philosophy of life; it implies understanding of one's own culture, including the perspectives gained by study of history and of other cultures; it implies acquaintance with the deep human wisdom treasured in the great religions of the world. Such studies provide the nurse with a frame of reference to deal with the society in which she lives and with the individuals—shaped by that society—whom she serves.

Strengthened by such an educational foundation, the nursing curriculum may effectively focus on the development of empathy itself. For the nurse to be able to extend herself in empathy, she must first have sufficient self-confidence. In Jersild's words, "To accept others, one must first accept oneself."[5] She must also be able to rise above her own problems, suspending for a time her own needs and desires in order to concentrate her whole attention on the patient and his problems.

Such concentration means bringing to bear all of her skill, all of her knowledge, and all of her compassion. To do so also implies an act of will on her part to sublimate or suspend her own self-concerns. It also implies use of the powers of imagination in an attempt to know what the patient feels as if "it were she experiencing it." As Einstein said, "Imagination is more important than knowledge."[6] It is the power that enables a person to enter into the feeling of another.[7]

Historically the concept of empathy, was derived from the term "Einfühlung" used by Lipp in his study of optical illusions.[8] Lipp used the word in describing the effect of a great painting upon a viewer. Through Einfühlung, (imagination and suspension of self-concern), the viewer was able to "enter into" the emotions expressed in the work of art. The term was later adapted to become empathy and is used by psychologists to denote such qualities as social perceptiveness, clinical intuition, insight into another's feeling, understanding, or even diagnostic competence.

The quality of empathy has also been singled out as the distinguishing characteristic of the mature person and of the mentally healthy person. Jersild, for example, states that compassion, which he associates closely with empathy, is the "ultimate expression" of maturity.[9] Katz[10] and Hoskins[11] not only associate the quality of empathy with mental health, but point out that impairment of ability to empathize is the fundamental psychic lesion of the psychotic.

In nursing mentally ill patients, one is struck by their egocentricity. Seclusiveness and withdrawal are common symptoms. Quite logically, therapeutic methods seem to consist mainly of helping the patient to gain release from his imprisoning self-concern by entering again into the feeling of others—i.e., by developing empathy. This objective appears to be the primary purpose, for example, of patient government, group therapy, and other resocialization methods.

To assist students or practitioners to develop empathy to the highest degree possible, it may be helpful to analyze the process into operational "steps." Although the word "steps" is used with intent to imply sequential development, it should be understood that strict adherence to an invariable sequence is not implied. These steps can be outlined as follows:

1. Acceptance of the self.
2. Exercise of the power of the will to concentrate on the patient's problem.
3. Identification with the patient and, through this, participation in his experience.
4. Toleration of anxiety.
5. Intellectual examination of the problem presented by the patient, including exploration of alternative possibilities.
6. Suspension of value judgments about the patient's feelings.
7. Full participation with the patient's feeling in its contextual relation to his life situation.

Because the above steps require a high order of both intellectual and emotional maturity, the time necessary for development of em-

32   Empathy

pathy and the extent to which it can be developed differs for individual nursing practitioners.

Many young students, for example, may find it extremely difficult to deal with sudden, overt emotion on the part of a patient, as the following incident illustrates:

Miss X, age 19, was in the hospital for evaluation of neurologic symptoms possibly indicative of a brain tumor. Diagnostic studies were negative for the presence of organic pathology. The physician stated that he felt that "something was bothering her psychologically," but the patient denied to him that she had any emotional problems.

On the second day that a nursing student (first semester sophomore) cared for Miss X, she was being prepared for discharge from the hospital. During the morning the patient had been quiet and non-communicative. Suddenly she began crying hysterically and throwing herself about in bed while mumbling, "I love somebody, and somebody don't love me . . . I might as well kill myself." The student seemed overwhelmed by the patient's behavior and remained silent as she stood by the bedside observing her.

In the conference discussion concerning the experience, the student stated, "It took me completely off guard. I didn't know what to say or do. I just wanted to cry, too." One student in the group stated, "The reason the patient reacted as she did is because they (the family) are old-family Portuguese, and they are emotional people." Another student commented that the episode showed "ridiculous behavior for a person of that age." Later, during an individual conference, the student told the instructor that she just "froze" because the incident recalled to her mind a similar personal problem which the student had recently experienced.

The reactions of these young students varied. One responded with sympathy ("I wanted to cry, too."). Another reacted in anger ("ridiculous behavior") and expressed a judgmental response. Still another attempted to explain the patient's emotion on a cultural basis. All of the reactions suggest a very early developmental stage in the ability to empathize—as might be expected of students beginning the sophomore year of college.

In the above example, one student's sympathetic reaction suggests the important distinction between empathy and sympathy. In response to the patient's distress, the student felt a similar type of distress, without, however, a clear conception of the patient's own situation. Rather than "entering into" the patient's emotional state, she reacted to it as a baffled, though sympathetic, onlooker.

The incident also illustrates the temptation inherent in many nursing situations for the nurses to withdraw rather than experience what may be traumatic and anxiety-provoking. The student in this incident did not yield to such temptation, but, rather, chose to remain with the patient despite severe emotional discomfort. This act of the will is one of the first steps in development of empathy.

The process of developing identification with the patient depends upon the practitioner's imaginative ability to sense what it is that the patient is feeling. Imagination has been defined as the power of the mind to engage in creative pursuits. It is the power to lift oneself over the barriers of self and situation in order to "experience" the situation of another.

In imaginatively entering the emotional situation of another person, the nurse exposes herself to the discomfort of anxiety. Often she attempts to avoid anxiety by avoiding the experience of the patient's distress. Both imaginative participation in another's situation and avoidance are illustrated in the following incident.

A student entered a patient's room and found her lying tensely in bed. She was quiet and pale. Earlier the student had talked with her and found her in a very happy mood; she had talked freely and seemed relaxed. Now she seemed to be scared to death.

Student Nurse: "What's the matter?"

Patient (starting to cry): "I've been in the hospital for three weeks. I've had so many needles—too many needles. I can't take any more. Yesterday they put a big needle here in my chest (bone marrow), it hurt so bad and now they are going to give me some more needles. I can't take it."

S. N.: "What are they going to do?"

P.: "They are going to give me some blood, here in my hand. How do they do it? How long will it take? Oh, I don't want any more needles."

Because the patient was severely anemic, the student knew the blood would help her to feel better and told her so. She also explained that the patient would feel pain only when the needle was inserted.

When the doctor and head nurse entered the room, the student could feel the patient tense up again.

Doctor: "Here we go—more needles." (The student's heart sank along with the patient's.)

The head nurse and the doctor proceeded with the insertion of the I.V. The student was making the other bed in the same room. The patient had started crying loudly, even screaming at intervals. The student continued making the bed furiously as an outlet for her own emotions.

Head Nurse: "Quiet, dear, this will only take a minute, Doctor, what is the difference between an angio-cath and an intro-cath? I've always wondered."

The patient continued screaming while the doctor educated the head nurse. Neither paid any attention to the patient.

34   Empathy

Not knowing "what to say" in an emotionally charged situation is itself anxiety-provoking for the nurse. There are times, however, when the best expression of empathy is a nonverbal one, as in the following incident.

A young primipara had carried her child to within two days of delivery. The doctor then told her her baby was dead. The student assigned to her care during labor had difficulty in dealing with her own feelings of sorrow at the terrible waste and ordeal this poor mother had to endure with nothing at the end. The student realized that the mother had to go through a period of grief and so she listened without comment as the patient related her feeling. But by a touch on her arm, by a cold cloth on her forehead and by rubbing her sore and aching back, the student communicated to her how she cared and how much she wanted to help.

The above example illustrates, too, the frequent necessity of subordinating one's own feelings of sorrow and grief in the interests of another. Maintaining this degree of control, the nurse is free to devote her time and energy to the patient's problem. She is aware of her own reactions and her own anxiety, but trusts her power to tolerate anxiety.

In short, however freely her emotion may flow toward the patient, there is a measure of her intellect which remains objective in order to consider the problem. It is as if a part of the nurse stands aside and observes the situation from an intellectual, detached point of view. As a result, in subtle ways, a nurse communicates to the patient that, while she is able to appreciate his experiences, she is at the same time capable of dealing with them.

The quality of empathy, as described above, implies a philosophy of life on the part of the nurse, a philosophy that fosters integrity, self-knowledge, self-acceptance, and commitment to others. It implies the ability to participate deeply in emotionally charged situations without being overwhelmed by them. It implies the ability to discover new dimensions in the self and to imaginatively experience the life-situations of others. A nurse who has acquired the ability to extend to her patients this remarkable quality of empathy offers a human service which is rare, precious, and needed in present-day nursing.

REFERENCES

1. Clemence, Sister Madeleine: Existentialism: A philosophy of commitment. Am. J. Nurs., *66,* 3:500-505, March, 1966.
2. Katz, R. L.: Empathy—Its Nature and Uses. New York, Macmillan, 1963.
3. Travelbee, J.: What's wrong with sympathy? Am. J. Nurs., *66,* 1:68, January, 1964.
4. Gross, M. L.: The Doctors. New York, Random House, 1966.
5. Jersild, A. T.: When Teachers Face Themselves. pp. 125-36. Bureau of Publications, Teachers College, Columbia University, 1955.
6. Einstein, A., as quoted on Frontispiece. *In* Osborn, A. F.: Applied Imagination. ed. 3. rev. New York, Charles Scribner's Sons, 1965.
7. Osborn, A. F.: Applied Imagination. ed. 3. rev. New York, Charles Scribner's Sons, 1965.
8. Lipp, T.: Zur Einfühlung. Leipzig, Engelmann, 1913.
9. Jersild, A. T.: *op. cit*
10. Katz, R. L.: *op. cit*
11. Hoskins, R. G.: The Biology of Schizophrenia. pp. 162-165. New York, W. W. Norton & Co., 1946.

BIBLIOGRAPHY

Barckley, V.: What can I say to the cancer patient? Nurs. Outlook, 6:318, June, 1958.

Bell, G. B., and Hall, H., Jr.: The relationship between leadership and empathy. J. Abnorm. Social Psychol., 49:156-57, 1954.

Brown, E. L.: Nursing for the Future. New York, Russell Sage Foundation, 1948.

Brunclik, H., Thurston and Feldhussen: The empathy inventory. Nurs. Outlook, 6:42, June, 1967.

Clemence, Sister Madeleine: Existentialism: A philosophy of commitment. Am. J. Nurs., 63:500, March, 1966.

Fivars, G., and Gosnell, D.: Nursing evaluation, the problem and the process. *In* Critical Incident Techniques. New York, Macmillan, 1966.

Gross, M. L.: The Doctors. New York, Random House, 1966.

Hatch, R. S.: An Evaluation of a Forced-Choice Differential Accuracy Approach to the Measurement of Supervisory Empathy. Englewood Cliffs, N.J., Prentice-Hall, 1962.

Hoskins, R. G.: The Biology of Schizophrenia. pp. 162-165. New York, W. W. Norton & Co., 1946.

Jersild, A. T.: When Teachers Face Themselves. pp. 125-36. Bureau of Publications, Teachers College, Columbia University, 1955.

Katz, R. L.: Empathy—Its Nature and Uses. New York, Macmillan, 1963.

Lipp, T.: Zur Einfühlung. Leipzig, Engelmann, 1913.

Mead, G. H.: Mind, Self and Society. Chicago, University of Chicago Press, 1934.

Noyes, A., Camp, W., and Van Sickel, M.: Psychiatric Nursing. p. 34. ed. 6. New York, Macmillan, 1964.

Osborn, A. F.: Applied Imagination. ed. 3. rev. New York, Charles Scribner's Sons, 1963.

Riker, A. P.: What nursing means to me. Nurs. Outlook, 12:23, February, 1964.

Speroff, B. J.: Empathy is important in nursing. Nurs. Outlook. 4, 6:326, June, 1956.

Travelbee, J.: What's wrong with sympathy? Am. J. Nurs., 64, 1:68, January, 1964.

Wilson, L.: This Stranger, My Son. New York, G. P. Putnam's Sons, 1968.

3

The Professional Nurse and Body Image

Catherine M. Norris

Professional nursing is carried out within the framework of a definition of illness and health, a definition of nursing and the needs and expectations of society. It is conducted within certain organizations or systems and within the knowledge available in the natural and social sciences.

The definition of illness and health used here is:

Health is a state of complete physical, mental and social well-being, and not merely the absence of disease and infirmity.* It involves maximizing the potential for living of which man is capable. Illness on the other hand is a maladaption in one or more spheres of function which interferes with a person's achieving his potential for wellness.

The definition of nursing used here is:

Nursing is a significant dynamic, therapeutic process† which involves a relationship between nurse and patient within which work is carried on in relation to identified goals, comfort and care, intervention in pathological processes, promotion of health and prevention of disease. Professional nursing is the planning, execution, supervision, evaluation, teaching, and organization of these activities among the several levels of nursing personnel to produce an environment and the conditions and skills that will accomplish the tasks of nursing.

Since World War II, during which many young men and women in the Armed Services learned about the kind of medical care available, more and more people have been asking for it. High-level wellness has been introduced as a goal for all people, and revolutionary advances

---

* World Health Organization. Preamble to Constitution.

† Nursing process is defined as a series of sequential goal-directed activities which nurse and patient undertake to work from point to point along a continuum toward the goal—the patient's potential for wellness.

in medical treatment promise greater health and longer life than ever before. The demands made upon the health professions and the government to achieve these goals have never been greater and the criticism in cases of failure has never been louder.

Within the many existing and emerging complex systems of health services there has been response to recently recognized medical needs even though the preparation of professional workers cannot keep up with the demand. Paramedical workers, including professional nurses, now have many functions that overlap with medicine. Professional nurses are expected to intervene in psychopathological and pathophysiological processes as never before.

The rate of discovery of knowledge will refine and change the ways in which nurses intervene in problems of health and illness. A theory of nursing needs to allow for examination and inclusion of this new knowledge.

One approach to the development of nursing theory is to describe the phenomena involved, thus providing a picture of the problems that need to be solved. In addition, one needs to categorize the problems in order to understand them and postulate therapeutic intervention, i.e., one must be able to conceptualize the problem. One also needs to be able to approach situations knowing that there are similarities among human phenomena. Any professional discipline would be impossible if each problem had to be approached as being completely different from every other problem. Some categorization may be done on the basis of meaning of events, but for all other categories the next step is to look for meaning. In psychiatry meanings would be in terms of psychiatric theory. Psychodynamics, an integral part of psychiatric theory, is not nursing theory, but it can be used to provide explanations for human phenomena. Other aspects of psychiatric theory—growth and development, personality structure, and psychopathology—help provide understanding of human behavioral phenomena, as well as concepts from the behavioral sciences of anthropology and sociology. If the nurse knows the related theory, knows her patient and knows the methodology of nursing, she initiates a nursing process that begins with sensitive observation and with skilled history-taking technics which provide data for assessment. This assessment may be in terms of predicting that certain phenomena will occur, or in terms of diagnosing the existence of a phenomenon. Nursing theory must go beyond this—it must guide action that will prevent the occurrence of certain behavioral phenomena or will intervene (control) therapeutically once they have occurred. This is still a distant goal for nursing and involves testing soundly formulated hypotheses about prevention or intervention in a variety of settings, with sufficient replication to warrant the statement of a theory of nursing and nursing therapy. Actually, nursing theory requires better description than we now have, as indicated by the paucity of literature in nursing concerning body image, weakness, fatigue, restlessness, and related phenomena with which nurses must constantly deal. This paper will concern itself with the phenomenon of body image.

Using this approach to body image, one would first describe problems which are already categorized broadly as threats to body image. Secondly, one would review the concept of body image as found in psychiatric theory—its development, its universality, its dynamic evolving nature. Increasing meaning would be provided by a description of the work involved in reworking or reorganizing the body image and integrating changes or events perceived as threats into the body scheme. A description of psychotherapeutic needs of patients who are trying to cope with body image problems would, hopefully, provide for increased understanding in this second phase of content development related to body image. Establishing relationships among body image problems, their meaning for the human organism, the needs they create, and the resultant healthy and maladaptive coping behavior is also part of the conceptual process.

A theory of nursing should also include recognition of the need to predict the occurrence of body image problems and assist in control of intervention at the levels of both prevention and cure.

WHAT IS BODY IMAGE?

The concept of body image has not been dealt with in an holistic way in the literature. By and large, theorists have been unable to integrate the concept of the person's body into the matrix of personality concepts called psychodynamic theory. The theory of body image, after more than a half-century of irregular and unsystematic treatment, consists of a series of typological measures that attempt to relate body type to personality type or other body-personality correlations; a small series of studies that attempt to link selected measures of physiological functioning to behavior; some explanations of behavior of persons whose body structure became distorted or mutilated; and a theory of psychosomatics that identifies meaningful linkages between body malfunctioning and personality malfunctioning. Very recently some workers—e.g., Lowen, Schutz—have taken the opposite approach to that of psychosomatic medicine and have become concerned with how the body image and body functioning affect emotional states.

Although many technics have been developed and used to study body image, most of the material found in the literature consists of reports of introspection, observations of patients, and anecdotes. Many relationships between behavior and body parts, e.g., ulcers and emotions, personality characteristics and arthritis are reported, but not within a whole body-behavior framework.

It should be noted that the differences between what is considered to be a healthy presentation of the body image and its pathological variants are not generally specified or known.

For the purposes of this paper a definition was developed after studying several others:

Body image is the constantly changing total of conscious and unconscious information, feelings and perceptions about one's body in space as different and apart from all others. It is a social creation, developed through the reflected perceptions about the surfaces of one's body and responses to sensations originating from the inner regions of the body as the individual copes with a kaleidoscopic variety of living activities. The body image is basic to identity and has been referred to as the somatic ego.

By and large there is considerable agreement that the body image or scheme functions as a standard or frame of reference, which influences the ways in which a person perceives himself and influences his ability to perform. We live as human beings with bodies. It is also fairly well agreed that the body image is developed slowly and is learned in the process of growth and development.

Ultimately, body image is an intrapersonal experience of the person's feelings and attitudes towards one's body and the way he organizes these experiences. Much of the auditing of the subjective experiences that go into making and modifying the body image is not conscious, and no one can describe his own total body image. However, it is not uncommon for a person to recognize in the body image of others characteristics to which he assigns meaning. A character trait such as "weak" may be assigned to someone with a receding chin. If a man is prematurely bald, he may be labelled as "virile"; if he has knock-knees, he is not to be taken seriously; if he is flat-footed, he may be "tactless" or even "not very bright." If he has a big nose, he may be labelled as a member of a "minority group." Certain kinds of posturing are called "effeminate" in men or "masculine" in women. Certain hair styles make the person observed a "hippie."

OPERATIONAL DEFINITION

The following outline constitutes an attempt to develop an operational definition of the concept "body image". It is an oversimplified definition of a very complex concept. This definition was created within the framework of the growth and development process. It is based on some of these ideas:

1. Body image is a social creation.
    a. Normality is judged by appearance, ways of gesturing or posturing, and other ways of using the body that are prescribed by society.
    b. Painful sanctions are imposed for deviations from normality, whether behavioral or structural.
    c. Approval and acceptance are given for normal appearance and proper behavior.
    d. Body image emerges out of an almost infinite variety and number of approvals and sanctions and an individual's response to them. Experience is integrated into the personality in terms of the satisfaction or dissatisfaction that the individual has had with it.
    e. Body development continually enlarges the individual's world, his mastery of it, his interaction with it, (including interpersonal interaction) and his ability to respond to the wide variety of experience it offers.
    f. This integration, which is largely unconscious, is constantly evolving and can be identified in the person's values, attitudes, and feelings about himself.
2. There is very close interdependence between body image and personality, ego, self-image and identity.
3. Body image is an important determinant of behavior.
4. The impact of any experience on the human being is determined by the interplay of its reality level or meanings, the level of conscious fantasy and feeling about it, and the unconsciously motivated fantasies and feelings.

STEPS IN THE DEVELOPMENT OF BODY IMAGE

1. At birth there is no physical body image except at the feeling level—comfort, discomfort, hunger, rage, pain, etc.
2. Mother is perceived as external source of comfort and discomfort—experienced but not interpreted by infant. Polyphasic rhythm of body functioning in terms of time cycle are learned in terms of mother's response to needs.
3. Exploring self, with an ever-increasing number of variables involved—sensory impressions, motility, kinesthetic and touch sensations, ego development and sociocultural stimuli; experiencing pleasure, pain, shame or doubt, with concomitant learning of body attitudes, values and boundaries.
4. Opportunities are provided for exploring and manipulating environment—bathing, eating, toys, tools, water play, snow play, jungle gym, and rhythmic activities, with concomitant learning of attitudes and values of power, pleasure, fear, doubt, helplessness, etc. Beginning of adaptation to diurnal sleep-rest pattern and other adult structured circadian rhythms.
5. Becoming aware of separateness of one's own body from mother and all others.
6. Opportunities for learning about various parts of body and their functions, to be discovered with joy and pride or to be hidden in shame.
7. Opportunities for learning mastery of the body—to do, to protect self, to protect others, with internalized feelings of pleasure, power, confidence which fosters self esteem, or to learn feelings of helplessness, pain, inadequacy, doubt and guilt.
8. Opportunities for manipulating self and tools of environment.
9. Learning to use and master environment—e.g., running, skipping, skating, swimming, with concomitant learning of pleasure, competence and worth, or feelings of inadequacy.
10. Learning to relate to others of the same sex, with concomitant feelings of pleasure, power, warmth, and anticipation, or pain, doubt and fear.
11. Opportunities for learning to audit or listen to the body with the potential for developing internalized feelings of pleasure and power.

12. Praise, blame, derogation or criticism in relation to body, body part, or usage of body or body part, with internalized pleasure or pain, doubt and guilt.

13. Comparative and competitive appraisal of body and its function at level of peer group, with concomitant learning of values and attitudes about the body as strong, competent and powerful, or weak and helpless.

14. Learning to relate to persons of the opposite sex, with concomitant learning of values, attitudes and use of the body.

15. Accepting one's body without undue preoccupation with its function, or the control or these functions, so that one is free for other living activities.

16. Recognizing the residuum of unresolved experiences, misconceptions, distortions and fears in relation to body image that persists from childhood.

17. Learning to see the personality as a whole, with less emphasis on the physical self and greater emphasis on the inner or psychic self, in preparation for aging and in developing mature acceptance of self and full human potential for living.

HOW DOES BODY IMAGE DEVELOP?

The psychoanalytic concept, typified by Freud, is the most complex of the theories formulated. In psychoanalytic theory the body is essentially divided into three areas or zones. The tools and tasks of these three areas, developing in succession—oral, anal, genital—are the focus of this theory. The success of the individual in coping with the changing demands of each area as it comes into its period of dominance is considered necessary to the development of a mature body image. If he is not able to integrate the functioning of each of these body zones in its turn into his total body scheme, his body image will retain some immature aspects. These immature images will interfere with securing adult satisfactions, which interference may be evidenced by personality disturbance. For example, in the anal phase, in which mastery of body and environment is the task, the child who does not learn who he is in relation to the world, how he can manipulate his environment, and how he can manage or control his body, may be left with an "all thumbs" body image, or he may rationalize that physical activity is for the common man and that esthetic activities are reserved for the elite.

Using the developmental approach, we can state that the body image develops pre- and postnatally by means of successive sequential steps in differentiation. Its goals are manipulation, mastery and control of relationships with self, others and environment, within a time-space context or rhythm. It is dynamic, i.e., everchanging, evolving, expanding or contracting, progressive or regressive, but goal-directed in terms of forming newer, more stable systems in the organism. As new neural functions develop they are integrated into the total individual, building on top of and inhibiting earlier and more primitive nervous structures. However, under stress, older ways of interpreting and functioning in relation to the body image may be revived. The human body image develops through sensory messages from the inner surface of the body and from the outer surface in contact with the environment. These sensations, which are received as the organism audits, experiments with, and manipulates the body and the environment, are of several kinds. They may be tactile, thermal or painful. Sensations come from the muscles, organs and nerves of the body in response to inner functioning or contact of the body with the environment. These experiences of the body may be interpreted in terms of feelings, view of self, by comparing and contrasting with other persons and comparing and contrasting with group or cultural value systems. Experiences, the use to which the organism puts them, and their storage in the form of memory, provide for a sense of body unity. Thus, each individual has a three-dimensional perception of form and position which functions as his somatic ego. Like the psychic ego, the somatic ego is developed as the result of experience (considering that the id is hereditary and the superego is culturally determined).

The infant receives many internal perceptions which he can only interpret as satisfying or painful. Many of these messages originate in the mucosa of the mouth and in the nervous structures of the body periphery. Severe maternal anxiety would be first experienced peripherally, but the full perception would be in the deep layers of the infant's body, with several organs potentially involved. The first component of body image to emerge, then, is the group of sensations felt in relation to the inner workings of the body and the way in which these workings communicate to the total organism. The second phase develops as the child explores the environment and works at mastering it. Impressions are made as to how one's body compares with others and whether one's body is attractive to others. With time, more stable impressions of sensation, mastery and normality are formed: i.e., the ego identity base being strong; there are more integrations with the psychic components of the ego, in which intellectual and emotional development are more in focus. The individual's intelligence, emotional health, social and interpersonal adequacy and general satisfactions in living will influence to a great extent his awareness of his body and his preoccupation with it. It is possible for many people to rather skillfully monitor or "listen" to their bodies without morbid preoccupation, while others are fully preoccupied with their bodies and get most of their satisfactions at this level. The healthy person is aware of how his body feels, how it works and the effect of his physical self on others. One teacher makes this point about a student:

> I have one very attractive little student. Others see her as little, but she has never in the world thought of herself as little. She is very short, but she is very capable and this does not seem to get in her way. Once there were two big patients slugging it out with each other and she rushed in and put her hands on each of their chests and said, "Now, stop it you guys!" And, fortunately, they stopped it. Several people talked to her about it; her interpretation was that she felt big enough to cope with it and she did.

THE DYNAMIC NATURE OF BODY IMAGE

In illness and health there is wide variety of messages about the body being constantly fed into the system, either for interpretation-acceptance with integration into the self or for rejection and revision. The infant responds to inner and outer experience at the sensory level with screaming, raging or cooing. Success in achieving comfort and relief from pain and anxiety prepares his body for the task of mastering the environment. Children in the two-to-four-year group, struggling with this task, are still uncertain of bodily boundaries and experience extreme apprehension about having their nails and hair cut. They have difficulty seeing body productions, namely feces, as separate, and given the chance, tend to resist having them flushed away.

After a sudden growth spurt, adolescents, not knowing how to manage their changed bodies, are very preoccupied with the changes in terms of cultural and social norms and attractiveness, and study their bodies, comparing various aspects of them with those of their peers.

An occasional maternity patient describes the experience of delivering a baby as having her insides torn out. We need to study this type of reaction and to determine what it means in terms of the acceptance of the newborn infant and his integration into the family, the relationships between husband and wife, and its influence on family planning.

Many people defend themselves against the physical processes of aging. We develop more and more technics for hiding wrinkles, preventing deformity, maintaining hair color, disguising obesity, and generally helping people to look younger. Hospitalization may be quite traumatic if the aging patient is unable to maintain what he considers to be his proper body image.

Every nurse is familiar with the disturbances in the person's body image following loss of a major part. A classic example is the phantom leg of the amputee patient. Although we may not be able to explain it on either a physiological or a psychological basis, we recognize it as a common phenomenon following amputation. It is so real that patients often act as if they still have both their legs, and end up falling to the floor, and we realize that this phantom may persist for years. We are somewhat aware that loss of certain other body parts—hair, teeth, one eye or both, the nose or a breast—necessitates adjustment of the person's body image. But, we are often not sure of how the patient perceives his body image as the result of the loss and of what the relationship of this perception is to his emotional experience.

We are less familiar with other events in which the body image of patients is disturbed. Patients' responses to these disturbances are less subject to recognition and study because the cause-and-effect aspect of the other events is not always as obvious as in the case of the loss of a limb. An obvious loss is only one experience in which a person's concept of his body image is affected. There are, in addition, surgical procedures in which the relationship of body parts is disturbed, e.g., colostomy, ileostomy, ureteroenterostomy or gastrostomy. Living with a colostomy a person can no longer ignore what he may have conceived as the dirty or unpleasant part of his bodily existence, for it is right under his very eyes and nose.

In other surgical procedures the loss of body parts, even if invisible to others, may necessitate a revision of the patient's body image. A woman often has a difficult time physically and emotionally after a hysterectomy. There is a wide variety of changes in perception of the body image which play a part in this emotional response. What does the loss of a lung, gallbladder, larynx or stomach do to the patient's image of his own body? It is the natural tendency among many nurses to assume that removal of the diseased organ is a complete solution to the patient's original problem.

The literature provides us with some evidence that repair procedures, such as are done in plastic surgery, may not produce the change in the body image that either the patient or surgeon assumed would occur. To what extent nurses could foster the hoped-for result, or how, is not known and this possibility has been little explored. For example, a patient feels inferior because he has an unusually large nose or ears that protrude to an abnormal extent. He goes to a plastic surgeon who does a plastic repair. The patient cannot reconstruct his body image to take in the improvements. He feels the same—inferior to others—as he felt before the surgery. How would the nurse go about studying this problem? How would she identify the steps in intervention? What are the risks in trying to help a patient change his concept of his body image?

We usually think of a surgical procedure when we think of the problem of integrating change in a body part into the total body scheme. Actually, equally dramatic physical changes occur in human pathophysiology. Can we, as nurses, study the various ways in which patients deal with changes in body size and proportion such as in the development of obesity, emaciation, acromegaly or gigantism? Other changes in the external surfaces of the body may be caused by the development of characteristics common to the opposite sex, as the development of mammary glands in men or hirsutism in women. People respond to color changes in the skin, such as in Addison's disease or chronic dermatitis. Skin texture also changes in such conditions as exfoliative and excoriative dermatitis, in thyroid conditions or in scar formation. In both atrophic and hypertrophic arthritis an almost infinite variety of changes, often grotesque, occur, not only in the joints but in the muscles, which atrophy for lack of use. Body posture may be distorted, and the face may take on the appearance of chronic suffering. Crippling changes occur in multiple sclerosis and Parkinson's disease.

Another problem of body image with which we are confronted is failure of a body part to function. Loss of function is usually accompanied by atrophy if the failure lasts a considerable period of time or is permanent. The rising rate of automobile accidents, along with military casualties, has increased the number of paraplegic patients. Nurses usually know a great deal more about the "acting out" behavior of the paraplegic than they do about how the patient's change in body image is perceived and interpreted. The increase in the number of older people among the population means that more patients are seen who have had cerebrovascular accidents with accompanying loss of function of one or more body parts.

Although heart attacks, asthmatic attacks and pneumonia do not leave a body part functionless, the symbolism of these diseases in terms of life and death may cause distorted notions concerning structure, function or significance. The organ may have a special image, even to the point of being independent of the body, with special needs and with a name of its own, such as "Burpy" or "Ticker."

Side effects of drug therapy such as moon face, hirsutism, striated skin, or changes in body contour can be very threatening to the body image.

An evolving social theme is that of violence. Both patients and nurses have problems dealing with the purposeless attacks on the body image that rape, shooting and knifing represent. In psychiatric nursing the schizophrenic patient often has a very poorly organized concept of his body. If he is asked to draw a picture of himself, he may draw parts of his body separate from his torso or place parts of the body in incorrect relationship to each other. He may deny that he has one or more body parts. We all know the patient who cannot eat because he "hasn't any stomach." We are familiar, too, with the patient who has anorexia nervosa, in which the maintenance of a particular kind of body image is a major component of the illness. In hypochondriasis, fantasies of somatic attack occur. In malingering there is conscious direction of concern to an organ or part through simulation of illness. Hysteria, a subconscious phenomenon, represents the dissociation of emotional content, displacement of the problems, isolation of a body target and introjection of the problem onto the organ that has become symbolic of the problem.

The patient who has tuberculosis and is isolated in the hospital receives the communication that his body is unacceptable and undesirable. This communication is reinforced by the amount of time he is actually left alone. The patient's input system picks these up in addition to whatever he feels and perceives to be happening in his chest. A patient whose condition is unavoidably malodorous may have considerable difficulty integrating this body concept into his total sense of identity.

We have been relating body images to illness and pathology, but as we become sensitive listeners we also become aware of the interactive nature of body parts and feelings in all interpersonal experience. There are literally thousands of idioms describing feeling behavior that people use every day. Nurses can learn to identify, by the theme in patients' use of body language, organs that feel, organs that are sensitive, or organs that may be possible targets for the individual under extreme stress. Many of these terms draw dramatic word pictures, such as "chicken-hearted," "yellow bellies," "lost my head," "blood-curdling," "jump out of my skin," "get my teeth into," "broken-hearted" and so on. Others, although not as pungent, are still descriptive of a certain physical experience such as "pain in the neck," "knees turned to water," "big mouth," "can't stomach any more," "have a belly full of," "knocked my eye out" or "put my finger on."

Intuitively, we are aware that body posture or functioning tells us a great deal concerning how a person feels about himself, how he feels today, how he approaches people, and how he functions. However, there have not been a great many systematic studies that document the manner in which behavior or feelings participates in shortening of muscles, in depositing or invading of muscle tissue by fatty tissue, in reducing function of the joints, or in affecting coordination of the body in action.

Nursing Implications

The body image problems of the patient, up to this point, have been identified essentially in terms of pathophysiological processes going on within him. We need to look, too, at some medical and nursing activities as also potentially threatening to people. For a few patients, especially children, the thermometer may be a threat. When we say, "I am going to *take* your temperature," one wonders whether this choice of words is purposeful or accidental. Other intrusive activities of nurses that might be threatening are enemata, catheterization, insertion of gastric tubes, intravenous infusion, intramuscular and subcutaneous injections, suctioning and the like.

Perhaps we should also study such intrusive diagnostic procedures as gastroscopy, bronchoscopy, sigmoidectomy, cystoscopy and dilatation and curettage in terms of the threat they may represent or the other effects they may leave on body image.

Another component of the mending and revising aspect of surgery is the nature of the threat or other experience that is posed by the "knife." Sutherland has demonstrated that the experience of cancer as a threat to the patient's body image cannot be separated from threat inherent in the curative measures—surgery and radiation.[1] Some of the postoperative emotional responses to artificial heart valves need to be explored from a body image point of view as well as from a physiological point of view. Such studies would help us deal with the problems of body image in the rapidly developing field of organ transplantation.

Nature of the Threat

Because the body image provides a base for identity, almost any change in body structure or function is experienced as a threat. This occurs even in normal growth; the maturing processes may be welcomed, but it still may be accompanied by the threat of new expectations and the threat of being found inadequate. This is particularly true of adolescence, in which we observe a great deal of comparing, testing, and experimenting in relation to particular changes and in relation to the whole body.

Psychiatric theory and research in body image indicate that serious threat to body image is related to many factors and that, in order to understand a particular patient's problem, one needs to construct for him a pattern of adaptation through study of the variables involved. The cultural values of youth, wholeness, normality and attractiveness enter into definition of threat. Dr. Martin Steinberg tells a story that illustrates how doctors may be caught up in a cultural bias about wholeness:

> One of our specialists is a man called Buerger and a disease was named after him—Buerger's Disease . . . hundreds of patients had come to us (with this disease) with the ever-present danger that they would lose the circulation in their legs. And there was always the question of trying as much as possible to keep the amputation rate low and save these legs. This was a tough clinic with hundreds of these patients. The nurse, however, refused

to accept this goal of keeping the legs. She took an awfully good look at it and finally convinced us that what we were doing was leading to the wrong goal; that just saving these legs wasn't good at all; that these people were now living without legs. They couldn't use them. They had legs and they got out of bed into chairs and had to be pushed around—but they had legs. She did the thinking and she said, 'No, this is not the right thing.' She got more people interested, and we began to realize that we're not talking about saving legs, we're talking about functions. It was much better to give somebody a prosthesis that he could use and get him functional than to have him stop everything he was doing . . .[2]

Some cultural groups do not allow the taking of pictures because of belief that the one who takes the picture is stealing the identity or spirit of the person being photographed. When you ask a Navajo Indian his name, he will never tell you, because to do so would be to allow you to take his name away from him. Then he would have to go look for another name. In some cultures, thieves are punished by cutting off one or more fingers. A person from such a culture who lost fingers in an accident would be especially traumatized because of the stigma attached. In our country we are committed to wholeness, beauty and health. As we learn more about disease and accident prevention it will be interesting to study changes in public attitudes toward those who do not meet the culturally determined criteria of health.

Threat is also related to the extent to which the individual's patterns of adaptation are interrupted. Each person develops patterns of behavior that meet his needs for security and does this within the framework of the requirements of his environment. These habits or patterns may depend heavily on certain organs of the body. If these organs become diseased or have to be removed the threat is greater than if an organ unimportant to the patient is affected. In one study of 3 women who had hysterectomies, data was collected about the meaning that the uterus and its removal had for patients.[3] The range of meaning is impressive: anxiety about the effect of the operation on sexual activity; anxiety over loss of sexual desire, inability to respond to spouse; fear of loss of sexual attractiveness; inability to have intercourse; expectation of painful intercourse and having to refuse spouse on this basis; fear that spouse would not obtain satisfaction because of damaged sexual organs; fear of loss of husband; fear of destruction of marriage; fear of loss of strength and ability to work; expectation of being invalided for a long time ("strength comes from womanly organs"); belief that one will never be the same again; concern for loss of childbearing capacity; fear of looking older and losing beauty or youth; fear of going insane; fear of becoming unable to control husband, with whom sex has been used as a bargaining point; fear of loss of independence from husband; fear of increased vulnerability; fear of development of personality changes; concern about loss of menstruation as a means of keeping body "cleaned out."

Ullman[4] gives recognition to the concept that one's patterns of adapting to the environment play an important role in perception of threat to the body image when he notes that if a stevedore becomes mildly aphasic he might have only minor anxiety about it, but a teacher who becomes mildly aphasic might panic. Thus, we observe that the degree to which loss of functional control creates loss of customary control of self, physical environment, time, and interpersonal field is very closely related to degree of threat. In the aging process, as well as the illness process, the prospect of still further loss mobilizes a great deal of anxiety.

The meaning that the curative procedure itself, particularly surgery, has for the patient is another variable among threats to the body image. Some patients feel that to sign a release for surgery is to sign away one's life. Others feel that to sign for general anesthesic is to sign away control of one's body, and render oneself absolutely helpless. There is also the fear of being cut, being in pain, and being mutilated.

The person who has limited coping abilities to deal with stress, and who is easily made to feel helpless and powerless, will experience greater threat with a change in his body image.

To understand the nature of the threat, then, one needs to know the pattern of adaptation, the value of this pattern for the particular individual, and what coping capacities he has.

Other people in some instances influence to a considerable extent a person's response to alteration in his body image. A study of 38 married colostomy patients who were from 5 to 13 years postoperative revealed that 25 of their spouses had never seen the colostomy or had seen it only initially.[5] Only 13 of these patients (16 were woman) were given body care that involved sight of the colostomy by their spouses after being discharged from the hospital. At least nine spouses had severe reactions to the colostomy, which included refusing to look at it, fainting, vomiting, or expressing disgust. Some patients concealed their colostomies because they felt their spouses couldn't take it.[6]

Keeping in mind the 3 sequential aspects of the development of the body image, one can recognize the identity threat to some extent because one knows what aspect of body image is of primary importance in each phase. For example, to a young child, a disfiguring illness would not be as threatening in itself as one that immobilizes him or takes away some aspect of self-mastery. A sixteen-year old who suffered disfigurement would be greatly threatened, because he is concerned with attractiveness and normality. In adults one would expect the threat to be balanced by satisfactions that emanate from the soma and satisfactions attained in the intellectual, spiritual, and social spheres of the psyche.

Other factors that influence the degree of threat include the extent or degree of change and the rate at which it occurs. One great and sudden change will cause a greater threat than numerous small changes over a period of time.

ADAPTATION TO ALTERATION IN BODY IMAGE

Adaptation to alteration in body size, function or structure, as has been noted, depends upon the nature of the threat, its meaning to the individual, his coping ability, the response from others significant to him, and the help available to him in undergoing change and to his family. If surgery is involved, adaptation really starts beforehand. In the study of colostomy patients cited earlier,[5] three patterns of family responses to the recommended surgery were identified. One type of family gave encouragement and support, hiding its own fears and anxieties to encourage the patient. Another type of family became threatening, attempting to force the patient into surgery immediately and warning of the dire consequences of delay. These families went into action at the point of emergency at which the diagnosis became known, rather than from the point at which the patient had symptoms. The third type of family became immobilized either from fright or illness of another family member and left the patient alone to make the decision and arrange for hospitalization. Also, included in this group is the uninterested, rejecting family. This study provided evidence that the family's preoperative pattern of behavior toward the patient indicates how they will behave toward him postoperatively. The groundwork is laid for postoperative healthy adaptation in the healthy preoperative patient-family relationship.

In elective surgery a preoperative adaptation task for the patient is to project himself into the experience ahead. Signs of potential maladaptation are absence of anxiety, joking about the surgery or matter-of-factness about it. A normal person is concerned and begins dealing with it. The serene patient who communicates that the surgery will bring an end to all difficulties, or that he will never miss the part to be removed, is anxious to such a degree that the anxiety is repressed, only to come to the fore later as panic or in some way to alter the postoperative course.

Accidents account for over 1,800,000 traumatic injuries per year. Thus, almost two million people experience some alteration in body image which cannot be prepared for in advance. One might expect that after the shock of trauma wears off, these patients would experience the attacks on their body images more sharply and acutely than would the person who elects surgery.

The patient often initiates the adaptive process by requesting to see the changed part of his body. He may not ask, but instead peeks a little more each time dressings are done; he studies the area, using a mirror. Being able to look at what has happened to the self is one step in coping with it. Victims of accidents or emergencies may have more difficulty at this point because of the lack of opportunity to "prepare." However, if the patient is still in a state of shock or has a concussion, he may accept change calmly, only to panic when he again has full use of his faculties.

Testing and experimenting with those persons significant to them may be the next steps for most patients in coping with change. Nurses, as persons significant in the patient's recovery, are often the first ones tested. Many nurses find this a difficult task and some misunderstand the patient's need to show "my operation." The patient may give the nurse a choice and ask, "Have you seen my operation?" or "Would you like to see my operation?"; or the patient may complain of pulling, itching or local pain, hoping to coerce the nurse into an examination. Other patients will raise their gowns and demand, "Look at my operation!" This even happens in social situations. There are probably two related problems operating in these patients. The afflicted part is a source of both fascination and revulsion. The patient can hardly tolerate the thought, sight or idea of the change in his body image, but cannot stop looking and exploring the significance of the change. Another explanation for this patient's behavior might be that he was really saying, "I don't know whether I'm as attractive or worth as much as I was. What do you think?" Hopefully, the patient will be able to take the next step up to testing with family and friends. This does not mean that showing is the only way of testing. Discussion and observation of the behavior of others is testing, too. The patient's expectation of rejection or his feelings of guilt over what happened to him may cause errors in perceiving the behavior of others, so that his pessimistic expectations seemingly are confirmed. Another patient problem in the early verbal-testing phase is questioning that pleads and beguiles the respondent into giving a positive or hopeful answer. It is important that any conversation about change in body image go well. As soon as emotionally laden material can be talked about, one step in acceptance has occurred; the subject is no longer too painful to mention.

If the body image change has been highly threatening to the patient, he may rage and grieve. This is a very normal reaction which may be necessary before hope and positive action can supplant it. Prolonged grief and rage, such as one may see in the adult paraplegic victim, may be very difficult to interrupt.

Denial is a common response also. It has been noted that this can occur preoperatively as a maladaptive response in surgical patients. The denying patient is headed for further such responses, some of which are reworked into a way of living. Feelings of emptiness, vague symptoms of illness such as weakness and fatigue, feelings of fragility, feelings of vulnerability, intractable pain, hypochondrical problems, psychosomatic conditions involving organ or system pathology, nervousness, obsession, or phobias are some of the conditions that may develop and persist as ways of coping with trauma, including trauma to the body image. Denial is often the result of repressed anxiety, but it may be related to altered perception. Ullman describes this kind of problem in patients after stroke, in which the patient is unaware of his illness.[6] The thinking of the patient goes "If I can't feel it, if it feels like it's missing, if I can't find it, then, indeed, it isn't mine, but must belong to somebody else."

In patients who have lost control of complex, coordinated neuromuscular activity, denial may be the only alternative to psychosocial death, psychosis, or succumbing to apathy and resignation. Shame is nearly always a response to threat in which control of self or one's

58   The Professional Nurse and Body Image

immediate space—e.g., the ability to manipulate a urinal, bed pan, meal tray etc.—is lost.

Time, as has been noted, is a factor in adaptation. It takes time to cope adequately with threats. However, if anxiety is high and support is low, pathological coping mechanisms go into operation early and are more difficult to alter than they are to prevent.

NURSING INTERVENTION

The content of other disciplines provides a general theoretical framework for understanding the development of body image, its dynamic nature, its importance to self-actualization, its socially and culturally determined facets, the variety of psychotic traumata that occur when the body is attacked, and the variety of coping and succumbing responses of which man is capable.

The nursing process that makes this content become meaningful and operational may be called nursing assessment, nursing examination or nursing history. Whatever we call it, the basic problem of this process is how to structure the nursing history, assessment or examination so that we elicit the information needed to make a nursing diagnosis.

The conceptual frame of reference for this examination has many dimensions. Cultural values and prejudices concerning wholeness, independence and attractiveness can be used to determine whether the patient feels isolated, excluded, stigmatized, helpless or ashamed. Knowledge about the patient's occupation, social group membership and his habitual ways of interacting can be used to decide to what extent his life is disrupted. Knowledge about a person's needs for inclusion, affection and control helps the nurse look at him in light of the attack on his body image. Knowledge about the patient's feelings of self-esteem and security, as well as operation of his methods of coping, is helpful in identifying actual and potential problems. Knowledge of family dynamics helps the nurse assess family solidarity—whether the family provides sustained support, or at the other extreme, is emotionally impoverished and cannot rise to any crisis. Knowledge of useful or nonuseful human coping activity helps the nurse to identify avoidance, compensation and problem solving. She should be able to recognize the grief that accompanies final, permanent and irrevocable loss, which may elicit rage or, oppositely, succumbing behavior. She will be helped greatly also if she recognizes that body image attack involves problems of altered appearance, discomfort, dependence, stigma, social isolation, action and movement limitation, vocational threat, deformity, and loss of control. Age is always a consideration, and the nurse also needs to be aware of the vast discrepancy between psychological, physiological and chronological age. It should not surprise her that some middle-aged spinsters grieve more deeply over a hysterectomy than do some young and newly married women. In all aspects of assessment the nurse should be aware of the patient's definition of the situation—his perception of what is to happen, or what has happened to him. Actually, the casual or laconic patient is the easiest to describe and diagnose, but most difficult to work with because of the effectiveness of his denial. The stroke patient, mentioned previously, who denies because of disordered perception and sensation is even more difficult to approach.

In the history taking process, usually the most useful attitude for the nurse to assume is to regard the patient as a person coping, in however inadequate a way, with what is to him an overwhelming experience. If the nurse labels the patient "disoriented" or "crazy," it may be difficult to identify coping mechanisms.

In relation to a patient's body image, the nurse should look for indications that his life roles are challenged, threatened or are meaningless; that the patient is questioning who he is; that he is experiencing strange bodily sensations, loss of feeling or contact, detachment or depersonalization, as if he were observing what is happening to him instead of experiencing it. Intellectualizing in which the patient is both very reasonable and logical is related to this observation. The nurse needs to ask about what she sees. If the nurse feels threatened by what she sees, she will be unable to explore its meaning with the patient. The nursing diagnosis needs to include an appraisal of the family's ability to support the patient, to tolerate stress, and to deal with all the realities of the situation. It needs to include the patient's reality orientation to his experience, the problems with which he is trying to cope and how he is trying to cope with them. The nursing diagnosis should include predictions insofar as possible, since this alerts others and sets up expectations.

The nursing care plan needs to include means of supporting family members and helping them develop the strengths needed to cope with the patient's problem. It also needs to include support of positive moves the patient makes and ways of dealing with his inadequate coping mechanisms. The need to express grief and rage to an accepting person cannot be ignored for the period immediately following an abrupt change in the body image. This period may be a long one if the loss is very great. Following this period, reinforcing hope and suggesting moves to compensate for the problem must be considered within the total plan.

The nursing therapy aspect of intervention in matters involving the body image is limited at present because of the need for more nursing research in this area. Valid nursing theory requires more adequate descriptions of patient response to body image threats. It must look for ways to characterize patients and their response to threat into some kind of typology, identifying the variables that provide for prediction, and then test situations in which nurses prevent or intervene in these problems.

REFERENCES

1. Sutherland, A. M.: Psychological impact of cancer and its therapy. Med. Clin. N. Am., *40*:705-72, 1956.
2. Conference on Preparation for Leadership in Psychiatric Nursing Service. p. 74. Teachers College, Columbia University, New York, Columbia University Press, 1963.
3. Drellich, M. G., Bieber, I., and Sutherland, A.: The psychological impact of cancer and cancer surgery. Cancer, *9*:1120-1126, 1956.
4. Ullman, M.: Disorders of body image after stroke. Am. J. Nurs., *64*:89-91, October, 1964.
5. Dyk, R. B., and Sutherland, A. M.: Adaptation of the spouse and other family members to the colostomy patient. Cancer, *9*:123, 1956.
6. Ullman, M.: Disorders of body image after stroke. Am. J. Nurs., *64*, 10:89-91, 1964.

BIBLIOGRAPHY

Abel, T. M.: Figure drawings and facial disfigurement. Am. J. Orthopsychiat., *23*:253-264, 1953.

Alexander, F.: Psychosomatic Medicine. New York, W. W. Norton & Co., 1950.

Angyal, A.: Experience of body-self in schizophrenia. Arch. Neurol. Psychiat., *35*:1029-1053, 1936.

Arnhoff, F., and Damianopolous, E.: Self body recognition and schizophrenia. J. Gen. Psychol., *70*:353-361, 1964.

Asch, S. E., and Witkin, H. A.: Studies in space orientation: 1. Perception of the upright with displaced visual fields. J. Exp. Psychol., *38*:325-337, 1948.

Asch, S. E., and Witkin, H. A.: Studies in space orientation. 2. Perception of the upright with displaced visual fields and with body tilted. J. Exp. Psychol., *38*:455-477, 1948.

Bailey, A. A., and Moersch, F. P.: Phantom limb. Canad. Med. Ass. J., *45*:37-42, 1941.

Baker, W. Y., and Smith, L. H.: Facial disfigurement and personality. J.A.M.A., *112*:301-304, 1939.

Bard, M.: The use of dependence for predicting psychogenic invalidism following radical mastectomy. J. Nerv. Men. Dis., *122*:152-160, 1955.

Bender, L., and Silver, A.: Body image problems of the brain damaged. J. Soc. Issues, *4*:84-89, 1948.

Bender, M. B.: Disorders in Perception. Springfield, Ill., Charles C Thomas, 1952.

Bennett, D. H.: Perception of upright in relation to body image. J. Ment. Sc., *102*:487-506, 1956.

Bibring, G. L.: Psychiatric principles in casework. Soc. Casework, *30*:230-235, 1949.

Bressler, F., Cohen, S. I., and Magnussen, F.: The problem of phantom breast and phantom pain. J. Nerv. Ment. Dis., *123*:181-187, 1956.

Bruch, H.: Falsification of bodily needs and body concept in schizophrenia. Arch. Gen. Psychiat., *6*:18-24, 1962.

Bychowski, F.: Disorders in body image in the clinical pictures of psychoses. J. Nerv. Ment. Dis., *97*:310-335, 1943.

Bibliography

Cath, S. H., Glud, E., and Blane, H. T.: The role of the body image in psychotherapy with the physically handicapped. Psychoanal. Rev., *44*:34-40, 1957.

Cleveland, S. E., Fisher, E., Reitman, E. E., and Rothaus, P.: Perception of body size in schizophrenia. Arch. Gen. Psychiat., 7:277-285, 1962.

Cohen, H., and Jones, H. W.: Reference of cardiac pain to a phantom left arm. Brit. Heart J., *5*:67-71, 1943.

Deutsch, F., *et al.:* Mind and the Sensory Gateways. New York, Basic Books, 1963.

Dixon, J. C.: The relation between perceived change in self and in other. J. Gen. Psychol., *73*:137-142, July, 1965.

Echols, D. H., and Colclough, J. A.: Abolition of painful phantom foot by resection of the sensory cortex. J.A.M.A., *134*:1476-1477, 1947.

Ewalt, J. R., Randall, G. C., and Morris, H. D.: The phantom limb. Psychosom. Med., *9*:118-123, 1947.

Fisher, S. M.: Body image and psychopathy. Arch. Gen. Psychiat., *10*:519-529, 1964.

Fisher, S., and Cleveland, S.: An approach to physiological reactivity in terms of a body image schema. Psychol. Rev., *64*:26-37, 1957.

Fisher, S. M., and Cleveland, S. E.: Body Image and Personality. New York, Van Nostrand, 1958.

Fisher, S. M., and Seidner, R.: Body experiences of schizophrenic, neurotic and normal women. J. Nerv. Ment. Dis., *137*:252-257, 1963.

Flew, A.: Body, Mind and Death. New York, Macmillan, 1968.

Freud, A.: The Role of Bodily Illness in the Mental Life of Children. *In* The Psychoanalytic Study of the Child. Vol. 7. pp. 69-81. New York, International Universities Press, 1952.

Garrett, J. F. (ed.): Psychological Aspects of Physical Disability. Federal Security Agency, Office of Vocational Rehabilitation, Series No. 210, Washington, D.C., 1952.

Garrett, J. F., and Levine, E. S. (eds.): Psychological Practices with the Physically Disabled. New York, Columbia University Press, 1962.

Hamerschlag, C. A., Fisher, S., Decrosse, J., *et al.:* Breast symptoms and patient delay: Psychological variables involved. Cancer, *17*:1480-1485, 1964.

Harvey, F.: Some social aspects in the care of patients undergoing breast surgery. Med. Soc. Work, *4*:99-110, 1955.
Heusner, A. P.: Phantom genitalia. Trans. Am. Neurol. Ass., *75*:128-134, 1950.
Hoffer, W., and Osmond, H.: Olfactory changes in schizophrenia. Am. J. Psychiat., *119*:72-75, 1962.
Hoffman, J.: Facial phantom phenomenon. J. Nerv. Ment. Dis., *122*:143-151, 1955.
Hoffner, W.: Mouth, hand and ego-integration. *In* Psychoanalytic Study of the Child. Vols. 3-4, pp. 49-56. New York, International Universities Press, 1949.
Horowitz, M. J., Duff, D. F., and Stratton, L. O.: Body-buffer zone: Exploration of personal space. Arch. Gen. Psychiat., *11*:651-656, 1964.
Jacobson, J. R.: A method of psychobiologic evaluation. Am. J. Psychiat., *101*:343-348, 1944.
Kolb, L. C.: Observations on somatic sensory extinction phenomenon and body scheme after unilateral resection of the posterior central gyrus. Trans. Am. Neurol. Ass., *75*:138-141, 1950.
─────: The Painful Phantom. Springfield, Ill., Charles C Thomas, 1964.
Kubie, L. S.: Motivation and rehabilitation. Psychiatry, *8*:69-78, 1945.
Levy, D. M.: Body interest in children and hypochondriasis. Am. J. Psychiat., *12*:295-315, 1932.
Linn, L.: Some developmental aspects of the body image. Int. J. Psychoanal., *36*:36-42, 1955.
Long, D. C.: Philosophical concept of a human body. J. Philosoph. Rev., *73*:321-337, 1964.
Lowen, A.: The Betrayal of the Body. New York, Macmillan, 1967.
McConnell, W. B.: The phantom double in pregnancy. Brit. J. Psychiat., *111*:67-69, 1965.
Meerloo, J. A. M.: Fate of one's face with some remarks on implications of plastic surgery. Psychiat. Quart., *30*:31-43, 1956.
Perls, F., *et al.:* Gestalt Therapy. New York, Dell, 1965.
Pinner, M., and Miller, B. F.: When Doctors Are Patients. New York, W. W. Norton & Co., 1952.
Pollack, M., and Goldfarb, W.: The face-hand test in schizophrenic children. Arch. Neurol. Psychiat., *77*:635-642, 1957.

Rubin, R.: Body image and self-esteem. Nurs. Outlook, *16*:20-23, June, 1968.
Saxvik, B. O.: Distortions of body image following destruction of a body part. Appl. Ther., 7:43-47, 1965.
Schaffer, J.: Persons and their bodies. Philos. Rev., *75*:59-77, 1966.
Schilder, P.: The Image and Appearance of the Human Body: Psychological Monograph. London, George Routledge & Sons, 1935.
Schontz, F. C.: Body concept disturbances of patients with hemiplegia. J. Clin. Psychol., *12*:293-295, 1956.
Schutz, W. C.: Joy: Theory and Methods for Developing Human Potential. New York, Grove, 1967.
Scott, W. C. M.: Some embryological neurological, psychiatric and psychoanalytic implications of the body scheme. Int. J. Psychoanal., *29*:141-155, 1948.
Secord, P. F., and Jourard, S. M.: The appraisal of body cathexis: Body cathexis and the self. J. Consult. Psychol., *17*:343-347, 1953.
Sedman, G., and Kenna, J. C.: Depersonalization and mood changes in schizophrenia. Brit. J. Psychiat., *109*:669-673, 1963.
Smythies, J. R.: The experience and description of the human body. Brain, *76*:132-145, 1953.
Thornton, G. R.: The effect upon judgments of personality traits of varying a single factor in a photograph. J. Soc. Psychol., *18*:127-148, 1943.
Tolstoy, L.: Death of Ivan Ilych. New York, Signet, 1960.
Traub, A. C., and Orbach, J.: Psychophysical studies of the body image: I. The adjustable body-distorting mirror. Arch. Gen. Psychiat., *11*:53-66, 1964.
Ullman, M.: Disorders of body image after stroke. Am. J. Nurs., *64*:89-91, 1964.
Updegraff, H. L., and Menninger, K. A.: Some psychoanalytic aspects of plastic surgery. Am. J. Surg., *25*:554-558, 1934.
Wapner, S., and Werner, H. (eds.): The Body Precept. New York, Random House, 1965.
Wright, B. A.: Physical Disability: A Psychological Approach. New York, Harper & Row, 1960.
Wright, G. H.: The names of the parts of the body; a linguistic approach to the study of the body image. Brain, *78*:188-210, 1956.

4

Shame

Silvia Lange

The following are everyday situations in nursing settings. Their common denominator is the emotion of shame.

A teenage girl with downcast eyes tells the school nurse that she is ashamed to tell her parents that she is pregnant.

A woman delays examination of a lump in her breast because of her horror of a possible mastectomy which would lessen her femininity.

A high school athlete, quadriplegic from a diving accident, flushes crimson as the nurse tends to his bowel and bladder needs.

The parents of a child with symptoms of mental retardation keep him hidden away in a back room from friends, other children and family.

A nursing student holds back tears of humiliation when the anxious surgeon snaps at her awkwardness.

A woman, severely beaten by her husband, asks him not to visit her so that he won't be embarrassed by the hospital staff.

A man returns to the hospital in DT's after repeatedly promising himself and the staff that he would never drink again.

"Can't *you* do anything *else* to stop my pain, nurse?"

A meeting is held on the psychiatric ward in which the staff members share their feelings of inadequacy, failure, guilt, and shame after a patient on pass has committed suicide.

A four-year-old on the pediatric unit wails in despair after soiling his bed in the night.

A man berates himself for crying with pain.

A nursing instructor feels that she has failed when her students do poorly on a nationwide, standardized test.

For many people the experience of illness is in itself shameful. The diagnosis, the medical treatment, the body changes, the reactions of family and friends, hospitalization, and the many contacts during nursing care all may precipitate feelings that range from social discomfort to embarrassment to abject humiliation. A sick person is a suffering person and very vulnerable. His whole life has been changed, at least temporarily, and he struggles with the resurgence of past experiences as he attempts to cope with present realities and to plan for the future.

The nurse is a central figure in his immediate life. Through sensitive and compassionate understanding and actions she can provide multiple opportunities for the patient to maintain his self-esteem and for him to share with, and explore with her, the aspects of his illness that threaten him. The nurse can develop her awareness of what shame means to individuals in all sorts of situations. In order to do so, she must be aware of her own feelings of shame in both her professional and her personal life. Shame leaves no one alone. Experience in observing illness, and daily contact with any group of patients, gives the nurse many opportunities to observe, analyze, and intervene therapeutically in the reactions of people being shamed and shaming others.

DEFINITION OF SHAME

Shame is only one emotion or affect among many, although it is central, complex, and interrelated with the others. Its importance in any person's life depends to a large extent on it's intensity, duration, and frequency. Shame is often mixed with other emotions; thus these emotions are experienced along with the shame. One can be afraid and feel ashamed of cowardice; one can feel humiliated and cover it up with anger; one can feel jealous and be ashamed of one's pettiness. Shame, guilt, and feelings of inferiority are often present together.

Shame and its synonyms are words used frequently but without precise definition. Webster defines shame as "Painful emotion excited by a consciousness of guilt, shortcoming, or impropriety."[1] Disgrace, humiliation, embarrassment, tragedy and guilt can all be expressed by "It's a shame." Other popular expressions include, "Shame on you!" "I was too embarrassed for words;" "A shameless hussy;" "I could have sunk through the floor." Children sing a mocking chant, "Shame, shame, double shame, everybody knows your name." A social blunder may be erased by the jingle, "It's better to burp and bear the shame, than squelch the belch and bear the pain." (Not everyone would agree.)

Tomkins wrote extensively on shame and stated:

> ...shame is the affect of indignity, of defeat, of transgression and of alienation.... shame strikes deepest into the heart of man...shame is felt as an inner torment, a sickness of soul. It does not matter whether the humiliated one has been shamed by derisive laughter or whether he mocks himself. In either event he feels himself naked, defeated, alienated, lacking in dignity or worth.[2]

The early psychoanalytic definition indicated that shame is a defense against exhibitionism and voyeurism: "I feel ashamed" means "I do not want to be seen."[3]

Threat of exposure is part of shame. Erikson stated:

> Shame supposes that one is completely exposed and conscious of being looked at—in a word, self-conscious. One is visible and not ready to be visible. That is why we dream of shame as a situation in which we are being stared at in a condition of incomplete dress, in night attire, "with one's pants down"... the destructiveness of shaming is balanced in some civilizations by devices for "saving face." Shaming exploits an increasing sense of being small, which paradoxically develops as the child stands up and as his awareness permits him to note the relative measure of size and power.[4]

Lynd regarded shame as being closely associated with self and therefore being a clue to a broader understanding of identity:

> "Experiences of shame....are experiences of exposure, exposure of peculiarly sensitive, intimate, vulnerable aspects of the self. The exposure may be to others but, whether others are or are not involved, it is always ....exposure to one's own eyes."[5]

The relation of physical exposure—nakedness—to shame is shown in the account of Adam and Eve, who felt shame after eating of the fruit of the tree of the knowledge of good and evil, and subsequently covered themselves from the sight of each other and from God. The German word from which our word "shame" is derived is part of a compound word relating to the genitals. However, experiences of shame involve much more than sexual exposure. The uncovering of weakness, failure, physical defect, passivity, misplaced confidence, and lack of recognition are all shameful experiences.

When urged to participate in a therapeutic speech group by reading a poem, a 28-year old woman rushed out of the room cursing and slamming the door. Later, she told the nurse she was very ashamed of not knowing how to read and that she usually covered this up by bluffing or getting angry. The nurse conveyed her impression that the patient was an intelligent person, and later was able to help make arrangements for special tutoring.

A teenage girl received severe burns of her breasts as the result of sunbathing in the nude. She delayed medical treatment because of her embarrassment about the location of the burn and because of her feelings of shame that she had been so stupid.

One cause of shame for a girl seeking a therapeutic abortion was that she had put her trust in a man who turned out to be the local Casanova. She was ashamed because she had been seduced by an unworthy man and felt so guilty that she could only consider abortion or suicide, and was ashamed that she must ask other people for help. She was embarrassed by her tears and her dependence.

A 77-year old woman was restless and anxious after emergency surgery until she confided that her chief concern was that the black from her recently-dyed hair was rubbing off on the pillowcase. The nurses were surprised that she had so much pride in her appearance at her age.

Hair, dentures, make-up, privacy, and toilet rituals are taken for granted until a person is plunged into the often bewildering, impersonal, and embarrassing hospital environment. In the home, a sudden visit by the public health nurse may precipitate feelings of exposure and shame regarding children who won't behave, an alcoholic husband, or even dishes piled in the sink.

Shameful experiences are characteristically sudden and unavoidable. The incident may appear trivial or inconsequential to others, but it can precipitate intense feelings of self-consciousness and personal failure. Another aspect of shame involves admitting to oneself parts of the self that have been unrecognized or unacceptable. Shame may occur when one deceives others into believing something about oneself that is not true. Feelings of shame for others may be acute. Children may be painfully ashamed of, and for, their parents, and parents may experience helpless feelings of shame for their children, whose behavior may reflect their own parental failures. Parents of hippies often demonstrate this.

The feelings and reactions that have been labeled as shame are often complex and difficult to distinguish from other feelings, such as anxiety, guilt, and inferiority. Shame and guilt are often linked as if they were synonymous. However, closer study has differentiated them. Although they may be operating in the same individual at the same time, they are considered to be overlapping, rather than identical, emotions. For instance, a girl may feel guilty about her promiscuity, ashamed of her frigidity, and inferior in regard to other girls. The young child who has difficulty with anal control feels bad, ashamed, and inferior.

Some of the differences between shame and guilt have been identified as the following:

1. Shame is generated when a goal or ideal is not being reached; guilt is more tied with transgression of a specific code or law.

2. Shame concerns the more basic, unalterable aspects of the self (appearance, intelligence, race) as compared to the ideal—the should-be's and the ought-to-be's; guilt concerns violations of social codes of behavior, cleanliness, politeness, and rules—the do's and the don'ts.

3. The unconscious, irrational threat in shame is abandonment; in guilt it is retaliation, mutilation, and castration.

4. Shame may involve the feeling of having loved the wrong person or being inadequate for the person one loves; guilt involves a feeling of wrong-doing toward a love object. Unconscious hostility is often part of guilt.

5. Shame results from tension between the ego and ego ideal; guilt stems from conflict between ego and superego.

6. Shame pertains to what one is—weak, inadequate. Guilt pertains to what one has done—bad things.

7. To be shameless is to be brazen, unblushing, insensitive to self and others—"bad"; to be guiltless is to be exonerated, innocent—"good."

8. Shame refers more to visual exposure; guilt occurs predominantly in reaction to verbal demands, prohibitions, and criticisms.

Is there feeling opposite to the feeling of shame? If this reaction stems from experiences of failure or as a defense against exposure, can self-confidence and pride be regarded on the other end of the continuum? Engel supports this view:

> Pride is the affect specially indicating success in living up to standards of the ego ideal. It pronounces satisfaction with the self, which feels correspondingly strengthened, loved, admired, and invulnerable. The person feeling pride is eager to display himself and to be seen . . . (Pride) is particularly related to all varieties of achievement, the various ways in which mastery is achieved in relation to the environment and to objects. The earliest expressions of pride are particularly related to the development and mastery of the body.[6]

72   Shame

In writing about the effort to maintain social poise, Goffman stated that the individual who senses that he is "in face" will typically respond with feelings of confidence and reassurance.[7] He can hold his head up high and openly present himself to others. According to him, poise is the capacity to suppress and conceal any tendency to become shamefaced during encounters with others.

Pride is as complex an emotion as shame and its consideration cannot be oversimplified. It ranges from compensatory measures for feelings of inadequacy and inferiority to genuine feelings of self-respect and accomplishment.

DESCRIPTION OF SHAME REACTIONS

Who needs to be told what it feels like to experience shame? Ranging from mild embarrassment to excruciating humiliation, the subjective feeling involves a sudden awareness of anxiety, a sense of painful self-consciousness, and the wish to hide or escape. Statements of self-blame and self-derogation may be made, along with other verbal reports that the person feels embarrassed, ashamed, or humiliated. The more intense the feeling, the less likely one is to report it or mention it.

Shame can be recognized by some characteristic body reactions which may be observed in oneself or others. These are the general signs of anxiety, with specific relevance to the state of being observed. Some signs are:

1. Complete or partial withdrawal from visual contact—lowering of the eyes, blinking, bowing the head, turning the back, avoiding eye contact, glancing up furtively, covering face with hands.

2. Sudden changes in skin color—blushing, blanching, flushing.

3. Nervous physical gestures, etc.—twisting of the fingers, nervously playing with hair or clothes, inspecting hands carefully, scuffing the feet, tremors, hesitating or vacillating manner, weak knees, tense muscles.

4. Difficulty with speech—stuttering, very soft voice, voice pitched very high or very low (or breaking), dryness of mouth, inability to speak, incoherence.

Modification and control of the reaction to shame are seen in the adult who abbreviates the response by quickly raising his eyes and head. The frozen face of chronic shame may look continually humble and bowed down. A person may assume an anti-shame posture, in which the head is tilted back with the chin jutted out to help himself obey the command against admitting shame: "Keep your chin up." The embarrassed laugh attempts to cover up the discomfort, as may the burst of anger.

The mixture of shame with other emotions may produce such facial expressions as the following: with fear—humble and terrified; with distress—sad and defeated; with excitement—eyes glancing around, although the head is bowed; with anger—tight jaw, lowered head, a frown.

Blushing is a reaction to the experience of shame that has been mentioned repeatedly in both classical and psychiatric literature. Usually related to sexual feelings, the sudden, involuntary flushing of the face is a common symptom. This reaction is generally not regarded as pathologic, although as erthyrophobia it may reach such proportions as to keep a person from social situations that are stimulating and shaming. Because blushing is an open signal of inner discomfort, the shaming situation may be compounded. There comes the wish to cover one's face, sink into the floor, or become invisible. Young male patients, especially those on orthopedic wards, exploit this phenomenon to the nth degree with young nursing students by means of a barrage of suggestive remarks, dirty jokes, and excessive compliments. Learning how to cope with this situation is a special kind of learning experience.

> A man frequently shifted attention away from himself in group therapy by observing correctly that the therapist was blushing. The therapist would then blush even deeper, but handled this matter-of-factly by saying, "Yes, and you know how to make it worse" and refocusing on the patient.

Another specific way of expressing and handling shame reactions is the use of hand-to-mouth movements, which restore social and psychic equilibrium.[8] Such things as playing with the mouth, biting on a pencil, thumb sucking, lip biting, and covering of the lower face serve to hide a quivering lip. Gum chewing, the cocktail glass, cigarette smoking, excessive cosmetics, and moustaches help to accomplish the same purpose. Rangel developed the following sequence of security operations:

1. Infant with its mouth and snout buried in the breast.
2. 1½-year-old in its mother's arms, when approached by a stranger, turning away and burrowing into his mother's shoulder.
3. Older child turning its face into a corner so as not to be seen.

4. Adult, unpoised, blushing, and wanting to cover or hide his face.[9]

THE DEVELOPMENT OF SHAME

Shame results from tension between the ego and the ego ideal. The ego ideal refers to standards, aspirations, and goals which are internalized through identification with the culture—specifically, with the parents. The parent can either be loving and reassuring or one who imposes his own ideals (often unachieved). In his ego ideal the child also includes qualities that he wishes that the parent did possess—such as beauty, wisdom, strength—as well as qualities of his own. Keys to the ego ideal include the answers to such questions as: What did you want to be when you grew up? What did your parents want you to be? Who was your childhood hero? Why? What is the ideal—be it girl, woman, wife, mother, or boy, man, husband, father—like? What is the ideal nurse like? If you had a magic wand, what about yourself would you change?

Shame, according to Engel, involves the discrepancy between the idealized self and the self as actually perceived.[10] The failure to achieve the standards stimulates a fear of abandonment as expressed by the reaction "I am not worthy." The susceptibility to shame is increased when the internal standards are too high or too perfectionistic. If parental figures demand too high a performance as the price for love, the "failing" person may feel that he is unlovable and, therefore, not deserving of attention and love. The feeling of utter worthlessness and being held in contempt with the threat of abandonment expresses the most extreme shame reaction. Lesser degrees involve less harsh and final judgments and so allow for greater potentiality of making good, regaining pride, and re-establishing a favorable opinion of oneself. Success in meeting the ego ideal results in pride.

Kaplan and Whitman developed a way of looking at shame as stemming from two origins—the positive ego ideal and the negative ego ideal.[11] The negative ego ideal includes the qualities that have been ridiculed, disparaged, and held in contempt. For instance, if courage in the face of physical pain is part of the positive ego ideal, then cowardice is part of the negative ego ideal. Therefore, shame can result when one falls short of his interalized aspirations, and also when he behaves or feels about himself in a way that approximates his negative ego ideal.

Beginning nursing students frequently experience embarrassment, humiliation, and a sense of personal failure by setting unrealistic goals for themselves as expert practitioners. They compare themselves unfavorably with more experienced students and R.N.'s and are mortified when they have to admit to a patient that they don't yet know how to do a simple procedure.

At times hospital staff members and instructors may add to this stress by shaming the student, either consciously or unwittingly, for her ineptitude and lack of knowledge. Nursing instructors can help students to deal with the situation more adequately, assisting them in sorting out their educational goals, discussing their assets and limitations, and talking about their ideals and the necessary steps to reach these goals.

Engel also considered disgust to be linked up with the development of shame.[12] Disgust is the affect that is a reaction against the oral and anal drives which are primarily involved in tasting swallowing, and smelling. Disgust contributes to the standards that are part of the ego ideal and the superego and that inculcate a special kind of guilt and shame. To be disgusted with oneself involves judging oneself as being dirty (fecally or sexually) and malodorous, therefore deserving only to be pushed away, segregated, and isolated. To feel disgusted with someone else is to see him as unclean, unacceptable, and/or unpleasant, and to wish to be rid of him.

Nurses need to come to grips with the reaction of disgust and learn to understand it in order to give nursing care to patients whose condition is repulsive. Sometimes disgust is an automatic response of some persons to such things as feces, vomit, or foul-smelling drainage. Other people are disgusted by obesity, disfigurement, emaciation, congenital anomalies, sexual deviations, lice, and body odor. Before the patient can be helped with his condition, the nurse must understand the basis of her own reactions and deal with them appropriately.

Shame is generally considered to be first experienced in regard to body function and image. The child feels ashamed of his weakness, smallness, nakedness, and lack of control, especially when compared with his parents. A derivative of this is feeling shame because of a deformity or disfigurement.

Shame for adults involves abstract concepts such as: the values of physical and mental health; intellectual performance; beauty; strength; sexual, vocational and monetary success and power; racial identification; national prestige; and socio-economic status. In any society there may be moral and ethical codes that conflict with these concepts, and the child may be presented with standards different from those of his parents, educators, peers, and the broader society. The ego ideal changes as new and different identifications are made; however, under stress, the individual generally returns to original constructs.

Ruesch identified some of the overall American values as being related to our pioneer and puritan heritage, with the virtues being those of toughness, resourcefulness, purpose, purity, equality, sociality, and change.[13] He recognized the powerful influence of the cultural group on the individual's feelings and behavior, with the degree of conformity being a common consideration. Competition and the need to win success are stimulated at an early age, when the American parent covertly requires and demands of his baby that he be larger, healthier, and more precocious than other children. Love is given conditionally to reward these achievements, which can be demonstrated in quantitative terms—number of hits in the Little League, number of Girl Scout cookies sold, how many A's on the report card, and how many dates a week. As a social group the hippies are challenging many of these values; they are interesting to study in relation to shame because of their questioning attitudes toward many traditional values. Ethnic groups that have not been assimilated may have different values.

In the development of the personality, some experiences are of special significance in relation to shame; one such is muscular control. According to Erikson, the child struggles with the problems of muscular control during the second stage of personality development—roughly, from the second to the fourth year. Achievement of self-control results in the feelings of autonomy, pride and self-esteem. Failure to do so results in shame, doubt, and diffuse anxiety.

Later, illness may reactivate conflict about bodily control and thereby impose stress, which complicates complete recovery. Such conflict is particularly characteristic of illnesses or treatments that radically change the body image and functioning. For instance, a colostomy is generally regarded by the patient as disgusting, ugly, and unnatural, despite preparation before surgery, and the task of regaining bowel control is closely linked with shame, humiliation, pride and self-esteem.

Child-rearing practices often involve shaming, particularly in relation to toilet training and the inculcation of appropriate social behavior. The control of bed wetting is often handled (or mishandled) through shaming technics.

If shaming is used extensively in the socialization of the expression of emotions, the individual may later experience shame in many situations in which a display of emotion takes place.[14] For instance, if a child is made to feel shame for his noisy excitement and laughter, he may later feel shame over any source of enjoyment and excitement, sexual or otherwise. If he is shamed because he has cried in distress, he may later feel shame whenever distressed by hunger, pain, fatigue, and frustration. This may pose particular problems during illness. The child may be shamed for expressing anger, contempt, fear, surprise, curiosity, and shame itself.

Tomkins emphasized the importance of child-rearing practices that are based on an "anti-shame" ideology.[15] Through attitude, word, and deed, parents can convey an attitude of respect and caring. They nurture the child with sympathy and understanding, so that he is helped to cope with discouragement and failure, and to learn ways to avoid defeat. Good socialization of shame experiences may: attenuate shame; allow the child to express, deal with, and reduce shame; increase trust; increase willingness and ability to offer sympathy and help to others and self; potentiate progress; develop physical courage; increase tolerance in problem solving; and aid in the achievement of identity. The nurse, especially in maternal-child and public health nursing, has many opportunities to help parents develop these attitudes toward their children.

As the child enters the latency or juvenile period, he shifts to his peers for recognition and for hope of inclusion in a peer group. Differences in background, abilities, maturation, and social standing help to create in-groups and out-groups. Ostracism becomes a powerful weapon, which the child seeks to avoid having directed against him. Disparagement and ridicule of others may develop at this time. Learned from parents who teach the child to notice the shortcomings of others, it can be a means of maintaining a shaky self-esteem by attacking and depreciating others. If used extensively, disparagement can interfere with correct appraisal of one's personal worth—everyone is "bad," including me.

Adolescence is also a crucial period in which shame is operative. Physical appearance, masculine and feminine identity, emancipation from dependence on parents, achievement in school and work, and comparisons with both the younger people's and older people's worlds—all may be shame-provoking. Loss of face, embarrassment, humiliation, exquisite sensitivity make this period a trial for many. The adolescent who becomes ill brings all his pride and shame to the treatment situation. This is one reason that nursing students find it particularly difficult and challenging to work with someone in this age bracket.

During the years of middle and old age, the individual may experience painful and devastating feelings of shame for what he has not accomplished, for becoming socially useless, and for failure of his physical and mental capacities. At their extreme these feelings may lead to suicide.

THE FUNCTION AND VALUE OF SHAME

Although it is generally considered a "negative" emotion, shame has both function and value. It can be regarded as an important message to oneself and can provide opportunities for further self-development.

Engel has divided emotions into two main categories—the drive-discharge affects (anger, love, tenderness, sexual excitement) and the signal-scanning affects (shame, guilt, sadness, hopelessness, contentment, joy, and pride.)[16] The latter fulfills a warning function—an evaluation of one's performance—a "how am I doing?" The judgment of "good," "bad," "pleasant," "unpleasant," "success" or "failure" is sent back as part of ego function, either to maintain present behavior or to make a shift.

The drive-discharge affect reaches a peak and is either discharged or blocked. In either case the emotion is then replaced by one of the signal-scanning affects, pleasurable or unpleasurable, depending upon the ego's evaluation of the consequences. A teacher might shout at a student in anger and feel ashamed that she had lost her temper and not "understood" the student. A nursing student may reach out in great tenderness and compassion to hold a sick toddler and then feel embarrassed and bewildered when the child screams.

Shame provides a warning to the ego that some impulse, thought, fantasy, or act has failed or will fail to meet the standards of the ego ideal. When the signal is effective, psychic processes or behavior, or both, maintain the standards. A twinge of shame at the dean's reception might prevent one from acting inappropriately and making a fool of himself. Ego defense mechanisms that prevent expression of the impulse may be used as well as activity directed toward accomplishment, creativity, and achievement.

If the signal is ineffective, the unpleasant affect of shame is felt with increasing intensity. Secondary psychic and behavior processes occur. An overwhelming sense of total personality failure may result in labeling oneself as a "slob," "fink," "jerk," "sucker," "weakling," or "square." In this way, shame may be reduced by lowered aspirations or expectations of self. Self-deprecation is one of the most destructive results of discrimination and ridicule, in that the person becomes deeply ashamed as he sees himself through the eyes of the prejudiced and accepts their evaluation as true.

Although shame-provoking experiences are characteristically painful, they may throw an unexpected light on who one really is and thus may point the way to a more complete understanding of who one might become. Such experiences may lead to a greater understanding of all men and how they live their lives.

In the trusting relationship there is a paradox regarding shame experiences. If you reveal yourself to someone you care about and he accepts you, there is a strengthening of the bond and a boost of self-esteem. However, rejection by one who is important is much more humiliating and shameful than is rejection by a mere acquaintance.

The act of sharing a "shameful" experience may in itself alleviate the fear of rejection, abandonment, and disgust. After all, everyone is human—and what's shameful about that? However, one of the most difficult aspects of dealing with shame is the private nature of the things one feels ashamed about. They are the very things one *wants* to hide and *not* talk about. Yet, when one is able to talk about it, there is a sense of relief and universality. People are just not so very different from one another in their dreams, fears, hopes, hates, lusts, and loves.

Perls has labeled shame and embarrassment as "quisling" emotions because, like the Norwegian collaborator who turned against his own country, these emotions tend to obstruct and restrict the individual's expression.[17] On the other hand, endurance, acceptance and expression of the shame will enable the person to bring the repressed material out, establish contact with and confidence in another, and discover with amazing relief that the facts behind the embarrassment were not so incriminating after all. Such liberation makes it possible for a person to experience the basic feelings of love, fear, hurt, anger, and trust.

Hank had repeatedly referred to things that he "couldn't talk about" in group therapy. The nurse received a phone call from a former friend of his, asking about his progress and inquiring if he were still getting cobalt treatments. This was new information. She decided to ask Hank about this in the group, knowing it would provide both support and pressure. He became very angry and refused to talk except to threaten to leave treatment. When he talked with the nurse privately, he maintained that the group wouldn't understand him. She expressed her concern for him whether or not he had cancer or had had treatment and encouraged him to take a chance.

Two days later Hank took a deep breath, asked the group to listen to him first and condemn him later, and confessed that to his deep shame he was a pathological liar. He had made an elaborate web of lies of which the cancer and treatment were only a small part. Instead of condemnation, the group applauded him for his courage and helped him to sort out his present problems. "I feel like a thousand-pound weight has been lifted," he said with relief.

Shame can either be a spur to accomplishment—an incentive that helps a person reach a higher level of achievement and self-esteem—or it can be an overwhelming reaction that results in progressive self-derogation, withdrawal and hopelessness, and may lead to suicide.

Shame in the Interpersonal Context

The cause and feelings of shame may be known only to the person with a secret shame, but generally other people are part of the experience of being exposed and shamed. In relating poise to shame, Rangell stated that these reactions occur only in the presence of others, for although anxiety may be present when one is alone, social threat and fear of ridicule are not. He stated:

> When one is alone, one can let oneself go, assume a posture of which one is not proud, examine in the mirror a skin blemish of which one might be ashamed, let one's stomach stick out, grimace at oneself, or squeeze a blackhead; unless, that is, one fantasies other persons as still present; in the absence of this, even the most unpoised and vulnerable can achieve a relaxed state when alone. In company and in a social setting such is not the case; a stiffening-up takes place and a certain armour, no matter how subtle, is assumed.[18]

The Function and Value of Shame

Lack of privacy in most hospital settings forces the patient to deal constantly with the threat of social disapproval at a time when he is poorly equipped to do so. Interaction with others raises the questions, "How will I do?" "Will I be accepted?" "Will my needs be met?" "Will I be welcomed, respected, noticed and listened to?" In the beginning of her clinical experiences, the nursing student is preoccupied with these questions pertaining to herself, and then she gradually shifts the focus to concentrate on the patient's needs. One student reported:

> I was to care for a two-year old boy who was in traction with synovitis of the hip. When I went in to become acquainted, I noticed that his father was there with the child. When I approached the youngster, I found that he did not wish to cooperate with me. He fought me and yelled for his father every step of the way. I usually get along very well with children, and I began to get embarrassed and to completely lose confidence in myself..... I lost my effectiveness altogether, and I became so "still" and unnatural that I never could communicate effectively with the child after that.[19]

Like anxiety, shame and embarrassment may be contagious. Therefore, considerable efforts are often exerted in order to protect oneself and others from recognizing these reactions.

Goffman stressed the importance of interpersonal situations in the precipitation of the sense of shame. Regarding all encounters as situations in which "face" is established, maintained, threatened, and recovered, he said:

> Should he sense that he is in wrong face or out of face, he is likely to feel ashamed and inferior because of what has happened to the activity on his account and because of what may happen to his reputation as a participant. Further, he may feel bad because he has relied on the encounter to support an image of self to which he has become emotionally attached and which he now feels threatened. Felt lack of judgmental support from the encounter may take him aback, confuse him, and momentarily incapacitate him as an interactant. His manner and bearing may falter, collapse, and crumble. He may become embarrassed and chagrined; he may become shamefaced.[20]

An incident reported by a nursing student illustrates this point:

> I had to do an abdominal perineal prep on this woman who was scheduled for surgery. She made many comments about how embarrassing it must be for me to do this procedure. When I said I wasn't she replied that a nurse would get used to doing it and would become hardened about

doing things like this so it would not bother her. I wasn't embarrassed at first, but as she continued to make comments of that sort, I became embarrassed and fumbled in my work.[21]

Tomkins has identified five different positions in relation to feeling shame and being shamed.[22]

1. I may feel shame for many things for which no one has shamed me. (Failure to achieve my own goals or violation of my own standards.)

2. I may not feel shame although another has tried to shame me. (if he expressed contempt of me, I may just get angry or contemptuous of him.)

3. I may be shamed by another person even though he didn't intend it. (The other person is so busy or preoccupied that he ignores me. Closely identified person—spouse, child—may produce shame by his behavior, which would shame you if you did it.)

4. I may feel ashamed because another expresses negative feelings toward me even though he doesn't intend to shame me as such. (If he is angry at me or distressed by me or frightened by me, I may feel shame for my behavior.)

5. I may feel shame because the other person is trying to shame me. (If I am doing the best I can and am satisfied but another says he is disgusted with me, I could feel shame.)

The last position was elaborated on by Leveton in discussing reproach and "shamesmanship."[23] Shaming can be a powerful interpersonal weapon, ranging all the way from tears to suicide on the part of the patient, and counterattack on the part of the therapist, by means of abandonment or inappropriate treatment.

The hypochondriacal patient, the depressed patient, and many families of schizophrenic patients use shame to an extensive degree. Hospital staffs may be demoralized by the master of reproach, who has the skill to elicit expectations and shame someone into trying to fulfill them unsuccessfully. Shaming tactics between staff members, nursing and medical, are also usually destructive.

Nonverbal aspects of the act of shaming another person include the derisive laugh, staring a person down, and using the shaming gesture—one forefinger stroking downward on the extended forefinger of the opposite hand.

Disparagement, when expressed openly and verbally, is called ridicule. Particularly vulnerable are people who deviate visibly from the norms of appearance or behavior. Wright, using many first-hand accounts of shame and humiliation, points out the devastating effects that taunting and ridicule can have on the child with a physical defect and suggests that he be given special preparation to avoid lasting damage to his self-esteem.[24] Ridicule from adults is generally more covert, though it may be expressed through curiosity, pity, ostracism, and oversolicitude.

A 13-year old boy who was extremely sensitive about his crippled legs from polio had always been overprotected. For the first time in his life he went downtown alone to a movie. As he was standing in front of the theater with a half-empty box of popcorn and his crutches, a passerby solicitously dropped a quarter in the box. On return to the hospital, the boy told the nurse about his humiliation and his fury. She listened with the feeling, "It *would* have to happen to *him*." After agreeing with him that it had been a well-meaning but very thoughtless gesture, she helped him cope with the situation by saying, "Well, at least it will pay for the popcorn the next time." He did go out alone again.

Two basic methods of handling shame situations are avoidance and correction. The person who seeks to avoid being shamed will conceal parts of the self he thinks are unacceptable, use cautious and ritualized behavior, conform socially, and keep away from "loaded" topics. Corrective efforts include acknowledging and challenging the shamer, seeking special achievement through acts that restore pride and self-confidence, maintaining a facade, denying that one has been shamed, and reacting with anger or joking.

To avoid shaming another person, an individual may provide physical and psychological privacy, keep away from touchy areas, explain why the other person need not be upset, utilize face-saving etiquette, overlook shortcomings and deviations, and use humor.

Once the situation has been precipitated, the shamer can attempt to correct it by helping the victim to restore face, apologizing and making amends, stating that he was joking or that the comment was meaningless or unintentional ("just my way"), stating that he was acting under the influence of another, and purposely ignoring shame reaction.

People are shamed by different things at different stages in their life. An experience that was humiliating at the time may be funny in retrospect.

When I was a beginning student, I was very anxious to be a good nurse and give "complete" nursing care. I was giving morning care to an elderly man who had had a stroke which left him somewhat disoriented as well as hemiplegic. He was in a six-bed ward with only curtains drawn to separate us from the other men. When it came time to "finish the bath," I realized that he didn't grasp what I meant. I lifted up the bath blanket and began diligently scrubbing away. He began to moan and groan so that the whole room could hear him. "What's the matter?" I asked, afraid that I was hurting him. "Oh lordy, oh, *lordy*," he shouted, "Does that feel good!" To make matters worse, he reached up and pinched my cheek, saying, "You delightful little devil, you!" I was very, very embarrassed—not wanting to stay with him and not wanting to leave the sanctuary of the curtained bed and face the other men. Later that night, I told my classmates in the dorm and they roared. I am still telling the story and can now laugh about it, too.

APPLICATION OF THE CONCEPT OF SHAME IN NURSING

The nurse must develop a sensitivity in relation to shame. Her knowledge of general socio-cultural values that affect patients must be used with an awareness of individual differences to minimize stereotyping. She needs to be alert to her own cultural background and biases so that she does not impose them on the patient or misinterpret his behavior. Some situations that would precipitate shame in the nurse might not in the patient, and the patient may be embarrassed by actions that are commonplace to the nurse, such as questions about elimination. Many nurses and other health team members come from a white, middle-class background. The common values that form their ego ideals might differ considerably from those of the patient who comes from another background.

This point is illustrated by Cahill in the description of the misunderstandings by nurses of the attitudes of Negro and Puerto Rican lower-class women toward illegitimacy.[25] The assumption that all unmarried mothers feel shame was often found to be a reflection of the nurse's value system but not that of the patient. Strenuous efforts to "protect" all such patients may be unwarranted and even possibly destructive.

General nursing actions related to shame are:
1. Avoid causing shame.
2. Give anticipatory help in situations in which shame is likely to occur.
3. Encourage the patient and family to share shame feelings and to deal with these constructively.
4. Minimize the need for shame in the nursing situation.

An example of this last approach:

A woman, severely injured in a hurricane, was having her clothes cut off in the emergency room. Increasingly anxious, she blushed and blurted out, "I wear falsies." "That's o.k.," the nurse replied, "I wear them, too." The patient was visibly relieved.

Nurses have the responsibility, opportunity, and privilege of helping people in crisis situations. Many times these situations involve radical shifts in ways of thinking, acting, and feeling because of the impact of illness and the necessity of altering patterns of living. Shame can be precipitated by almost any situation.

A person's perception of himself and of the situation determine whether shame is precipitated. Some common nursing situations in which shame can be anticipated and dealt with are:

1. Modesty situations
   a. Lack of privacy and exposure of the body during physical nursing procedures (enemas, catheterization, bathing)
   b. Elimination and reactions to loss of bowel and bladder control
   c. The obstetrical situation, with exposure of the genitals and discussion of the reproductive cycle
2. Regressive behavior under stress
   a. Anger
   b. Crying
   c. Loss of control during anesthesia, toxic reactions, or alcohol intoxication
3. Reactions of the patient and his family to critical situations such as:
   a. Loss of limbs and/or other disfigurement, especially of the face
   b. Mental retardation, mental illness
   c. Adjustment to physical disability, immobility and/or enforced dependence (such as being in traction)
   d. Suicide or unsuccessful suicide attempt of a family member
   e. Venereal disease and genitourinary conditions
   f. Congenital defects
4. Body changes
   a. In adolescence
   b. In the aging process

Many more could be added. Therapeutic failures and disturbed staff relations may be shame-producing for the nurse.

86   Shame

The following examples illustrate the application of the concept of shame in three major clinical areas—medical-surgical, maternal-child, and psychiatric nursing. Shame is viewed from three different perspectives: shame that comes from changes in body functioning, shame that comes from failure to meet social values, and shame that results from another's behavior.

Shame that results from changes in body functioning. For example paralysis, whether from a cerebral-vascular accident or an external injury to the spinal cord, presents complex problems. Along with grief, fear, bewilderment, anger, and denial, the patient may experience shame. This is often related to his extreme dependence, interruption of ability to care for bowel and bladder needs, lack of ability to control muscles of locomotion and speech, loss of sexual function, and impaired control over emotional expression. The nurse needs to consider the impact of illness on the person in order to help him utilize rehabilitation opportunities to the fullest.

Application of the concept of shame would include the following:

1. The nurse explores her own experiences, backgrounds, and feelings in regard to radical changes in body functioning and dependency.

2. The patient may be experiencing many emotional reactions, some of which may be shame, embarrassment, and disgust in relation to changes in his body image and lack of control over functioning and temporary dependency. The intensity depends on his unique personality and plans for the future.

3. Anger, denial, and withdrawal may be used to reduce feelings of shame, inadequacy, and despair.

4. Regaining personal control over body functions increases self-esteem and decreases shame. The nurse helps the patient by giving expert physical care, by encouraging maximal decision-making by the patient, and by teaching self-help skills.

5. Shame can be felt for another and can be precipitated in interpersonal contacts. The nurse includes the family and members of the nursing team in her understanding of the dynamics of shame for this patient.

6. Mastery of a shameful experience may lead to further personal development and a sense of pride. The nurse helps the patient to cope with his limitations and to develop alternate ways to maintain self-esteem. She may provide contact with other patients who have made a good adjustment to their condition. This helps both persons.

Shame that comes from failure to meet social values. A typical situation calling for an understanding of shame in relation to social values is that of the premature infant. Viewing the birth of a premature infant as an acute emotional crisis in a family, Kaplan and Maron expressed that the mother often experiences a deep sense of failure because she has a small, weak, often ugly baby, who barely holds on to life.[26] Such babies rarely inspire pride; congratulations, if any, are cautious. The mother feels useless, helpless, and undeserving of even being in the hospital. In her shame she avoids the nursery and the baby.

From this research it was determined that a definite pattern of psychological tasks must be accomplished in order for the mother to master the situation, so that she can provide a future healthy mother-child relationship. One task for the mother is to face and acknowledge the fact of her failure to deliver a normal, full-term baby. If she is not able to do so, it is all the harder for her to use the time with her baby in a psychologically productive way. A possible lifetime of misery and emotional disturbance for the family may result.

The nurse can help the mother of the premature (or birth-injured) infant admit, express, and come to grips with her feelings of failure and shame. Awareness of the following may be useful:

1. Part of the positive ego ideal of most women is that they will be able to deliver healthy, normal babies of which they can be proud. Part of the negative ego ideal would be inability to do so, this inability being a reflection on them as women, wives and mothers.

2. Along with feelings of inadequacy and shame, the mother may experience anger, distress, fear and guilt, which she directs at others, including her family and the medical and nursing staff, in an effort to reduce anxiety.

3. Because shame may be lessened by recognition and sharing, the nurse provides opportunities for the mother and father to talk about the baby and to express disappointment and grief without further shaming. Both privacy and companionship should be provided for.

4. Shame can be decreased, and self-esteem increased by opportunities for achievement that will relate to the shameful experience. The nurse may provide appropriate opportunities for the mother to participate in the care of the baby.

5. Feelings of shame can be reactivated—the nurse should be alert to this possibility in subsequent pregnancies of this mother. Also, the

mother may attempt to compensate for her initial failure by overprotection, and she may need help in allowing the child to grow up as a normal person with normal needs.

6. If the premature infant has other congenital anomalies or is brain damaged, the nurse should recognize the long-term needs in regard to helping the family and child make an optimal adjustment in terms of self-esteem and accomplishment without shame.

Shame as the result of another's behavior or condition. In examining the effects of the husband's mental illness upon the family, Yarrow *el al* reported that wives of hospitalized mentally ill men expect the illness to be stigmatized.[27] Wives are quoted as saying, "I'm not ashamed, but people who don't know the hospital would take the wrong attitude toward it." . . . "I live in a horror—a perfect horror—that some people will make a crack about it to Jim (child) and suppose after George gets out everything is going well and somebody throws it up in his face. That would ruin everything." "At first I was a little ashamed, but now I'm getting to understand it better . . . Of course, I have cut out seeing all but a couple of our friends . . . in fact, Joe asked me not to tell his friends . . ." This study presented much fascinating data about this difficult situation and indicated in summary that the wives are generally subject to conflicting emotions as to whether they can communicate with others about the husband's illness—they need help and understanding, but are generally unwilling to reveal the nature of the illness and the anxieties associated with it.

Nurses could help the members of the family as well as the designated patient with feelings of shame, failure, and stigma. Some ideas are:

1. Mental illness is still a stigmatized condition in this country which often produces feeling of shame in the individual and his family. This may result in a delay of treatment.

2. Part of the ego ideal is that one will marry a happy, stable, productive mate. Mental illness in a spouse may produce feelings of failure, guilt, and shame.

3. It is difficult and painful to talk about shameful experiences, even with professional people who are offering help.

4. The nurse should look at her own feelings, background and experiences in relation to mental illness and determine if she views it as shameful, embarrassing, or frightening. She must discover whether

she tends to blame or shame the family members for the patient's condition.

5. Family members of hospitalized psychiatric patients may express feelings of shame, resentment, anger, and inadequacy to the patient and toward the staff. The nurse can refrain from retaliating and can help them to develop more realistic expectations of themselves, of others, and of treatment.

6. Loss of self-esteem and feelings of inadequacy, shame, and guilt are common feelings among patients with mental illness. Their feelings are particularly related to depression and may precipitate suicide attempts. The nurse interacts with the patient and his family in such a way as to mobilize ego assets, restore and maintain self-esteem, and regain confidence. She creates a therapeutic environment to foster this.

Application of the concept of shame is useful in examining the educational process—from how a nursing student moves from being flustered and embarrassed by her first bed bath to being an experienced nurse coping with the complex reactions in which the feelings of patient-nurse-physician are intimately entwined. The nurse should develop her own ego ideal for nursing, which will help her to achieve maximal satisfaction under the common stressful situations in which shame, inadequacy, guilt, and helplessness play a part.

Basic Assumptions Regarding the Application of the Concept of Shame in Nursing

General Application:
1. Shame is a complex, common reaction which occurs in a wide variety of situations throughout life. Many people seeking medical attention may experience feelings of shame because of the illness, the necessary treatment, and the changes in patterns of living.

2. The experiences of shame one has had in the process of growing up play a significant part in behavior regarding self-esteem, self-confidence, guilt, doubt, disgust, poise, ability to persevere, and ability to cope with failure.

3. Shame reactions can be identified by subjective feelings, verbal descriptions, and nonverbal behavior, with varying degrees of intensity and significance.

4. Shame occurs in an interpersonal context—it can be precipitated, intensified, relieved, or resolved through communication.

Nurse-patient-physician relationships may be influenced by shame.

5. The professional nurse is expected to be able to cope with her own feelings of shame, guilt, disgust, and inadequacy so that she will be able to anticipate, recognize and intervene in shame reactions with patients and families when it is deemed appropriate.

Specific nursing intervention:

1. General nursing action related to shame involves maintaining the dignity and self-esteem of the individual through both obvious and subtle means—verbally and nonverbally. Basic to such action is an attitude of not blaming and not shaming the patient for being the person he is and by helping him to be more of the person he wants to be. It includes common courtesies, such as knocking on the door, providing privacy, calling a person by name, and encouraging individuality.

2. Specific verbal intervention includes the nurse helping the patient under the appropriate circumstances in the following sequence:

   a. The nurse, recognizing that the patient is experiencing shame, encourages him to acknowledge it to her or, at least, to one other person.
   b. The nurse helps the patient to determine the reason for the shame—in what way does the patient feel inadequate, humiliated, and a failure?
   c. The nurse draws the patient's attention to the relationship between the reason and his ego ideal—in what ways did he fall short of this ideal or come close to the negative ego ideal? How did he acquire this expectation? Is it still appropriate? Was it ever appropriate? What does he want to do?
   d. If the patient decides that the goal is still desirable and worth working toward, the nurse helps him to determine what steps can be taken to approximate the goal more closely.
   e. If he decides that his previous ego ideal was inappropriate, skewed, or incomplete, the nurse helps him to determine what he does want for himself and what is possible.
   f. If it is determined that the patient was shamed through the behavior of the nurse, other staff members, or institutional practices, the nurse will act to make amends and avoid such behavior in the future. She will also try to evaluate accurate-

ly when it enhances the patient's self-esteem more not to discuss the situation.

3. The nurse can apply the concept of shame to herself in order to increase her own understanding of self, so that she can be a happier and more productive person, professionally and personally.

REFERENCES

1. Webster's New Collegiate Dictionary. p. 777. Springfield, Mass., G. & C. Merriam, 1958.
2. Tomkins, S. S.: Affect, Imagery, Consciousness. Vol. 2. pp. 6-118. New York, Springer, 1963.
3. Hinsie, L. E., and Campbell, R. J.: Psychiatric Dictionary. p. 677. New York, Oxford University Press, 1960.
4. Erikson, E., Kluckhohn, C., Murray, H. A., and Schneider, D. M.: Personality, in Nature, Society, and Culture. p. 200. New York, Alfred A. Knopf, 1959.
5. Lynd, H. M.: On Shame and the Search for Identity. pp. 27-28. New York, Science Editions, 1962.
6. Engel, G. L.: Psychological Development in Health and Disease. pp. 177-8. Philadelphia, W. B. Saunders, 1962.
7. Goffman, E.: On facework. Psychiatry, *18*:213-231, 1955.
8. Rangell, L.: The psychology of poise. Int. J. Psychoanal., *35*:317, 1954.
9. *Ibid*, p. 325.
10. Engel, *op. cit.*, p. 170.
11. Kaplan, S., and Whitman, R.: The negative ego-ideal. Int. J. Psychoanal., *5*:183-87, 1965.
12. Engel, *op. cit.*, pp. 172-3.
13. Ruesch, J., and Bateson, G.: Communication: The Social Matrix of Psychiatry. pp. 97-8. New York, W. W. Norton & Co., 1951.
14. Tomkins, *op. cit.*, pp. 227-8.
15. *Ibid.*, pp. 305-317.
16. Engel, *op. cit.*, p. 128.
17. Perle, F. S.: Ego, Hunger and Aggression. p. 178. San Francisco, Orbit Graphic Arts, 1966.
18. Rangell, *op. cit.*, p. 315.
19. Seman, M. A.: A Survey of Stressful and Satisfying Incidents of Nursing Students During Pediatric Clinical Experience. p. 83. Master's Thesis, University of Washington, 1964.
20. Goffman, *op. cit.*, p. 215.
21. Yasuda, P. M.: Some Factors Contributing to Interpersonal Relationship Problems Experienced by First-Year Nursing Students with Medical and Surgical Patients in a Selected General Hospital. p. 42. Master's Thesis, University of Washington, 1958.
22. Tomkins, *op. cit.*, pp. 154-155.

23. Leveton, A.: Reproach: The art of shamesmanship. Brit. J. Med. Psychol., *35*:101-111, 1962.
24. Wright, B. A.: Physical Disability—A Psychological Approach. pp. 242-50. New York, Harper & Brothers, 1960.
25. Cahill, I. D.: Facts and fallacies about illegitimacy. Nurs. Forum, *4,* 1:39-55, 1965.
26. Kaplan, D. M., and Mason, E. A.: Maternal reactions to premature birth viewed as an acute emotional disorder. *In* Parad, H. J. (ed.): Crisis Intervention: Selected Readings. p. 122. New York, Family Association of America, 1965.
27. Yarrow, M. R., Clausen, J., and Robbins, P.: Personality and family-community. *In* Smelser, J., and Smelser, S. (eds.): Personality and Social Systems. p. 397. New York, John Wiley & Sons, 1963.

5

Grief and Mourning

Carolyn E. Carlson

Mr. Hall is an energetic 50-year old businessman who is striving to become a vice-president of his company. He has always been very athletic, playing handball or tennis or running at least an hour a day. He is married, has three children, and has always been a good provider. He and his family have recently moved into a $50,000 home. Mr. and Mrs. Hall entertain often, and both enjoy the luxury of gourmet foods.

Suddenly, the lives of the members of the Hall family have changed. Mr. Hall is in the hospital because he had a massive coronary occlusion. He has been placed on a strict diet, and his activities have been severely curtailed. He has been told that he must make drastic changes in his life, for the time being, and, perhaps, permanently.

Kim Chandler is a model and an actress. She has put off marriage because of her career. Her primary asset in relating to the world is her beautiful body. Now she is in the hospital for a breast biopsy. The result of her biopsy—malignant.

Mr. Jensen is a 70-year-old, widowed, retired gentlemen who presently finds his world restricted to a nursing home. His sight is poor, and he has extreme difficulty in walking. Those few friends who are still living find it difficult to get out to visit him. His two children, who are unable to care for him, visit once or twice a month.

Sally is a 19-year-old student of nursing. She has been caring for a child dying of cancer. She has never before known anyone who died. "Why does it have to happen? I should be able to do something. No one should suffer like this. I thought I would always be able to help any patient. I can't tolerate feeling so helpless."

All of the people mentioned have in their own private worlds, been subjected to tremendous losses. Most can never be what they once were; they can never again do what they once did so well and so easily, or see themselves as they once did. Mere words seem so inadequate to convey the agony, sorrow and the absolute despair of these persons.

Despite the tragedy, something can usually be done to reduce the impact of such losses, or to help people adjust to the losses that have so drastically disrupted their lives.

Professional nurses come in contact with a population that has a high incidence of loss experience. They encounter patients and families who are in various stages of the loss, grief, and mourning sequence. The patient or family may be anticipating a loss or responding to a recent or past loss. The significance of the losses varies in different persons; thus their responses will differ. Therefore, understanding of normal grief and mourning, and possession of the ability to recognize behavior indicative of loss and to identify events that precipitate the experience of losses, are essential for nursing practice. Nurses may then intervene so as to prevent or reduce loss, to help the individual make best use of his resources to adjust to losses that are inevitable, and to elicit necessary help for the person whose behavior is recognized as nonadaptive or maladaptive.

DEFINITIONS

Grief is a word that is in almost everyone's vocabulary. Through usage, it has acquired many meanings; however, it most often is used to describe suffering, sorrow, failure.

Grief, as discussed here, includes the series of emotional responses that follow the perception, or anticipation, of a loss of one or more valued or significant objects. These responses often include helplessness, loneliness, hopelessness, sadness, guilt, anger and the like.

Mourning refers to the psychological processes that follow a loss of a significant or valued object, or that follow the realization that such a loss may occur. These processes usually lead to giving up the lost object.[1] Mourning, therefore, includes the processes that are necessary to overcome the subjective state of grief.

Object loss is used in its broadest sense. Objects include people, possessions, a job, status, home, ideals, parts and processes of the body and the like.[2] Value or significance of an object varies from one person to another.

Loss of a valued object refers to any situation in which the valued object is rendered inaccessible to the person or is altered in such a way that it no longer has the qualities that were valued.

Engel,[3] a psychiatrist who has studied grief, poses the question, "Is Grief a Disease?" He strongly supports the affirmative, because grief has an etiology, involves suffering and impairment of functioning, and is manifested in a discrete syndrome.

Engel[4] compares object loss and mourning to the wound and wound healing. Object loss is similar to the infliction of a wound and the process of mourning is similar to the process of wound healing. It might be added that grief is analagous to pain and other subjective discomfort from the wound. Just as the processes of wound healing serve to remove the wound and its associated pain, so the processes of mourning overcome the valued object loss and the subjective states of grief.

ILLNESS, TREATMENT, AND LOSS OF VALUED OBJECTS

Grief and mourning are generally thought of as phenomena that follow the death of a loved person. Certainly, the death of a loved one is a profound loss and is usually, if not always, followed by grief and mourning. However, many other losses are equally painful, or at least painful enough to be followed by a period of grief and mourning. Anyone who has had to relinquish a pet dog or cat either through death or by other means will certainly agree with this.

Potential and actual losses occur in all our lives; however, the probability of a significant loss increases for those who are ill. It seems safe to assume that anyone who has perceived himself as ill, or who is hospitalized, will experience the loss of some, and probably numerous, objects that he values. These may be temporary or permanent losses. Also, some may be more severe or significant than others. The severity and duration of the loss naturally affect the intensity of the grief reaction and the length of the time necessary for the mourning processes.

Many of the losses experienced during illness are quite obvious. The amputation of limbs, the removal of an eye or other organs are easily recognized as significant losses. Disturbances in perceptual capacities might also represent a loss to the individual, i.e., difficulties in hearing or seeing. A diagnosis of terminal illness represents impending loss of a most highly valued object—life itself. A patient with chronic heart disease related that she had experienced the feelings of grief and had gone through the processes of mourning because she had been forced to give up the dreams that she had had for her future.

Often overlooked are the losses of self-worth that frequently follow the realization that reproductive functions have passed or are threatened. These losses may be experienced in many events, such as in undergoing a hysterectomy or prostatectomy. They also may occur during the normal process of menopause.

Illness of any nature is usually accompanied by physical, emotional and social changes that are likely to interfere with an individual's ability to function as he did in health. Responsibilities may have to be relinquished. A husband and father may lose his ability to work and provide for his family. He may be unable to participate in his usual social and recreational activities. A mother's losses might include inability to care for her children, to plan and cook meals, to shop, to socialize and to concentrate. A child may no longer be able to run and jump, play ball, achieve in school. According to Rochlin,[5] any threat to self-esteem constitutes a loss to the individual.

Changes in usual control of body functioning, such as loss of bowel control in diarrhea and incontinence, or loss of the ability to walk, can also be perceived as significant losses. Control of physical, emotional and social processes is highly valued by most individuals and by society. Any prolonged and significant loss of control can lead to a grief response.

Hospitalization and treatment suggest more potential losses to the patient. Most significant of these, perhaps, is the loss of individuality and respect and, sometimes, of identity. The patient entering the hospital is often stripped of everything that he has except a name bracelet, a diagnosis and a few personal belongings. He has a room and a gown like everyone else, and becomes just another patient on the ward. He is referred to as the coronary in room 300. Moreover, the patient's established behavioral patterns are altered by illness or treatment, and there is the possibility that he will experience a loss.

Situations of this kind must always be taken into consideration if the nurse is to prevent or ameliorate object losses.

Individual Variations

Although object losses may be the same, the significance often varies from person to person. Many factors influence the reactions to the actual losses that the ill person experiences. Previous experiences are closely intertwined with other factors that determine the significance of losses that occur during illness. For example, patterns of living have developed through past experience. These patterns vary in importance for each person. Alterations in these established patterns of living affect individuals in different ways, depending upon the significance of the pattern to the person, the needs the patterns serve, and the extent of the alteration. For example, two patients who are deprived of food for a few hours in order that diagnostic tests may be carried out are likely to respond differently if their food and eating habits differ in meaning and significance.

A male patient was hospitalized for diagnostic tests. He was a refugee from Hungary who had experienced severe starvation and had witnessed several deaths from starvation. To this man food meant security, safety, well-being. The first day that he was deprived of food for tests was an experience of horror for this man and his family. The nurse described him as being in absolute panic. She described the family's behavior as similar to that which is observed when a patient is dying. Later, the staff found out that the patient and family did believe that the patient was dying. To them, deprivation of food was equated with death.

Another patient who experiences the same deprivation of food for tests eats only because he knows he has to in order to live. He is hungry during the time that food is withheld, but is not particularly disturbed by the state of affairs. He knows that the food deprivation is only temporary, and he finds other activities to occupy his time.

This example illustrates that there are pronounced differences in the significance of established behavioral patterns among individuals. These individual differences indicate the importance of nursing assessment and understanding of patient behavior.

A person's perceptual capacities also affect his experience of loss. For example, perception of losses of any nature may vary owing to distortion of sensory input. Ego defense mechanisms such as denial can contribute to distortions of, or absence of, awareness of real or potential losses.

Anyone who has suffered significant losses in the past may perceive additional losses differently from the individual who has not had such an experience. One who has been given false hope in the past may perceive a loss more quickly than one who had not had such disappointing experiences, and he may refuse to accept hope and reassurance. For example:

Mr. J., a 29 year old husband and father, rushed his wife to the hospital because of her rapidly deteriorating strength and an increase in many vague symptoms. He was terribly worried because she looked very ill. Doctors and nurses attempted to reassure him that his wife was responding favorably to treatment and would be all right. He said he knew this wasn't true and begged them to do something. His wife died within 24 hours. Mr. J. had been disappointed too many times before to be able to hope and perceived the loss of his wife before it occurred. When he was a youngster, his older sister died of cancer. Shortly after that his favorite aunt also died. Both times he had been convinced that they would get well. He could not be convinced again.

SIGNS AND SYMPTOMS OF GRIEF

The research conducted by Lindemann[6] is considered to be a classic on the subject of grief and mourning. He has studied neurotics, relatives of patients who died in the hospital, bereaved disaster victims and relatives of military casualties. He found a definite syndrome with psychological and somatic symptomatology that usually follows the loss of a loved one through death. The syndrome includes the following reactions: the person who has experienced the loss has sensations of somatic distress, such as tightness in the throat, an empty feeling in the abdomen, loss of appetite and loss of strength. These sensations may last from 20 minutes to an hour at a time. Similar symptoms often occur when a patient is told that his illness is terminal. They are often precipitated by sympathy from visitors or any reference to the loss. The individual has a tendency to avoid these unpleasant sensations at all cost.

A man who was told that he had cancer and had only a few months to live refused to see any visitors until shortly before his death. Perhaps this was an attempt to avoid the sensations associated with the anticipated loss.

The sensorium is also altered. There is usually at least a slight sense of unreality and an increased emotional distance from people. In cases of loss through death there is intense preoccupation with the image of the deceased. The deceased may become an imaginary companion to the one who is experiencing the loss. Similarly, a lost body part may be imagined to remain intact and the person who has lost the body part is often emotionally distant from people for a period of time.

Preoccupation with feelings of guilt is another common symptom in the syndrome. The person searches desperately for evidence of his failure "to do right." This feeling of guilt is often expressed in verbal self-accusations. For example:

> The mother of a nurse was critically injured in an automobile accident. Her daughter cared for her 16 hours a day, every day for several weeks. The mother remained comatose and eventually died.
>
> Weeks later, the daughter continued to go over everything she had done while caring for her mother. She was searching for signs and symptoms that might have been there that she did not see. She wondered if she had done the wrong thing in caring for her mother.
>
> When she described this process several months later she said that she considered herself extremely fortunate to have taken a course in graduate school in which she studied the processes of grief and mourning. This helped her to understand that what she experienced was normal. She realized that she would have experienced guilt if she had not cared for her mother.

Another individual, also a nurse, expressed the wish that her husband had died in an airplane crash instead of from pneumonia. She kept reliving the events that preceded the death, torturing herself with the thought that perhaps she was at fault for not having recognized the seriousness of his symptoms.

A common response to the suffering imposed by illness and treatment is, "Why has this happened to me? What have I done to be punished in this way?" Often, patients reach the conclusion that they are experiencing the consequences of sins of omission or commission and become preoccupied with things that they should have done or should not have done. Along with the somatic distress, altered sensorium, and feeling of guilt, there is also loss of warmth in relationships with others, and there are changes in daily activities.

Relationships with others are characterized by irritability, anger and the desire not to be bothered. These reactions are generally disturbing to the bereaved; one common reaction is of fear of loss of mental equilibrium, e.g., "I felt as if I were going out of my mind—as if I were going to explode." When the sufferer tries to overcome this loss of warmth, formal and stiff interactions with others result.

Changes in daily activities are characterized by restlessness, aimless motions, inability to initiate and maintain organized patterns of activity, and nervous speech; however, it is not uncommon for the

Grief and Mourning

bereaved to attempt to cling to the daily routines and at least go through the motions. Engel[7] states that the interruptions in automatic responses in living increase the awareness of the bereaved person's dependence on the deceased. This is accompanied by feelings of impotence, helplessness and loss.

A 29-year-old widow, 3 months after her husbands' death, said: "He was so strong and we had such a good marriage. We had everything planned for how we were going to work together to help the children develop their potential. Now I don't know if I can manage. The children are such a big responsibility. I don't know who I am. He was such a part of me. I don't know what is part of him and what is part of me. I don't know how I can go on. It is so lonely without him."

STAGES OF GRIEF AND MOURNING

Engel[8] reports three stages of grief and mourning: Shock and disbelief, developing awareness of the loss, and restitution. These stages follow the loss of any valued object. Understanding of the experiences and behavior that occur during these three stages will be helpful to the nurse as she makes an assessment of behavior and plans her intervention.

Shock and Disbelief

During this stage, which immediately follows the loss, the person experiences stunned numbness and refuses to accept or comprehend what has happened. He looks and acts as if he is out of contact with what is happening around him. He may accept the loss intellectually while denying the emotional impact in an attempt to protect himself from feelings that are overwhelming. In such instances he may busily make arrangements, attempt to comfort others and appear to be managing everything appropriately.

This phase may not follow a loss that was anticipated, because in such cases, shock often is experienced prior to the loss.

Developing Awareness of the Loss

Generally, the shock phase is short-lived, and the reality of the loss penetrates the consciousness with increasing frequency. Awareness of the loss leads to pain, anguish, emptiness and acute sadness. Helplessness, hopelessness and anxiety are also intertwined with these feelings. The individual views the environment as frustrating and empty without the valued object. Such frustration may lead to anger and aggression directed towards anything or anyone that might be held responsible for the loss. Guilt results if the person finds himself to blame for the loss.

The desire and need to cry are very intense at this time. Crying seems to indicate regression to a more helpless, childlike state, as well as acknowledgment of the loss. Usually, crying leads to support from others.

Some people find it difficult or impossible to cry, even when they feel the desire to do so. If the person cannot cry because of cultural restrictions, he is likely to cry inwardly or when he is alone. Inability to cry at all often indicates that the person's relationship with the lost object was highly ambivalent or contained opposing feelings such as love and hate. Such an instance is serious because it is accompanied by undue guilt, which can interfere with the normal process of mourning.

Restitution

The rites and rituals associated with mourning that are institutionalized in society initiate recovery from the loss. When death is involved, these rites and rituals include the gathering of people who share the loss. Support is given to those most affected by the loss. The funeral serves to reinforce the reality of death. Religious beliefs help some persons, inasmuch as they may provide the basis for expecting a reunion with the lost person after death.

The main work of mourning occurs intrapsychically. Several steps must be taken once the mourner has accepted the reality of the death.

First, he must cope with the painful absence of the lost person which feels like a defect in the psychic self. He is not able to replace the lost relationship with new ones but often accepts passive, dependent relationship with old, established objects. Often he becomes much more aware of his body, as evidenced by bodily sensations and pain. Bodily discomfort is often similar to symptoms that the deceased experienced. He maintains an attachment to the lost person in this way and also may relieve any guilt feelings that he may have. In healthy mourning, such discomforts are usually brief.

For a while there is tremendous preoccupation with the lost person, as indicated by repetitive talk about memories of him. The lost one becomes idealized; thus negative feelings are repressed. During this time the mourner often vacillates between feelings of guilt, remorse, and fear. He may be preoccupied with the belief that he was responsible for the loss.

The idealization eventually leads to detachment of the lost person from the self, because the person becomes an intellectual memory. Also, the mourner begins to identify with positive qualities of the lost person.

Eventually, after many months, the mourner becomes less and less preoccupied with the lost person, and he is able to remember the lost relationship more realistically and comfortably. He is able to become interested in new objects. The final resolution of grief and mourning is indicated when the person is again able to allow himself enjoyment and pleasure.

Obviously, the loss of objects other than valued persons are not followed by exactly the same responses as those that follow death. For example, some of the identification processes that follow the loss of a person are unlikely to be present following other losses. For the most part, however, the subjective responses and processes of resolution are similar. As has been stated, the degree and length of mourning processes vary in accordance with the significance of the loss to the person.

Crate[9] has used Engel's phases of grief and mourning as a model of adaptation to chronic illness. Chronic illness involves permanent loss of physical capacities and loss of habitual ways of relating to the world. In the phase of disbelief the patient denies the condition that threatens him. He may become involved in diversional activities, refuse to follow a treatment plan, and even refuse to accept the diagnosis. On the other hand, he may accept the illness intellectually but not emotionally. When denial can no longer be maintained, awareness of the illness and its implications begins. The patient often reacts to threats of dependence and feels guilt for being incapacitated. This state of affairs is likely to result in anger, which may be directed at numerous objects, including himself.

In the process of healthy adaptation, the patient begins to reorganize relationships with people who are significant to him. These people begin to relate to the patient as an ill person and can offer understanding. When the patient begins to cope with the consequences of his illness and treatment, he identifies with others who have similar difficulties and alters his self-concept. He becomes able to accept himself with his incapacity. Initially, he may be self-deprecating; however, resolution occurs when he has respect for himself, can think of himself as a person with an illness that limits his abilities, and can allow himself to depend on others. An excellent and moving account of personal grief and mourning is found in *A Grief Observed,* by C. S. Lewis. Lewis describes his life following the death of his wife.[10]

PATHOLOGICAL MOURNING

A significant loss is not always followed by the growth that often accompanies healthy mourning. Unsuccessful mourning or unresolved grief can take many forms, as described by Engel.[11] Prolonged denial of the death or other loss is one form. This reaction represents an exaggeration of the denial that occurs in normal mourning and is considered to be a psychotic response. Reality is rejected, and the person continues to behave as if the loss had never happened.

Denial of the significance of the loss is another unsuccessful response. Mourning cannot take place because of the strength of the denial. Psychotic depression, a manic reaction, and other disorders are some likely outcomes of this type of response.

In playing down the effects of the loss on him the bereaved may project these effects onto another mourner. He expects this other mourner to assume the role of the lost object. This form is called use of a vicarious object. If the vicarious object fails to assume the role of the lost object, or leaves, depression may result. Thaler[12] reports that when depression results, the loss has to the bereaved a special meaning that is unrelated to the actual loss. He himself is not aware of the special meaning, and an outsider cannot understand the meaning. The loss is experienced as catastrophic and the depression is extremely debilitating.

VARIATIONS IN EXPRESSION OF NORMAL GRIEF AND MOURNING

It is extremely important for the nurse to keep in mind that individuals vary considerably in the ways that they express feelings.

When she makes an assessment of behavior, it is necessary for her to consider everything that she knows about the patient and his past experiences, and how these influence the present situation and the resulting behavior of the patient. Only then can she begin to understand what the patient is experiencing and begin to plan her intervention.

Every cultural or ethnic group has definite expectations of how a person who has experienced the loss of a loved one should behave. Volkart and Michael[13] report that conventional grief and mourning behavior varies greatly from one culture to another. The expectations vary considerably in different parts of the country, and probably in large part are the result of the tendency of various ethnic groups to congregate in particular communities. Such groups often reinforce and perpetuate the rites and rituals that were expected and practiced in their home countries.

Increased mobility in the United States has resulted in the dissolution of many of the close-knit groups and communities of people with varied backgrounds and different expectations and norms. Unless one is cognizant of these variations, it is often impossible to be accurate in assessing individual behavior.

Because of differences in expectations about how an individual should behave when bereaved, there is a tendency to misinterpret behavior and to make quick evaluative judgments such as: "He's not even crying. He must not have cared." . . . "She's acting so hysterical trying to make us think that she loved him." . . . "She is so controlled at work that she is not grieving normally—she's heading for trouble." How can one know what an individual's behavior means without considering that person's cultural, ethnic, religious backgrounds and the like? The fact that the stoic finds it important to avoid expressions of feelings in public does not mean that his feelings are not expressed in private.

Too often, judgments about a person's grief and mourning are made on the basis of only a short interaction with, or observation of, a person.

A woman was seen at work by a friend only a week after her son had died. The friend talked to her for about five minutes about her son. Afterwards, the friend expressed concern because the woman was not mourning properly. Her concern was based on the fact that the woman was able to carry on a conversation about her son without crying: "She even smiled and laughed a few times."

In this example the friend had no idea how the bereaved mother behaved at home or in other situations. It was found out later that this woman spent many hours crying, usually, when she was at home alone or with persons who were closest to her. Work was a relief to her because she was busy and was able to "pull herself together" for that amount of time.

At the time of the actual loss, it is sometimes difficult for an observer to recognize that the loss has taken place. For example, a wife may experience many losses of valued aspects of her relationship with her terminally ill husband, before he is lost to her through death. As his condition deteriorates, he and his wife are forced to relinquish activities that have been very important to them. In such a case, much grief and mourning have occurred prior to death; thus the response to the death is quite different from what it is when death is sudden. The above situation might be called anticipatory grief and mourning; however, it seems that the response is to an actual loss rather than to an anticipated one.

NURSING RESPONSIBILITIES FOR ASSESSMENT AND INTERVENTION

The following discussion is based on the belief that a primary function of the nurse in grief and mourning is to assist patients in maintaining behavioral stability.

Effective nursing intervention in situations in which patients or family members are experiencing grief and mourning requires accurate assessment of behavior so as to determine the emotions the person is experiencing and which phase of mourning he has entered into. Only then can appropriate nursing intervention be planned and carried out.

Anticipation of Losses

The more knowledge the nurse has of the person, the more accurate and specific she can be in her assessment. Realization of which objects are most significant or highly valued by the individual enhances her ability to determine the effect of various losses on him. Perhaps she may be able to prevent some of them from occurring.

The nurse can usually assume that life itself is highly valued by most individuals, but what about the less dramatic losses? How can the nurse learn the significance of these things, people, and events to the individual? There are, of course, many ways.

Knowledge of a person's typical behavior in health gives clues to the things that are important to him. This knowledge can be gained by listening to the topics that he discusses, observing his present behavior for rituals from which he does not deviate, and for objects to which he relates most frequently and intently. Such information can also be elicited from family members and friends. Generalizations about groups of people, such as ethnic, religious and age groups, etc., can be helpful in understanding behavior as long as the nurse avoids stereotyping and keeps the individual in focus.

Evaluation of objects significant to the person will make it possible for the nurse to prevent or reduce some losses by helping the person to maintain his relationships with significant objects, in so far as this is possible.

When a significant loss is anticipated and cannot be prevented (e.g., amputation of a leg because of gangrene) the nurse can intervene to help the patient prepare himself for the loss. This can be done by spending time with the patient and allowing him to express his feelings about the impending loss, and by helping him to maintain as much stability as possible in the rest of his life. Doll play is useful for children, in helping them to express feelings and adjust to impending losses such as amputations. The nurse should remember that grief and mourning begin before the actual loss has occurred.

When death is anticipated, it is essential to give the afflicted person the opportunity to talk about it if he wishes. Often a conspiracy of silence exists among nursing personnel when it has been determined that a patient has a terminal illness. Many are uncomfortable with the subject because of their own fears of death. As a result, the topic is ignored, and frequently the patient is too.

Some patients may wish to talk about death, others do not. Feifel[14] believes that the dying wish to talk about their thoughts and feelings about death, and that they deserve the opportunity to express themselves without censure.

Saunders[15] has found that fewer than half of the terminally ill openly discuss death. The point is that if a person chooses to talk about his thoughts he should at least have an interested listener. Ideally, the nurse, doctor and family are interested and concerned listeners. To listen adequately usually requires that the listener has considered his own thoughts and feelings about death to the extent that he does not have to avoid or flee from any encounter with the topic.

The Family

The family is an important focus of nursing intervention in the hospital and community. The aim of intervention in this case is to help the patient's family prepare for (and adjust to) losses, and to assist them in helping him cope with present or impending losses.

Whenever possible, the family should be incorporated in planning patient care, for family members are usually important resources affecting the patient's ability to cope with stress. Whether the impending loss be life itself, a part or process of the body, a job or a valued role, and whether the patient be a child or an adult, involvement of the family in his care can facilitate his adjustment to loss.

It must be remembered that family members frequently are experiencing or anticipating losses. In the home losses may include death, loss of a job, changes in family roles, and/or a child leaving home. When illness is involved, the family may face the death of a family member, permanent changes in relationships because of debilitating disease, and so on.

Perhaps one of the most difficult situations in which the nurse is called upon to intervene effectively is one involving the dying child and his parents. Studies have been done on the reactions and needs of parents of the dying child. Bozeman[16] found that three needs were most frequently expressed by parents facing such a situation: (1) tangible services such as transportation and housekeeping; (2) temporary escapes from the oppressive awareness of the illness and the approaching loss; and (3) emotional support to bolster their functioning in the face of the horror of the situation.

The nurse can help to meet these needs by allowing the parents to decide upon the time they will spend with the child, letting them provide some of the care, keeping them informed of the progress of the illness and the treatment plans, giving them opportunities away from the child to express their feelings and concerns. Hopefully then, the parents will be more comfortable in relating to the child. The parents' comfort or discomfort is usually reflected in the child's behavior.

Ujhely[17] points out the importance of helping the family members cope with their impending loss in a way that allows them to continue to carry out other family responsibilities. It may be necessary for them to deny the reality of impending death in order to be able to function. They frequently need support in avoiding emotional expression.

The family needs time to adjust to anticipated death or actual death or to other losses. The members need the support of an interested person who is willing to listen to them as they struggle to adjust. Expression of feelings to the nurse may make it easier for the family to work them out with the patient.[18] At times, especially if a death has occurred, it is very important that the family be allowed privacy so that they can express their grief openly.[19]

The Patient

The nurse encounters at least two types of situations involving patients and their losses. First is the situation in which the nurse anticipates the loss, or is at least aware that there has been a significant loss. In the second type of situation, she is unaware that a loss has occurred. When she is aware of the loss, she has the advantage of anticipating that the patient's subsequent behavior may indicate that he is experiencing grief and mourning. She is "tuned in," so to speak.

The second type of situation, in which the nurse is unaware that the patient has experienced a loss, requires that she begin by making an overall assessment of the patient's behavior. If the patient has experienced loss, the nurse's ability to recognize behavioral manifestations of grief and mourning should lead her to recognize it and trace it back to its cause.

In both types of situations, the nurse bases her intervention on the behavior of the patient, and thus needs skill in determining the meaning of behavioral cues.

This skill includes the realization that different people express any one feeling in many different behavioral acts. There is no specific formula for determining if an individual is experiencing anxiety, anger, guilt, and the like. There are many ways in which to show feelings, and an equal number of ways to hide them. The nurse must then depend upon generalizations about grief and mourning, and close observation of how a particular individual expresses his feelings, in order to determine if he is experiencing grief and mourning.

The nurse observes that Mr. M., who has had a leg amputated, is very quiet and withdrawn, speaking only when asked a question. He is stooped over and moves very slowly. This represents a decided change in Mr. M's behavior. Immediately following the amputation, Mr. M. had been quite active and talkative, smiling and laughing frequently. He did a lot of reading and his conversations focused on his plan to resume all of his previous activities. He talked about his future life as if nothing had happened. Based on her knowledge of grief and mourning, the patient's response to the medical plan and her understanding of him, the nurse considers that the patient may be becoming increasingly aware of the reality of the loss of his leg and the emotional impact of the loss. He is no longer able to deny the trauma that has occurred. The nurse knows that the patient can seldom talk about feelings. The family has told her this, and she has observed that the patient has never talked about how he feels since he has been in the hospital. She brings this knowledge to bear in her plan for intervention.

In most situations in which the patient is attempting to adjust to an anticipated or actual loss, the nurse's primary function is to support him in his coping with the loss. She allows the patient to deny his loss but does *not* reinforce the denial. She listens intently to the patient as he denies his illness but neither agrees with him nor argues with him. As stated by Crate,[20] the patient needs to be assured that the nurse can be depended upon to represent reality, even though there are aspects of reality that he is presently unable to accept.

In addition to supporting the patient's coping mechanisms, the nurse manipulates the environment in such a way as to help him to maintain as much of his usual life activity as possible. In this way she may prevent additional loss.

It is important that the nurse recognize pathological responses to loss; that is, instances in which the patient does not progress from denial to awareness of the loss. When she has identified such a problem, she should bring it to the attention of the physician. Together they can decide on a course of action, such as calling in a psychiatric nurse-specialist or psychiatrist.

Caring for patients who are responding to profound losses requires attributes such as patience, tolerance, and acceptance in the nurse. Acceptance of the patient and his right to his feelings often requires the nurse to have tolerance of angry verbal attacks directed at her, and patience, as he gradually goes through the processes of mourning in his own way.

The most important thing to remember in caring for one who is losing, or has lost, something he values highly, is to keep him from feeling alone and abandoned. If genuine concern is communicated to the patient, it is unlikely that these feelings will occur.

In summary, nursing intervention for persons experiencing grief and mourning includes:

1. Supporting the patient's coping mechanisms.
2. Allowing the patient to express feelings when he wishes.
3. Manipulating the environment to allow the patient to continue as many usual daily activities as possible. (Preventing other losses).
4. Providing privacy when needed.
5. Incorporating the family in the plan of care. (Maintaining resources).
6. Preventing feelings of abandonment.
7. Recognizing maladaptive mourning and evaluating necessity for other types of intervention.

The information needed to understand grief and mourning is readily available in the literature. Skills necessary for the assessment of significant objects and of the behavioral manifestations of grief and mourning can be developed through supervised practice in describing and analyzing verbal and nonverbal behavior. Perhaps the greatest potential obstacle to effective nursing intervention in situations involving death or other significant losses is the nurse's own fear of these. Death and incurable disease are losses that are generally very difficult for the nurse to accept. Her own needs can result in denial of death or withdrawal from terminally ill patients.[21] There is no magic formula that will take away the nurse's fear of death and other losses; however, awareness of her feelings and needs can help her to take constructive action to cope with them, rather than running away from them. Kasper[22] in his paper on "The Doctor and Death" states his belief that the physician can help the dying patient if he is aware of his own fears, weaknesses and hopes. Such awareness will help him to accept his failure and disillusionment. He can then function as a comforter, offering hope without promising life. Certainly, this also applies to nurses.

The nursing student should be encouraged to note her attitudes and feelings about patients and their conditions early in her educational program and to share them with others when she can. The sharing offers comfort, for the student usually finds that others have similar feelings and attitudes.

It is also important for the student to emphasize what she can do for a patient, rather than what she is unable to do for him. In other words, the student needs to learn to set realistic expectations for herself. She may not be able to prevent death; however, she can help the patient to maintain his feeling of self-worth, respect and dignity.

Probably the most useful way to help the nursing student give effective care to patients who have experienced significant losses is to expose her to an effective model. Ideally, the nurse instructor will serve as this role model for the student, rather than merely as an information giver.

REFERENCES

1. Bowlby, J.: Processes of mourning. Int. J. Psychoanal., *42*:317-340, 1961.
2. Engel, G. L.: Is grief a disease? Psychosom. Med., *23*:18-22, 1961.
3. Engel, G. L.: Is grief a disease? Psychosom. Med., *23*:18, 1961.
4. Engel, G. L.: Psychological Development in Health and Disease. p. 273. Philadelphia, W. B. Saunders, 1962.
5. Rochlin, G.: The dread of abandonment: A contribution to the etiology of the loss complex and to depression. Psychoanal. Stud. Child., *16*:451-470, 1961.
6. Lindemann, E.: Symptomatology and management of acute grief. *In* Fulton, R. L. (ed.): Death and Identity. pp. 187-199. New York, John Wiley & Sons, 1965.
7. Engel, G. L.: Grief and grieving. Am. J. Nurs., *64,* 9:94, 1964.
8. Engel, G. L.: Psychological Development in Health and Disease. pp. 273-280. Philadelphia, W. B. Saunders, 1962.
9. Crate, M.: Nursing functions in adaptation to chronic illness. Am. J. Nurs., *65,* 10:72-76, 1965.
10. Lewis, C. S.: A Grief Observed. London, Faber & Faber, 1964.
11. Engel, G. L., *op. cit.,* pp. 279-280.
12. Thaler, O. F.: Grief and depression. Nurs. Forum, *5,* 2:9-22, 1966.
13. Volkart, E., and Michael, S. T.: Bereavement and mental health, *In* Fulton, R. (ed.): Death and Identity. pp. 272-293. New York, John Wiley & Sons, 1965.
14. Feifel, H.: Attitudes toward death in some normal and mentally ill populations. *In* Feifel, H. (ed.): The Meaning of Death. New York, McGraw-Hill, 1959.
15. Saunders, C.: The last stages of life. Am. J. Nurs., *65,* 3:70-75, 1965.
16. Bozeman, M. F., *et al.:* Psychological impact of cancer and its treatment. The adaptation of mothers to the threatened loss of their children through leukemia. Part I. Cancer, *8*:10, 1955.
17. Ujhely, G. B.: Grief and depression: Implications for prevention and therapeutic nursing care. Nurs. Forum, *5,* 2:23-25, 1966.
18. Crate, M., *op. cit.,* p. 75.
19. Engel, G. L.: Grief and grieving. Am. J. Nurs., *64,* 9:98, 1964.
20. Crate, M., *op. cit.,* p. 74.

21. Smith, S.: The Psychology of illness. Nurs. Forum, *3*, 1:35-47, 1964.
22. Kasper, A. M.: The doctor and death. *In* Feifel, H. (ed.): The Meaning of Death. p. 270. New York, McGraw-Hill, 1959.

BIBLIOGRAPHY

Bowlby, J.: Processes of mourning. Int. J. Psychoanal. *42*:317-340, 1961.

Bozeman, M. F., *et al.:* Psychological impact of cancer and its treatment. The adaptation of mothers to the threatened loss of their children through leukemia. Part I. Cancer, *8*:1-19, 1955.

Crate, M. A.: Nursing functions in adaptation to chronic illness. Am. J. Nurs., *65*, 10:72-76, 1965.

Engel, G. L.: Grief and grieving. Am. J. Nurs., *64*, 9:93-98, September, 1964.

——: Is grief a disease. Psychosom. Med., *23*, 1:18-22, 1961.

——: Psychological Development in Health and Disease. Philadelphia, W. B. Saunders, 1962.

Feifel, H.: Attitudes toward death in some normal and mentally ill populations. *In* The Meaning of Death. New York, McGraw-Hill, 1959.

Lindemann, E.: Symptomatology and management of acute grief. *In* Fulton, R. (ed.): Death and Identity. New York, John Wiley & Sons, 1965.

Rochlin, G.: The dread of abandonment: A contribution to the etiology of the loss complex and to depression. Psychoanal. Stud. Child., *16*:451-470, 1961.

Saunders, C.: The last stages of life. Am. J. Nurs., *65*, 3:70-75, March, 1965.

Smith, S.: The psychology of illness. Nurs. Forum, *3*, 1:35-47, 1964.

Thaler, O. F.: Grief and depression. Nurs. Forum, *5*, 2:9-22, 1966.

Ujhely, G. B.: Grief and depression—Implications for prevention and therapeutic nursing care. Nurs. Forum, *5*, 2:23-35, 1966.

Volkart, E. H., and Michael, S. T.: Bereavement and mental health. *In* Fulton, R. (ed.): Death and Identity. pp. 272-293. New York, John Wiley & Sons, 1965.

6

Trust in the Nurse-Patient Relationship

Mary Durand Thomas

Trust, which can bridge the gap between patient and nurse, is fundamental to full attainment of the purpose of nursing. The nurse, in assisting a person in his movement toward health, observes, diagnoses, intervenes and evaluates the results. But her observations, upon which the remainder of the nursing process is based, are inaccurate and incomplete unless they are made in a relationship of mutual trust. For it is improbable that the patient who believes the nurse to be untrustworthy will share with her his true thoughts and feelings. Their interactions would then be a mere facade rather than a productive encounter between two trusting persons.

But helping the patient to trust is warranted on the basis of a broader consideration: the nursing goal of health promotion. For trust has been called "the cornerstone of a healthy personality"[1] because it allows the person to be open to and accepting of himself, thus furthering constructive growth.

DEFINITIONS OF TRUST AND MISTRUST

What is this "trust" that is so crucial? It has been described as "a global undifferentiated attitude, a contentment and confidence which stems from a deep assumption that life is pleasant and will not become unmanageable." The trusting person "operates on the tacit assumption that situations ... will be of a piece with the stable known world." He expects that people and situations will be good and that their hostility, danger or undependability have to be demonstrated.[2] On the other hand, the person whose trust is impaired is one "who expects bad from every new situation and to whom the kindness and dependability of people must be demonstrated."[3] This impairment has been variously termed mistrust[4] and suspicion.[5]

Crucial to the development of an operational definition are the effects of trust and mistrust on behavior. Thus the person who trusts:

1. Is comfortable with an increasing awareness of himself, his goals and his motivations.
2. Is able to share this awareness with appropriate people.
3. Accepts others who deviate from his own ways of thinking, feeling, and acting without intense needs to change them.
4. Accepts new experiences.
5. Demonstrates a consistency betwen words and actions that lasts over time.
6. Is able to delay gratification.

Conversely, the person who mistrusts:

1. Is uncomfortable with any awareness of himself, his goals and his motivations.
2. Is unable to share this awareness with appropriate people and, as a result, demonstrates various manifestations of loneliness.
3. Does not accept others who deviate from his own ways of thinking, feeling, and acting; but instead he often attempts to manipulate others to behave in ways familiar to him.
4. Avoids new experiences.
5. Demonstrates inconsistency in words and actions over time.
6. Is unable to delay gratification.

The nurse in her interactions with patients, can use these behaviors as a measure of the extent to which both she and the patient tend toward trust or mistrust. One caveat should be offered, however. Neither the nurse nor the patient is ever completely trusting or completely mistrusting. Rather, each person may be considered to be somewhere on a continuum between the extremes.

As can be noted from the effects of trust on behavior, two reciprocal aspects are implied: "reasonable trustfulness as far as others are concerned and a simple sense of trustworthiness as far as oneself is concerned."[6] Thus, as a person is more self-accepting, he is more accepting of others who have different ways of behaving. And the degree to which a person is open to his own feelings and motivations influences the degree of his behavioral consistency as seen by others. Similarly, the person who mistrusts will usually be seen as untrustworthy by others. Unable to delay gratification because he is not sure his needs will be met and unable to accept awareness of himself, he avoids new experiences, is less accepting of others and demonstrates inconsistent behavior.

Trust and mistrust may be seen to be related to those behaviors frequently termed interdependence and dependency respectively. For the trusting person—who can accept himself, others, and new experiences, who is capable of consistency and delayed gratification—can participate in relationships that are genuinely interdependent. Conversely, the mistrusting person—concerned that his needs will not be met, unable to communicate awareness of self, and not trusting others to meet his needs—demonstrates behavior that is termed dependency.

Before looking at trust and mistrust in nurse-patient interactions, it may be well to define the relationship between trust and gullibility. Is the gullible person one who tends to be too trusting? As a matter of fact, gullibility is more closely related to mistrust than to trust. The gullible person, not open to what he really believes and feels, accepts others' interpretations of events as though they were his own. As he moves from situation to situation and from person to person, accepting interpretations of others, his behavior can be seen as inconsistent and forsaking of his own trustworthiness.

TRUSTWORTHINESS IN THE NURSE

Before the nurse can assist the patient to trust, she must be trustworthy. She may assess the extent of this attribute in herself by comparing her behavior in the nurse-patient encounter with the operational definitions of trust and mistrust. How comfortable is she with increasing awareness of herself? Is she able to share this awareness with others? How accepting is she of others who think, feel and act differently from her? Is she open to new experiences? Is there a consistency in her words and actions within a situation and from one situation to another? Is she able to delay gratification while working toward a goal? The extent to which these questions can be affirmatively answered is an indication of her ability to trust.

In nurse-patient interactions, there are two common situations in which the nurse may feel her trustworthiness is at stake. When asked a question by the patient, the nurse, fearful of losing his trust, may hesitate to admit to a lack of knowledge. But trust is not measured by the vastness of her knowledge. Instead, a reply of "I don't know, but I'll try to find out" could indicate that she is a person who does not attempt bluff but answers honestly—she is someone who can be trusted.

Another test of trust occurs when the patient says "I want to talk to you about something, but I don't want you to tell anyone." Because she is pleased that the patient has singled her out and hopes to gain his trust, the nurse may agree not to convey the information. But if she learns something that should be shared with other health team members, she can be caught in a dilemma: she must either bely his trust or prove untrustworthy in her nursing role. On the other hand, the nurse could respond: "If you tell me about something that is important for your care, I would want to share it with other nurses or with your physician." There is an obvious risk that the patient may be reticent about sharing the information, or may withhold it. But what is of greater importance in this encounter is that he has had the opportunity to learn that his nurse is honest and that what she does will be consistent with what she says.

This is not to imply that the nurse always would, or should, trust her co-workers. She may enter a work situation expecting to trust only to find that she has to reconsider another person's behavior. For example, she may see a co-worker has mishandled information shared about patients in the past. She then learns of a patient's minor infringement of a policy that was instituted for the protection of all patients. Would she want to share this information with her co-worker, knowing that the possible consequence would be some punitive response, such as stereotyping the patient as a "rule-breaker"? Unfortunately, there are no established answers; rather, a judgment appropriate to each situation must be rendered. However, being gullible or naive about another's behavior should not be confused with being trusting, and being singled out by a patient should not be equated with being trustworthy.

PREVIOUS DEVELOPMENT OF TRUST

The nurse's trustworthiness establishes the degree of trust possible in the nurse-patient relationship. But even the nurse who believes she is reliable may find—to her disappointment and irritation—that she has not gained the patient's trust. It is useful to remember that the most accepting and consistent nurse may be seen as untrustworthy by a patient whose prior experiences have led him to be mistrusting.

What are these previous experiences that have taught him to trust or to mistrust? During the first year or year and one half of life the infant is learning to trust both himself and others in the world around him. As his internal world becomes differentiated from his external world, "he is constantly testing the coherence, continuity and dependability of both."[7] This testing occurs through his felt experiences within his environment. For example, as he learns to control and adapt his movements he is gradually able to trust his own body. Similarly, his repeated experience of being hungry, communicating discomfort, and feeling comfort pursuant to nursing, assures the baby that the world is a dependable place.

The experience of mutuality implicit in such incidents is a critical element in his learning to trust. For it is in

> *getting what is given,* and in learning to *get somebody to do* for him what he wishes to have done, [that] the baby . . . develops the necessary groundwork to *get to be* the giver . . . Where this mutual regulation fails, the situation falls apart into a variety of attempts to control by duress rather than by reciprocity.[8]

Through all of his experiences the baby is thus learning to what degree he can trust himself and his environment. If he receives consistent understanding and love from his parents, he is helped to develop a basic trust. If, on the other hand, he frequently experiences his parents' indifference, lack of understanding or annoyance, his trust will be impaired and his tendency will be toward mistrust and loneliness.

Although the individual's most poignant encounter with trust and mistrust occurs as he is beginning his existence in the world, other situations later in life present the encounter in new forms. The child who finds himself alone in a dark room at night may wonder whether someone will come if he calls out; when a child or an adult gives a gift or extends himself to another person in some way, he may find that the other person reacts in an unexpected way; his ability to trust himself and to trust his expectations of others may be called into question. Thus all persons, through continuing tests of their mastery of trust, find opportunities for the further development of this trust.

HELPING THE PATIENT TO TRUST

It has been noted that one of these opportunities for developing a mutually trusting relationship occurs in the nurse-patient relationship. However, as she provides patients with opportunities for learning to trust her, even the best-intentioned nurse may find her task difficult when confronted by the patient who cannot trust himself, others, or the future. Some examples of patient situations will be discussed in order to view possible nursing intervention.

The Patient Who Attempts to Prove his Expectations

The mistrusting patient, without being aware of it, may create situations that prove his expectations.

Mrs. Adams was such a patient. After having been paraplegic for four years, she was admitted to the hospital for treatment of infected decubiti. She repeatedly said to members of the nursing staff: "You don't really want to take care of me . . . Nobody in the past wanted to and you'd rather not." Even though a nurse had cared for her several times, Mrs. Adams would still give specific instructions for turning the Stryker frame and caring for her decubiti. Her behavior indicated a lack of acceptance of others as well as the expectations that others would neither accept nor care for her. Rather than anticipating good from this experience of hospitalization, she expected that it would be like other situations in which she had perceived others as not caring.

A nurse in this situation could easily have become angry and not wanted to care for Mrs. Adams, thus actualizing the expectations and increasing the patient's loneliness. Instead one nurse responded: "Have you noticed something that seems to mean I don't want to care for you?" Mrs. Adams was able only to say that she *knew* nobody would want to care for her even before she came to the hospital. Over an interval of several days similar conversations occurred, and each time the patient repeated the instructions for her care, the nurse asked such questions as "Are you wondering if I'll do this correctly?" Eventually the patient said: "You know, before I came in, I was sure nobody would want to wash out these sores, but I guess that really hasn't been true."

The nurse did not say to the patient "You can trust me;" for when the patient expects people to be untrustworthy, such statements are meaningless. Instead she manifested her trustworthiness by her consistent acceptance.

The Patient Who Says that Everything Is Fine

Entering Mr. Davis' room, the nurse found him sitting in the chair, glumly looking out the window. In response to her question, he said that everything was "fine." The following conversation ensued:
Nurse: You don't look like you're feeling fine. You seem sad to me.
Mr. Davis: No. (pause) Well, yes . . . I am blue.
Nurse: Can you tell me what's wrong?
Mr. Davis: (talked at length of the restrictiveness of his diabetic diet and of having to attend classes with other diabetics) I know the doctor wants me to stay, but I'm thinking about leaving.
Nurse: Has it been that difficult for you?
Mr. Davis: (again talked of the restrictive diet) The doctor wants me to lose about 30 pounds and get my insulin regulated so that I won't have complications.
Nurse: But you don't know if it's worth it?
Mr. Davis: That's it. I enjoy eating and I've always just taken extra insulin.
Nurse: And so the change is hard to make.
Mr. Davis: It sure is.
Nurse: What have you heard about possible complications in the classes that you've been attending?
Mr. Davis: (discussed some complications) They do sound bad to me but it means giving up so much. (pause) Maybe it's worth it. I guess I'll stick it out for a while.

The nurse in this interaction noted the inconsistency between what Mr. Davis said and what he indicated nonverbally. He was unable to share his thoughts and feelings until she demonstrated by her responses that she would accept them. She also observed his difficulty in delaying present gratification for a future goal. While she helped him to become aware of, and to discuss, his feelings about the present restrictions, she was also encouraging him to trust that "sufficient satisfaction . . . [would be] sufficiently predictable to make waiting and 'working' worthwhile."[9]

The Patient Who Compares Notes

A patient who suspects that others are not trustworthy may attempt to verify his suspicion by "comparing notes." He may raise an identical question with a number of nurses and watch for any apparent or real inconsistencies. Or, information received from personnel may be compared either with what other patients have been told or with what has actually occurred. For example:

Mr. Carnes, a patient in a tuberculosis ward, kept a list of patients who had been allowed passes from the ward, which privilege he correlated with their length of hospitalization. Inasmuch as he had been admitted prior to many of the patients on the list and yet had been unable to leave the ward, he was quite vexed and perplexed. A nurse, noting his frequent inquiries, said: "How come you've been wondering about how long people have been here?"
Mr. Carnes: A lot of them haven't been here as long as I have—and they're getting passes.
Nurse: And you're feeling left out?
Mr. Carnes: Well, sure. A guy has the right to get out if other people do. But the doc says I can't go yet.
Nurse: Do you understand why not?
Mr. Carnes: Well, he said my kids would get my TB germs if I didn't wait for a while. But some of these guys have kids and they've gone out.

The nurse continued discussing with the patient his feelings and the reasons why his progress could not be compared with the progress of other patients on the basis of length of stay.

When the nurse shares her observations of the patient's behavior with him in such situations, he can be helped to discuss his expectations. Apparent contradictions may become clarified in the conversation, and real inconsistencies can be discussed with other personnel.

The Patients with Whom the Nurse Has Brief Contact

Because learning to trust is a slow process, it may seem an irrelevant consideration for the nurse who has only brief contact with patients. It is true that this nurse may rarely have the satisfaction of seeing growth in the mistrusting patient's ability to trust her. But she *can* provide the opportunity for him to trust and can know that at least she has not reinforced his mistrust.

CONCLUSION

Helping a patient learn to trust is a difficult, time-consuming process, which demands trustworthiness and effort on the part of the nurse. But such a relationship is essential to the entire nursing process. By experiencing the openness of trust, a patient is more able to share with the nurse his true feelings, which in turn allows for greater accuracy in nursing observations and diagnoses and increased effectiveness in interventions. And it is by developing trust as a bridge in such a relationship that the nurse can assist the patient in moving toward health.

REFERENCES

1. The eight stages in the life cycle of man. *In* Youth and the life cycle: An interview with Erik H. Erikson. Children, 7:45, March-April, 1960.
2. Baldwin, A.: Behavior and Development in Childhood. p. 547. New York, Dryden Press, 1965.
3. *Ibid.*
4. Erikson, E. H.: Growth and crises of the "healthy personality." *In* Kluckhohn, C., and Murray, H. A. (eds.): Personality in Nature, Society and Culture. p. 190. New York, Alfred A. Knopf, 1953.
5. Deutsch, M.: Trust and suspicion. J. Conflict Resolution, 2:267, September, 1958.
6. Erikson, E. H., *op. cit.,* p. 190.
7. Lynd, H. M.: On Shame and the Search for Identity. p. 45. New York, Harcourt, Brace & Co., 1958.
8. Erikson, E. H., *op. cit.,* p. 192.
9. Erikson, E. H.: The problem of ego identity. J. Am. Psychoanal. Ass., 4:97, January, 1956.

BIBLIOGRAPHY

Baldwin, A. L.: Behavior and Development in Childhood. New York, Dryden Press, 1955.
Bettelheim, B.: The Empty Fortress: Infantile Autism and the Birth of Self. New York, The Free Press, 1967.
Deutsch, M.: Trust and suspicion. J. Conflict Resolution, 2:265-279, September, 1958.
Dittman, L. L.: A child's sense of trust. Am. J. Nurs., 66:91-93, January, 1966.
Erikson, E. H.: Growth and crises of the "healthy personality." *In* Kluckhohn, C., and Murray, H. A. (eds.): Personality in Nature, Society and Culture. pp. 185-225. New York, Alfred A. Knopf, 1953.
___ : Growth and crises of the "healthy personality." *In* Symposium on the Healthy Personality. Supplement 2: Problems of Infancy and Childhood. pp. 91-146. New York, Josiah Mach, Jr. Foundation, 1950.
___ : On the sense of inner identity. *In* Health and Human Relations. pp. 124-143. New York, Blakiston, 1953.
___ : The problem of ego identity. J. Am. Psychoanal. Ass. 4:56-121, January, 1956.
___ : Wholeness and totality—A psychiatric contribution. *In* Friedrich, C. J. (ed.): Totalitarianism, Proceedings of a conference held at the American Academy of Arts and Sciences, March, 1953. pp. 156-171. Cambridge, Mass., Harvard University Press, 1954.
Gibb, J. R.: Climate for trust formation. *In* Bradford, L. P., Gibb, J. R., and Benne, K. D. (eds.): T-Group Theory and Laboratory Method: Innovation in Re-education. pp. 279-309. New York, John Wiley & Sons, 1964.
Jourard, S. M.: The Transparent Self: Self-Disclosure and Well-Being. Princeton, Van Nostrand, 1964.
Lynd, H. M.: On Shame and the Search for Identity. New York, Harcourt, Brace & Co., 1958.
Maier, H. W.: Three Theories of Child Development. New York, Harper & Row, 1965.
Midcentury White House Conference on Children and Youth. A Healthy Personality for Every Child. Washington, D.C., Health Publications Institute, 1951.

Satir, V.: Conjoint Family Therapy: A Guide to Theory and Technique. Palo Alto, Science and Behavior Books, 1964.
Vanden Bergh, R. L.: Loneliness—Its symptoms, dynamics and therapy. Psychiat. Quart., 37:466-475, July, 1963.
Weigert, E.: Loneliness and trust—Basic factors of human existence. Psychiatry, 23:121-131, May, 1960.
Werner, A. M.: Learning to trust. In Burd, S. F., and Marshall, M. A. (eds.): Some Clinical Approaches to Psychiatric Nursing. pp. 73-76. New York, Macmillan, 1963.
Youth and the Life Cycle: An Interview with Erik H. Erikson. Children, 7:43-49, March-April, 1960.

7
Humor in Nursing

Vera M. Robinson

In the May, 1964 issue of *RN*, this ancedote appeared:

The talkative new graduate had bored us for most of the lunch hour with her ideas about "empathy" and "total patient care." Finally, Mrs. B., an old-timer snorted: "You and your empathy! Just how do you establish it with the patient?" "That's easy," said the neophyte airly, "Just put yourself in bed with him."

Convinced of the value of humor, having expounded at length about the lack of it in nursing practice and nursing education, I find myself, like that talkative new graduate, "in bed" with a concept. I am faced with the reality of my desire to establish that humor does have an important and unexploited place in nursing.

The concept of humor has been explored by man from as far back in time as he could express himself in writing, and probably long before that. Humor has been discussed from the points of view of philosophers, psychologists, psychoanalysts, anthropologists, sociologists, physiologists, dramatists, playwrights, poets, prose writers, satirists, comedians, educators, child development specialists, industrial management specialists, and others, ad infinitum. Ralph Piddington comments in *The Psychology of Laughter* that "probably no human reaction has given rise to so many conflicting opinions as those found in works dealing with laughter."[1]

A simple definition that is universally accepted is as difficult to find as is a universal theory of humor.

One cannot begin to study humor without encountering a myriad of related or integral ideas about such behavior as wit, laughter, joking, comedy, kidding, teasing, clowning, mimicking, satire, and so on. Certainly, humor includes all of these.

Adding to the complexity of this elusive concept is the fact that, like the clock that stops when one takes it apart to see what makes it tick, humor also loses its impact when it is analyzed. E. B. White says that humor "can be dissected, as a frog can, but the thing dies in the process and the innards are discouraging to any but the pure scientific mind."[2] Martin Grotjahn in *Beyond Laughter* apologizes because his book is "not funny." Laughter, he says, "has a tendency to disappear when we focus our intellect on it and try to understand it." But, he goes on, "there remains, however, the hope that we may laugh even more merrily and with greater inner freedom when we understand laughter better."[3]

Spurred on by Grotjahn to rise above the physical burden (the verbosity, the theories and the definition) in my pursuit of humor, I found myself hit with its emotional impact as well. My initial review of the literature brought forth such devastating analyses as "fear is the basis of much of America's humor" and definitions that dwelled on "aggression, hostility and sadism . . . depression, narcissism, and masochism."[4,5] I was suddenly faced with a horrible thought: had I simply been finding a permissible outlet for my own hostility in asserting that humor is synonymous with healthy, has therapeutic value, and is an excellent catalyst in learning? For a time, I worried that my strong belief in the use of humor and laughter as a constructive force might not survive as I struggled in "that bed," fending off the grasping arms and groping hands of hostility and aggression.

Continuing my research brought back my perspective. Certainly one would agree that humor is a socially acceptable outlet for hostility and aggression, but, even in this context, it is still a constructive and useful mechanism. As a relief for tension and a way of coping with stress, it is a most beneficial agent. But beyond that, I have felt that the need to laugh and, thus, the need for humor, is as basic as the need for love, security, or faith, and that it should be added to this list of basic needs. One of the infant's first reactions to people is a smile. We pay outrageous prices for comedians to entertain us. The sense of humor is valued as an admirable characteristic of personality and a sign of maturity. No adult would really ever admit that he does not have a sense of humor.

Further reading reassured me.

> Laughter is a way of human communication which is essentially and exclusively human. It can be used to express an unending variety of emotions. It is based on guiltfree release of aggression and any release makes us perhaps

a little better and more capable of understanding one another, ourselves and life. What is learned with laughter is learned well. Laughter gives freedom, and freedom gives laughter. He who understands the comic begins to understand humanity and the struggle for freedom and happiness.[6]

My interest in the concept of humor arose originally from two mental health concerns: one involved facilitating students' adaptation to the stresses encountered in nursing, the other, providing a therapeutic milieu within the hospital setting to foster patients' ability to cope with the stresses of illness and hospitalization. One of the mechanisms that has been observed in both situations is the use of humor.

If we accept the premise that all human behavior is purposeful, has meaning, and can be understood, then it behooves us to look at humor in the same manner as we do other kinds of behavior. What purpose does it serve? What meaning does it have for the individual? When is it a constructive element and when is it not? Can the use of humor be developed and cultivated as a tool in communication and interpersonal relationships? These are some of the questions that need to be answered in applying the concept of humor to nursing.

DEFINITION

The definitions of humor are many and varied, and some authors simply solve the problem by not defining it. The archaic definition of humor (umor) is that of "moisture, vapor." In medieval physiology, humor referred to the four principal fluids of the body: blood, phlegm, cholor (yellow bile) and melancholy (black bile). As any one of these fluids predominated, it determined man's health or temperament or mood. A just balance made up a good compound called "good humor"; a preponderance of any one of the four made up a bad compound called "ill humor." We still speak of a person's "good humor" implying that he has a sense of well-being and a readiness to laugh.

Most definitions also include the idea that it is the unexpected shock, the sudden twist, the incongruous, ludicrous note that creates the humor. Often it points up a familiar dilemma or weakness that strikes home because it is common to all of us. Thus, humor has been defined as the frank enjoyment of the imperfect that generates some physical response such as smiling or laughter.

For the purpose of this discussion, I will use this working definition—simply, humor is that which produces laughter. And both humor and laughter will be used in a generic sense to encompass all the other related words or ideas.

THE NATURE OF HUMOR

William Fry in *Sweet Madness* calls humor a paradox of abstractions and says that it is related to play. Both humor and play involve smiling and laughter; both are interpersonal interaction communications; both are sensitive to what he calls the spontaneity-thoughtfulness balance. When we become too thoughtful or self-conscious about either play or humor, we lose it. There is a correlation between the development of humor and play, all the way from childhood through adulthood. Fry feels that the transition from the child's humor to an adult form of humor requires some psychological level of maturation and achievement of the ability to abstract and conceptualize.[7]

Yet the element of childhood play persists even in adult humor. Freud speaks of the "infantile" factor in the comic who reduces himself to a child and makes us discover the child in ourselves. The pleasure comes from being the onlooker and not the victim.[8]

With maturity, however, comes not only the comfort received from laughing at the minor distresses of others, but also the ability to laugh at one's own minor misfortunes. This implies the attainment to some degree of the power of objectivity—of seeing ourselves as others see us.

> There develops also a "larger humour" says William McDougall, "which finds occasion for laughter in those defects and shortcomings which are common to all men; such humor, including in its objects the laugher himself, does not wound, as does the lower, simpler form of laughter; for it brings a bond of fellowship between him who laughs and all his fellows, inviting all men, without discrimination, to share in the genial exercise."[9]

Humor, Freud says, has something liberating about it. It has grandeur and elevation. The grandeur lies in the "triumph of narcissism, the victorious assertion of the ego's invulnerability." The main thing is the intention that humor carries out, whether the person is acting in relation to the self or other people. It means, "Look! here is the world, which seems so dangerous! It is nothing but a game for children—just worth making a jest about."[10]

The humor that we see in our culture, then, seems to range on a continuum from a "laughing at" to a "laughing with."

THE PURPOSE OF HUMOR

Why does man need humor? Why does he laugh? These questions also have intrigued writers over the centuries, and the answers are many and varied: so that he may not cry; for relief; to give and receive delight; to decrease social distance; to satisfy repressed impulses; to dissipate hostility; to assert superiority. For whatever reason, it becomes apparent that humor is a pleasure upon which mankind pounces at the slightest excuse for indulging in it.[11] It also appears that humor serves "a myriad of communicative functions." William Fry agrees with Freud that a joke has a host of "unconscious chords," which sound in the audience's mind no less loudly than does the explicit joke. This, he says, proves the vital link between humor and life. "By these bridges of the unconscious the stream between humor and life is crossed and recrossed, and there is found to be ample traffic from shore to shore."[12]

In Nursing Situations

Within the health setting, humor is usually an indirect form of communication. It is subordinated to the formal communication patterns of the hospital; when used, it is casual and generally inconspicuosly blended into the flow of events. However, it serves a valuable purpose in "promoting the continued harmony of a social relation at the same time that important messages are conveyed."[13] It often has the over-all effect of diminishing discomfort and managing some of the "delicate situations" that occur. One reason for this is that humor is a familiar pattern of communication which both nurses and patients bring with them into the health setting.

Although humor serves a multitude of purposes, it is used predominantly in nursing situations:

1. To establish warm interpersonal relationships.
2. To relieve anxiety, stress, and tension.
3. To release anger, hostility and aggression in a socially acceptable way.

4. To avoid or deny feelings that are too painful and too stressful to deal with at the time.

5. To facilitate the process of learning.

Any one, or any combination, of these purposes may be operating in any given humorous situation. There are many factors, as in all interaction, that will affect the dynamics of the situation, and there are many technics of humor which can be used. However, the primary concern in evaluating the usefulness of the humor in a situation should be the needs that are being served rather than the type, technic or content of the humor. Humor is healthy when it deals with immediate issues and helps the individual handle realities. It becomes destructive and dysfunctional when it abets pathological denial of reality: when it becomes a means of running-away-from the difficulties of living rather than an easing-of the-way-to dealing with, them.

Establishing relationships

"To laugh, or to occasion laughter through humor and wit, is to invite those present to come close . . . it aims at decreasing social distance."[14] Humor is used frequently in hospital settings to break the ice, to reduce fear of the unfamiliar, and encourage the sense of trust, to establish a feeling of cameraderie, of friendship. It says to the patient, or colleague, or student: "You can trust me. Relax, I am a friend. This isn't such a terrible place." It sets a tone, whether in the classroom or the ward setting, for a cohesiveness, a team spirit, a working together in a therapeutic atmosphere. Sometimes it consists of the telling of a joke; sometimes, teasing or jocular talk; sometimes, a practical joke; sometimes, a situation joke that develops spontaneously out of the interaction.

Humor among colleagues relaxes the rigidity of the social structure without upsetting it. A group of beginning students were assigned to their first experience on a new ward. An x-ray orderly had at one time accidentally mispronounced the head nurse's name (which was Westrack) and continued this friendly interplay each time he came to the ward. With a blank innocent expression, he would say something like "Mrs. Beartrack" and she would groan. When this occurred on the students' first morning, it delighted them and helped to set a tone of warmth in which they, as low men on the totem pole in the hospital hierachy, immediately felt comfortable.

On admission to the hospital, which is a strange and unknown environment, the patient may joke with the nurse about all "the hotel service" he'll be getting, and about the "pretty nurses" who will take care of him. In some instances, the nurse can initiate such joking to set the tone for a more relaxed atmosphere, much as a dinner speaker does with his typical introductory joke. Sociologist Rose Laub Coser, who did a study of the social structure of a hospital ward, believes that the contribution humor makes to social economy within the institution of the hospital should be stressed. "In such a shifting and threatening milieu," she points out, "a story well told, which, in a few minutes, entertains, reassures, conveys information, releases tension, and draws people more closely together, may have more to contribute than carefully planned lectures and discussions toward the security of the frightened sick."[15]

Relief of anxiety, stress, tension

Anxiety is perhaps one of the most common sources of discomfort that prompts the use of humor. Anxiety is, of course, inherent in all five of the needs listed as being possibly amenable to alleviation by the use of humor, but in some situations it is the predominant theme.

The focus of humorous get-well cards and the myriad of jokes and cartoons about illness, hospitals, doctors, and nurses attest to the attempts by patients to use humor in dealing with anxiety-provoking, stressful situations.

In Coser's study of the hospital ward she observed that there was much jocular talk among patients and that it consisted mainly of jocular griping. This talk seemed to relate to three areas of anxiety: about the self, about adjustment to a rigid routine, and about submission to a rigid authority structure.[16] Humor, used as a means of allaying the anxiety, preserving the self against the pressure of the routine and the patient's low status, has a liberating effect and fosters triumph over weakness. The use of jocular talk (and particularly the jocular gripe) transforms the individual complaint or experience into a shared or collective one. "It's better than hotel service. Where else can you get fresh ice water at 5:30 in the morning?" is a typical example of such a jocular gripe regarding a common annoyance to patients.

The intimate procedures to which the patient is subjected are also a subject for jokes. Humor seems to provide a way to manage the anxiety, shame, embarrassment, and tension stemming from elimination procedures; jokes about bedpans, bathrooms, enemas, and so on are numerous.

One student was told a joke by a patient about a nurse who worked in a hospital where the call lights above the doors were red when turned on. When the nurse went to take her driver's test, she went through a red light and her response to the policeman was, "Oh, I thought it was just another patient wanting a bedpan."

Bedpan humor raises the question of regression in the service of the ego. Under stress, primary drives, normally under control in the healthy individual, may take over and need to be channeled through a socially acceptable medium such as humor. In a recent study investigating the reflection of group anxiety in art, a collection of French political cartoons done during the Franco-Prussian War (1870-71) was analyzed. When the war outlook seemed bleak, the cartoons showed a frank regression to oral, anal and sexual levels. As the war situation improved, the maturity level of the cartoons rose.[17]

In a study done on a gynecological ward, Joan Emerson found it was usually the staff who initiated the jokes around the pelvic examination. It seemed to be "an institutionalized way the staff coaxed the patients to put up with affronts to their dignity."[18]

The male patient who feels powerless, or feels that his body image has been injured, or is concerned about his masculinity, often responds with sexually-oriented jokes and joking with the nurses. This type of bravado—by means of which the patient may feel he is relating to the nurse as a man, rather than as a patient—asserts his masculinity. He also feels he can assert his superiority over the situation if it makes the nurse embarrassed and uncomfortable. The nurse who does not recognize that the patient's behavior is defensive and useful to him at this point may begin to wonder what she has done to encourage such a situation, and she may become defensive herself and less effective in her role. When she is able to perceive the reason for the patient's behavior and respond with banter, she can then recognize impending threats to his ego, and also meet his need for ego support in other ways.

Students in their initial reactions to the "reality shocks" of nursing make frequent use of humor to relieve the anxiety and stress. As James Thurber once said, humor is often emotional chaos remembered in tranquility. The delightful old "Probie" cartoons in RN, ("Quick, pick it up off the floor before it gets unsterile") often pinpointed these stresses.

A type of humor often used is macabre, grim humor, described by Freud as gallows humor in his famous story of the rogue who was being led to the gallows. It was on a Monday, and the prisoner remarked, "Well, this week's beginning nicely."[19] Although pity is initiated for the condemned man, his stoic jibe releases the listener from having to suppress the painful emotion of pity and instead he uses the emotional energy to laugh.

This bravado in the face of death was described in *Experiment Perilous,* in which sociologist Rene Fox reports what happened on a small experimental ward. Because of the gravity of the diseases with which the physicians had to deal, under the constant threat of failure and death, and because of the problems and uncertainties involved, which could be coped with only by trial-and-error methods, they evolved a highly patterned and intricate form of humor as a way of handling their stresses. As one physician said, "Our humour is a kind of protective device. If we were to talk seriously all the time and act like a bunch of Sir Galahads or something, we just couldn't take all this."[20] They joked about the uncertainties, about their inability to "cure" patients, and about possible impending deaths; they made bets about the unknown.

This type of joking is so characteristic of physicians that it is generally referred to as "medical humor." In the earliest years of their medical training, physicians learn that an effective and appropriate way to handle their reactions to death and other stressful or emotionally provocative professional situations is to joke with their colleagues about them in a look-it-in-the-face-and-laugh manner. The student nurse often uses this type of humor in stress situations also.

The hospital is a place in which staff must deal with problems (such as death) from which other people in society attempt to insulate themselves.[21] Humor is a technic used to neutralize the significance of this emotionally charged event. Although personnel joke among themselves, they rarely joke about death with a patient or visitors. Sometimes a patient himself initiates this type of humor. For example, "How's my blood pressure? Do you think I'll live?" Or this ancedote:

> The doctor was visiting his 90-year-old patient. She asked him, "Do you think I'll get well?" He answered sadly, "I hope so—but we doctors aren't

magicians. We can't make our patients younger." Her eyes twinkled. "But Doctor," she said, "I don't ask you to make me younger. I want you to help me get older."[22]

Another source of great anxiety to both patient and health team is the operating room; here, too, humor is a frequent mechanism for relieving tension. A cartoon that appeared in *The Saturday Evening Post* some years ago pictured an operating room with six gowned and masked persons standing around an empty operating room table, and the surgeon saying "Come, come, now, one of you must be the patient."

In an operating room there is usually much jocular talk ("Do I have to work with you again?") and even telling of jokes. Following an operation, during which the surgeon had interspersed his explanations to student nurses observing the procedure with several jokes, the surgeon commented: "Well, I guess you learned a few things today, including some new jokes."

The reaction of students to humor in this strained situation varies greatly, depending upon their own anxiety, which may be increased rather than lessened if the humor disgusts or embarrasses them because it is too macabre or risqûe.

The following situation joke amused a group of students one day. It was used by the nursing instructor to relieve the tension of a student who had arrived late because of an accident with her car, and had missed the surgery she was scheduled to observe. Instructor: "I'm so glad to see you. I heard you had an accident." Student: "I'm really sorry. I'm really sorry I'm late, but I'm so shook up." Instructor: "Well, that's all right. We'll just put you in the Recovery Room for today."

When anxiety or tension is too high, however, any attempt at humor falls flat. Enjoyment of the comic cannot emerge when there is a "release of distressing affects," Freud says.[23] If there is great pain or high anxiety and the person is himself a victim, all his energy is needed to ward off the danger, and the comic effect is lost. Anxiety must be mastered or controlled before reference to it may be enjoyed in the comic or humorous situation.

Jacob Levine says that a basic element in all humor is anxiety, and that a joke seems funny only if it arouses anxiety and at the same time relieves it. He believes there are three types of reactions to a joke: (1) if it evokes no anxiety, the listener is indifferent to it; (2) if it evokes anxiety and immediately dispels it, he finds it funny; (3) if it arouses anxiety without dissipating it, he reacts with disgust, shame, embarrassment or horror.[24] For example, when an elderly, dying patient moaned in pain, "Oh, God, dear God," an intern stepped behind a screen and said, "This is God. What do you want?" Everyone on the ward reacted with disgust rather than laughter, because for them the anxiety was not relieved, although for the intern it was an unfortunate attempt to relieve his feelings of helplessness in the situation.

Relieving hostility and aggression

Within the hospital society, there are many sources of frustration and anger, but, as in society in general, their outward expression is usually looked upon with disfavor. Civilization, says Freud, has caused repression of many basic impulses, and joking is a socially acceptable way of satisfying these instincts. By making light of the forbidden impulse, the joke or cartoon releases the inner tension and permits momentary gratification. The unconscious source of the person's tension is so disguised in the joke that it is usually not disturbing. Because sex and aggression are basic instincts that create more conflict in our culture than almost any others, they seem to be the basis for much of our humor.

The rigidity of hospital routines and their dehumanizing effects often make the patient angry. But he knows that to be openly hostile is contrary to the "good" patient role and might alienate the staff upon whom he relies for care. Therefore, a jocular gripe provides an outlet and acceptably performs the function of complaint. Humor is a safety valve. Comments like "Where else can you get ice water at 5:30 a.m." or "I'll have to go home to get a rest," are such evidences of frustration. The patient's anger at his illness is also often revealed and dissipated by the use of humor: e.g., the patient who referred to his colostomy as "Old Stinky."

The staff within the health setting may also use humor as a way of handling their own reactions to the frustrations of the work situation, as in the following incident:

A physician had ordered all stools to be saved on a patient who had been admitted for tests and observation. The nursing staff believed those that were filled with barium and the patient's enema returns were not valuable and disposed of them. The doctor, upset at this decision, re-wrote the order to read, "Save everything that emits from the anal canal." The nurses then proceeded to send buckets of enema returns to the lab, and also took a large plastic bag used for linen, filled it with air, and labeled it "fresh flatus."

For the nurses who felt rebuffed that their judgment had not been accepted, this practical joke was an outlet for relieving their anger. As the word spread throughout the hospital, other personnel who laughed at the incident vicariously relieved some of *their* own pent-up frustration. Whether or not the physician involved wanted to "take a joke" like this one, the social pressure was on him to be a "good sport" and laugh with the others, which he did. Thus the mechanism served to restore communication in the physician-nurse relationship, and to prevent either an outbreak of undisguised hostility or the bottling up of frustrations. Coser says that in a hospital, the "give and take of support through humor helps the participants to live up to role expectations and to overcome the contradictions and ambiguities inherent in the complex social structure, and thereby to contribute to its maintenance."[25]

Kaplan and Boyd studied the social functions of humor on an open psychiatric ward of the "therapeutic community" type, and observed patients' use of humor to express hostility.[26] When the humor was directed toward the staff, it served as a morale booster among the patients. When expressed toward "civilians," it functioned to decrease the distance and the difference between them. The expression of hostile humor toward other patients served to forestall deviant behavior by imposing a negative sanction. However, much of the humor directed by members of the therapeutic community toward other patients served to enhance the group's solidarity and comradeship, functioning almost as an initiation rite for their "in" group and providing members with each other's support. Self-deprecating humor on the other hand, was used by a patient either to deny the seriousness of his illness or to "accomodate" the staff. However, it was felt that this self-ridicule permitted the person for the first time to take a detached view of himself and his problem; this recognition is the sine qua non of the therapeutic process.

William Fry describes not only how humor and play are related, but also shows the relationship between play and fighting, which, he says may explain somewhat the frequent association of aggression and hostility with humor. Smiling and laughter are unconscious, non-verbal communication signals of aggressivity-passivity behavior in the social hierarchy, with humor being the territory in which these interactions can be carried out.

Certain figures of speech in our language demonstrate these: a disarming smile, a winning smile, weak with laughter, a triumphant laugh, "Smile when you say that" and the like. The joke teller is the dominant one; the joke is his weapon; laughter is the sign of victory. The audience is submissive; their laughter is the sign of their acceptance of defeat. "I give up," they say. In a joke orgy the pecking order changes and the dominant role is passed on as each new joke is told.

It is difficult sometimes to determine, in play and fighting, the point at which one stops and the other begins, as, for example, in animal play. The participants, however, must determine that they are playing, not fighting, and therefore, they must set up a "play frame," which says "This is play, it is not real." There must be meta-communications, cues to convey the message that "This slap is in fun, not in anger," although the slap itself is real.

The same kind of meta-communication occurs in humor. It says "This is a joke, it is not for real." Thus the stage is set for the punch line, to which the surprised listener reacts with laughter.

The term, "punch line," is related to fighting; in burlesque, it is called the "sock line." Its origin? From Punchinello, the medieval Italian comedy figure. We all know of Punch and Judy puppet shows and *Punch*, the English humorous weekly. Probably all derive from Punchinello, which comes from the Italian word, polcino, for chicken. Thus Punch, the cocky rooster, an honored figure in the tradition of comedy, reveals some truths about ourselves as represented by life in a barnyard.

What is the purpose, then, of the punch line? Fry says it is "to snatch some of the implicit materials" from within innumerable themes within the joke and "project it into the workaday world" or reality.[27]

In *On Aggression*, Konrad Lorenz also deals with the relationship between aggression and humor. He believes that, along with knowledge, humor is one of civilization's great hopes for reducing man's aggressive drive to a tolerable measure. He sees humor as exerting an influence on social behavior that is analagous to moral responsibility, that it tends to make the world a more honest, and thus a better place. Even at its most intense, laughter, he says, is "never in danger of regressing and causing the primal aggressive behavior to break through. Barking dogs may occasionally bite, but laughing men hardly ever shoot."[28]

Denial

> "And if I laugh at any mortal thing,
> 'Tis that I may not weep."
> Lord Byron

In many instances, humor is used to deny or avoid pain and distress. The "cut-up" who does not stop long enough to allow himself to feel often falls into this category. When the stress is too great, a person may use this mechanism for self-preservation until he is able emotionally to deal with the source of the stress. The nurse who makes jokes and laughs about a long, tiring night of emergencies and deaths, or the senior who regales the new freshman with the gory details of an autopsy, are examples of humor that are primarily denial of affect, although they combine elements of hostility.

Freud has said that in humor the ego refuses to be distressed by reality. In fact, the trauma becomes an occasion for it to gain pleasure. This rejection of reality and regression to the pleasure principle to ward off suffering is also characteristic of other more pathological methods used by the human mind, namely, neurosis, psychoses, intoxication, and so on. Humor, however, manages to achieve this escape effect "without overstepping the bounds of mental health."[29] The difference seems to be, Freud says, that the superego indulges the child in us and, like a good parent, is lenient, understanding, forgiving and kind.

McDougall believes that laughter has "survival value." When we laugh, it is not that we are pleased, he says, but rather that the ridiculous situations would otherwise displease us, be painful or distressing, because mankind is endowed with primitive sympathetic tendencies. This emotional contagion is the cement of society, but it also involves a great disadvantage in that we share the mishaps of others. This excess of sympathetic distress would destroy the individual if there were no antidote such as laughter.[30]

The humorous get-well cards on the market today may indicate this society's inability to handle the concepts inherent in illness—among them, fear of death, loss of control and so on. The funny card is a denial of real feelings, according to Norris, a "cover it up with a laugh" or an expression of helplessness, even though the person sending it is very concerned about the patient. It may be sending a message that says "I hope that you are not really ill, therefore, that this lighthearted card is appropriate...."[31]

Humor in the Nursing Care Plan

The use of humor was incorporated into a written nursing care plan for an elderly widow who, following major surgery, had become depressed, lethargic, and unwilling to participate in her own care. In a team conference, the nursing staff recognized, first of all, that, because she was without family and probably quite lonely, she needed to be shown a great deal of attention so that she would feel someone cared. As the discussion proceeded, several cues led the staff to decide to try an approach of joking, teasing, and humor with her, rather than solicitousness.

The student who had given the patient morning care after surgery had handed her a wet washcloth and said, "Would you like to wash off your face before breakfast?" The patient had replied very soberly, "No, I don't want to wash it off," as she took the cloth and washed. The student had not realized until the same thing happened the next day that the patient was teasing her.

One of the graduate nurses had come to the room to take an apical pulse. The patient's roommate mentioned that the patient was an active member of the local Senior Citizen's Club and loved to play shuffleboard. The patient said, "I won't play anymore." The nurse tried to reassure her without success. After taking the apical pulse, the nurse remarked, "I can tell you're a shuffleboard player from your heartbeat." The patient looked surprised, then burst into laughter.

The team passed on their plan to personnel on the evening and night shifts who also used a joking approach with the patient throughout the next week. A nurse would tease her about running a race as she walked down the hall or about giving her a speeding ticket. When the patient grumbled "Is it?" to the head nurse's "Good morning" the head nurse threatened to hang her by her heels if she didn't smile. The patient announced she would "cry like I did the first time I was hung by the heels," and then she laughed.

The patient began to respond to the extra attention and to participate more actively in her care. Her spirits improved and soon she was initiating the humor. By the end of the week, she was asking to go home.

The use of humor as a nursing intervention is in contrast to traditional psychiatric nursing approaches to the depressed patient. Why did it prove successful in this situation? There seemed to be two main factors: first, the life style of the patient, and, secondly, the tone or climate of the ward.

A friend of the patient described her as the "cut-up" of the Senior Citizen's Club, who had always had a "good sense of humor." Humor has been described as a strengthening and coping mechanism.[32] Apparently, in this patient's life, the mechanism had been an active one, and the staff picked up the cues so that she might respond to it. Also, her depression was not so severe that all affect was frozen, and thus she was able to respond.[33] The additional attention she received, with the warmth and camaraderie the humor conveyed, may have added to the success of the approach.

Secondly, humor was used extensively as a form of communication by the nursing team on the ward, which set the tone for the patients to express their feelings in this way. The head nurse also used humor, joking and teasing with her patients as she made rounds. This seemed to be her most comfortable way of communicating. Through it she was able to ascertain their needs, give them the feeling she was concerned about them, yet reassure them that their being in the hospital wasn't so deadly serious an event.

The nursing team also used humor to relieve their own anxieties and stresses. Besides the usual bantering and teasing, the blackboard in the locker room next to the nurse's station became a daily source of humor, with the graduates, student nurses and aides all contributing cartoons. One chalk drawing showed bedraggled, weary students on night duty with the dates of their service crossed off each morning and the instructor with wings and a jump suit hovering over. Another was of a student on "Preops" struggling with a syringe twice as big as herself, with patients running in all directions and the student saying, "But it's only 1 cc. of each."

In summary, the use of humor on this ward was a therapeutic force. It created a warm climate. It promoted good staff interpersonal relationships. The warmth was transmitted to the patients, who in turn were able to use humor as a method of relieving the stresses of hospitalization. Yet the use of humor was controlled: the realistic needs of patients were not lost in the laughter, and the humor could be turned off when it was not effective.

The patient's response to humor must always be carefully evaluated. "Not many unsuccessful jokes occur in hospitals, but, when they do occur, it is because 'some implicit message which may be unsuitable for direct communication is stripped of its camouflage.'"[34]

An enema was ordered for a young male patient who had had a hemorrhoidectomy and was going home. The nurse, who felt she had had a good relationship with him, thought she would tease him, and brought into the room a huge milk bucket and the largest piece of hose she could find. The patient took one look, ran to the bathroom, and refused to come out, apparently frightened and unable to see the joke.

The patient in this instance may have been reacting to the embarrassment of the intimate procedure or to the anticipation of discomfort. Very often the young to middle-age adult reacts to illness and hospitalization with a higher level of anxiety. To young, work-oriented members of society, illness may be so serious a threat that they find humor totally unacceptable, and it falls flat. Conversely, the older patient who has faced many crises and, perhaps, has dealt with prospects of decreasing good health, can take more in his stride and needs the lightness of humor to see him through the not-so-hopeful last years.

A 70-year-old gentleman was having a Levin tube inserted. Finally, after much discomfort and gagging, it was in place. The patient lay against the pillows exhausted. The instructor said, "There, how's that? Better now?" He looked up, slowly grinned, and said "Oh, yes, it has a marvelous flavor."

Humor to Facilitate Learning

Humor in the learning situation, between teacher and student, can serve all of the purposes described above—establishing warmth, relieving stress, releasing anger, avoiding feeling—and in addition it can enhance the learning. "What is learned with laughter is learned well."[35]

Role-playing in the classroom, for example, before students go on the wards, helps to relieve the anxiety and make the anticipated situation less frightening. It is interesting that children in their play seem to deal with anxiety-producing aspects of life—playing house, cops and robbers, cowboys and Indians. Dealing in advance with a serious situation in a play fashion says, "See, it's not such a frightening business."

When such procedures as admission and preoperative care were role-played in a classroom, at first in a very negative way, the students laughed uproariously. When they were done again, this time in a positive manner, the class seemed to progress more comfortably and with much less anxiety. The learning, in addition, I believe, was reinforced by the humorous presentation which the students will remember.

The planned use of humor in their lectures is an art that can be cultivated by instructors. Whiting and Harrel both describe technics one can learn to add humor to one's writing or speaking even though he may not possess a spark of natural humor.[36,37] We regard the humorist, Hoffman says, "like the poet, as born, and not made, but this isn't quite true. Humor can be cultivated. It is made up of confidence, independence, boldness and observation."[38]

Making use of situation humor in the classroom adds to an instructor's humanness. The instructor who can relate some of her own humorous experiences as a student or staff nurse helps the student, who usually has unrealistic expectations of herself, to relax. It's easier as a student to laugh at your own mistakes if the teacher can laugh at hers.

In a letter to the editor, a reader of the *American Journal of Nursing* commented on the "Time Off" page: "With this page I relax.... Before I'm through I realize that for every earthshaking problem in nursing, there is a humorous counterpart... this page makes my idiosyncrasies easier for me to accept, my own 'booboos' easier to laugh about."[39]

Students' imitations and mimicking of instructors and hospital staff, not only in private, but at school parties with the subjects of the humor present, are a combination of affectionate teasing, acceptable expression of hostility and relief of tension. The student who can initiate humor comfortably with the faculty gives evidence of an interpersonal skill that will be reflected in her ability to relate to other people.

The value of laughter in all of education has been aptly stated by Kenneth Eble in *The Perfect Education.*

> Learning begins in delight and flourishes in wonder.... Parents... must laugh greatly. For children, solemnity is like a whole pane of glass in an abandoned building. Solemnity invites shattering... But why laughter? Because laughter is giving and recognizing. It forces a physical giving that releases for a moment the very self. And if we did not recognize some rugged corner of ourselves, some flawed reality, we would not laugh. Such giving is necessary to prepare the self to learn... Parents can hardly do better than respond to their children's sense of absurdity, to let physical

ticklings grow into wit, to let wit grow into a sense of the world as it is and as it should be.[40]

Laughter makes parenthood bearable, and it creates the very air in which learning thrives.... Surely the thing that drives hundreds of bright, laughing college students out of the colleges of education is the solemnity of their utterances as well as their behavior.[41]

Education ... (should) keep us alive and hopeful ... and lead us to laugh in the face of heaven or hell. For serious as our strivings are, they should never be so serious that we cannot lean back and laugh at the absurdity of our being and doing. Education should teach us to play the wise fool rather than turn us into the solemn ass.[42]

How often have we in nursing education commented about the students' decreasing amount of involvement, the apathy that begins to set in by the second year, the fact that somehow, the young, eager, enthusiastic student we see as a freshman has disappeared by the time she is ready to graduate. Have we destroyed her motivation for learning and her eagerness for nursing by our "solemnity" and adherence to the "seriousness" of this nursing business? Might not the cultivation of humor and laughter in the classroom enhance the learning, foster the student-teacher relationship, and provide the vehicle for developing the student's ability to relate in a warm and "human" way to her patients and colleagues? Although we usually include in any list of characteristics essential for a nurse that of a sense of humor, do we do anything realistic to maintain it or develop it? Or do we squelch it in the process of her nursing education? Is humor the missing element in nursing?

> The Perception of the Comic is a tie of sympathy with other men, a pledge of sanity. We must learn by laughter as well as by tears and terror.
> Ralph Waldo Emerson

REFERENCES

1. Piddington, R.: The Psychology of Laughter: A study in Social Adaptation. p. 9. New York, Gamut Press, 1963.
2. White, E. B.: Some remarks on humor. The Second Tree from the Corner. New York, Harper & Brothers, 1954. In Enck, J. J., Forter, E. T., and Whitley, A.: The Comic in Theory and Practice. p. 102. New York, Appleton-Century-Crofts. 1960.
3. Grotjahn, M.: Beyond Laughter. p. vii. New York, McGraw-Hill, 1957.
4. Newhart, B.: An Evening of Humor with Bob Newhart. Colorado College Symposium on Humor, January 10, 1966.
5. Grotjahn, *op. cit.,* p. 33.
6. Grotjahn, *op. cit.,* p. viii-ix.
7. Fry, W. F. J.: Sweet Madness. A Study of Humor. Palo Alto, Pacific Books, 1963.
8. Freud, S.: Jokes and their relation to the unconscious. *In* Strachey, J. (ed.): The Complete Psychological Works of Sigmund Freud, Vol. 8. London, Hogarth Press, 1960.
9. McDougall, W.: The instinct of laughter. *In* An Introduction to Social Psychology. p. 395. New York, University Paperbacks, Barnes and Noble, 1963.
10. Freud, S.: Humor. *In* Strachey, J. (ed.): The Complete Psychological Works of Sigmund Freud. Vol. 21. pp. 161-166. London, Hogarth Press, 1960.
11. Bergson, H.: Laughter. In Enck, J. J.: The Comic in Theory and Practice. *op. cit.,* p. 58.
12. Fry, *op. cit.,* p. 67.
13. Emerson, J.: Social Functions of Humor in a Hospital Setting. p. 47. Unpublished dissertation, University of California at Berkeley, 1964.
14. Coser, R. L.: Some social functions of laughter. *In* Skipper, J. K., Jr., and Leonard, R. C. (eds.): Social Interaction and Patient Care. p. 293. Philadelphia, J. B. Lippincott, 1965.
15. *Ibid,* p. 304.
16. *Ibid,* p. 295.
17. Stuart, I. R.: Primary and secondary process as reflections of catastrophe: The political cartoon as an instrument of group emotional dynamics. J. Soc. Psychol., *64*:231-9, December, 1964.

18. Emerson, *op. cit.*, p. 238.
19. Freud, *op. cit.*, p. 161, and p. 229.
20. Fox, R. C.: Experiment Perilous. pp. 76-77. Glencoe, Ill., The Free Press, A. Corporation, 1959.
21. Emerson, *op. cit.*, p. 240.
22. Robinson, R.: More candles for her cake. R.N., 27:57, August, 1964.
23. Freud, *op. cit.*, p. 228.
24. Levine, J.: Responses to humor. Scient. Am., 194:31-35, February, 1956.
25. Coser, R. L.: Laughter among colleagues. Psychiatry, 23:81-95, February, 1960.
26. Kaplan, H., and Boyd, I. H.: The social functions of humor on an open psychiatric ward. Psychiat. Quart., 39:502-515, July, 1965.
27. Fry, W., *op. cit.*, p. 152.
28. Lorenz, Konrad: On Aggression. p. 294. New York, Harcourt, Brace & World, 1966.
29. Freud, *op. cit.*, p. 163.
30. McDougall, *op. cit.*, pp. 389-392.
31. Norris, C.: Greetings from the lonely crowd. Nurs. Forum, 1:73-82, Winter, 1961-62.
32. Otto, H. A.: Treatment and family strengths. Canada's Mental Health, 14, 1:1-6, January-February, 1966.
33. Nussbaum, K., and Michaux, W. W.: Response to humor in depression: A predictor and evaluator of patient change. Psychiat. Quart., 37:527-539, July, 1963.
34. Emerson, *op. cit.*, p. 150.
35. Grotjahn, *op. cit.*, p. ix.
36. Whiting, P. H.: How to Speak and Write With Humor. New York, McGraw Hill, 1959.
37. Harral, S.: When It's Laughter You're After. Norman, Oklahoma, University of Oklahoma Press, 1965.
38. Hoffmann, W. J.: Public speaking for business men. *In* Whiting, P. H.: How to Speak and Write with Humor. p. vii. New York, McGraw-Hill, 1959.
39. Time Off. Am. J. Nurs., 65, 9:240, September, 1965.
40. Eble. K. E.: A Perfect Education. pp. 3-4. New York, Macmillan, 1966.

41. *Ibid*, p. 15.
42. *Ibid*, p. 214.

ADDITIONAL READINGS

Bergler, E.: Laughter and the Sense of Humor. New York, Intercontinental Medical Book Corp., 1956.

Brown, J.: Perennially Yours, Probie. New York, Springer Publishing Co., 1958.

Eastman, M.: The Sense of Humor. New York, Charles Scribner's Sons, 1922.

———: Enjoyment of Laughter. New York, Simon and Schuster, 1936.

Eisenbud, J.: The oral side of humor. Psychoanal. Rev., 51:37-73, Spring, 1964.

Enck, J. J., Porter, E., Whitley, A.: The Comic in Theory and Practice. New York, Appleton-Century-Crofts, 1960.

Flugel, J. C.: Humor and laughter. In Gardiner, L. (ed.): Handbook of Social Psychology. Cambridge, Mass., Addison-Wesly, 1954.

Goodrich, A. T., Henry, J., and Goodrich, D. W.: Laughter in psychiatric staff conferences; A sociopsychiatric analysis. Am. J. Orthopsychiat., 24:175-184, 1954.

Harms, E.: The development of humor. J. Abnorm. Social Psychol., 38:351-369, 1943.

Mirams, S. W. P.: Humor as an element in mental health. New Zeal. Med. J., 60:144-146, April, 1961.

Obrdlik, A. J.: Gallows humor—a sociological phenomenon. Am. J. Sociol. 47:709-716, March, 1942.

O'Connell, W.: The adaptive functions of wit and humor. J. Abnorm. Social Psychol., 61:263-270, 1960.

———: Resignation humor and wit. Psychoanal. Rev., 51:49-56, Spring, 1964.

———: Multidimensional investigation of freudian humor. Psychiat. Quart., 38:97-108, January, 1964.

Pearson, G.A.: A child's humor. Nurs. Science, 3:95-108, April, 1965.

Tarachow, S.: Ambiguity and human imperfections. J. Am. Psychoanal. Ass., 13:85-101, January, 1965.

Vargas, M. J.: Uses of humor in group psychotherapy. Group Psychotherapy, 14:198-203, September-December, 1961.

Wolfenstein, M.: Children's Humor. Glencoe, Ill., The Free Press, 1954.

8

Listening

Lucille M. Wilson

The nurse's ability to work toward the solution of nursing problems depends to a large extent on her ability to recognize needs expressed in patients' statements and questions. Lack of recognition may arise from a variety of inner factors over which nurses can learn to develop some degree of conscious control by identifying their feelings concerning the patient and his problems. Barriers to communication also may arise from sources within the patient which render him emotionally incapable of verbally expressing his needs. Because a patient's willingness to verbalize is highly dependent upon the nurse's response to what he says, reflective listening on her part plays a major role in facilitating her recognition of patients' verbally expressed needs.

Reflective Listening may be described as a process that involves the listener's conscious or unconscious assessment and selection of clues from the auditory influx of data, his interweaving and interconnecting of this data with his own existing psychic organization, and his resultant behavioral responses. Hearing, as distinguished from listening, denotes mere reception of auditory stimuli. Listening denotes a voluntary effort to comprehend.[1] Reflective listening implies an integral relation between verbalization, listening and response, as well as a creative, progressive relationship between participants that depends on their listening abilities.

The purpose of this chapter is to present a conceptual analysis of the phases of listening in order to help the nurse examine and improve her listening technic. The table on the conceptual analysis presents the phases of listening, together with listening behavior that can be identified as positive and negative during each phase.

Table 8-1. Conceptual Analysis of Listening

Listening Phase	Negative	Positive
1. *Purposes*: Goals, needs, and functions of participants.	Unawareness of conscious and unconscious purposes of self and other.	Awareness of the conscious and unconscious purposes of self and other.
2. *Emotion*: Feelings and expectations toward self, other and situation.	Unawareness of emotional influences. Lack of control of feelings.	Knowledge and awareness of emotional influences. Control of feelings.
3. *Attention*: Degrees of attention to internal and to environmental data.	Unconscious or incomplete attention. Bored or uninterested appearance. Faked attention. No eye contact or steady eye contact. Untimely and inappropriate interruption. Frequent requests for repetition of what has been said. Easily distracted. Creates distraction.	Careful conscious attention. Interest, concentration. Appropriate posture, gestures and facial expression. Frequent eye contact. Control of environmental distractions. Control of preoccupying and distracting personal factors.
4. *Verbal reception*: Influx of spoken words is experienced.		

5. *Assessment*: Conscious or unconscious recognition. Identification, assessment *and selection* of content in relation to goals, needs, functions, feelings and expectations.	Inaccurate interpretation of symbols. No significance attached to vocal clues. Confusion as to central and supporting ideas.	Accurate interpretation of symbols. Awareness of implications of vocal clues: (1) choice, timing and context of words, (2) tone, tempo, volume, pitch and inflection of voice. Discrimination between main ideas and details. Awareness of selectivity in communication.
6. *Response*: Expression of reaction stimulated by selection of content and by reorganization of feelings.	Mechanical, passive, non-comprehending response. Indiscriminate response. Frequent interruption.	Goal-directed, active, comprehending response. Appropriate withholding of verbal response.
Influx of respondent's own words is experienced.		Awareness of effect of own response.
The expression may be understood or misunderstood.	Defective feedback. Prevents feedback.	Provision of feedback.
7. *Satisfaction*: A degree of satisfaction is experienced.	No validation of response.	Confirmed understanding of response.

[155]

The phases shown in the model (table on listening) can be understood to imply a spiraling sequential development in which the final phase, successfully completed, can lead in turn to an initial phase at a higher level. That is to say, the satisfaction associated with a validated response can result in improved mutual understanding of the participants' purposes and feelings involved in communicatio . This, in turn may result in fuller verbalization, keener attention, n re discerning assessment and so forth.

The remainder of this chapter will present a more detailed discussion, together with clinical nursing illustrations of the listening phases. The illustrations have been derived from nursing students' structured reports of their verbal interactions with patients and their reactions to these episodes.

PURPOSE

Both participants in a speaking-listening episode enter into the situation with conscious and unconscious purposes. Such purposes are related to individual goals and needs, as well as to the roles and functions of the participants. It is imperative that the person receiving a verbally transmitted message assume responsibility for determining the purpose of that message—and that he recognize the nature and intensity of his own purpose in getting the message.

The well established mental health concept, "all behavior is meaningful, is purposeful and can be understood,"[2] implies that the meaning of what a person says is related to his motivations. He may or may not be aware of his motives. He may or may not be able to communicate his motives. The listener, on the other hand, may or may not be able to understand the person's message in terms of purpose. Whether or not he understands is based not only on the clarity of the message, and on his own knowledge and appreciation of the context within which the message is delivered, but also on his willingness to strive toward clarification of the message and its purpose. Such effort may be useless, however, without awareness that what goes on at the nonverbal level can often impart more meaning than spoken words. In the following example the student nurse worked toward clarification while recognizing the purpose revealed by the patient on both verbal and nonverbal levels.

The patient was a 49 year old woman scheduled for an exploratory laparotomy.

Patient: *I'm* an *old* hand at surgery. (Quick, loud voice).
Student: Oh?
P.: Yes, I've had ten operations—all major. I guess this operation shouldn't scare me. (Jerky flow of words. Brushes hair back from face with hand).
S.: Those ten operations didn't frighten you, but this one does.
P.: That's right. The last three were done to remove tumors. I always felt that everything would be all-right—even for the last three. And everything *was* all-right—no cancer. (Clasps and unclasps hands. Tone, pitch and flow of words vary).
S.: You are doubtful about the outcome of *this* operation, though.
P.: Oh yes. The doctor discovered a mass on my kidney when he examined me a week ago. He said that another operation is in order—this one. (Brushes hair from face. Has been shifting position in bed. Frowns). I should be used to operations now. . . . It's silly for me to be scared. (Brief nervous laugh. Sighs. Shifts position).

The student recorded that by not laughing with her, but by listening seriously and empathetically, she could help convey that "no, your fears are not silly." The conversation continued:

Patient: I don't believe *you* think its silly. The other nurses that I've tried to talk to yesterday and today tell me (Mockingly): "Oh, you'll bounce back again," "You'll get along fine," "You have great stamina," "You're a great worry wart, but you'll be o.k.," "You cross your bridges before you come to them." (Speaking more slowly and smoothly). You're not saying things like that.
Student: This surprises you.
Patient: You bet it does. I really am worried—silly or not. That mass on my kidney could very well be cancer. The doctor said it is possible. He doesn't know—that's why he's doing this operation. I don't know. The nurses don't know. Nobody knows until tomorrow. I just have to wait. It might *not* be cancer—but its a worry. Its been a long week. (Brief pause). I feel a lot easier. You're easy to talk to. (Seemed more calm. Less body movement.).

Purposes are inherent in the participants' felt or perceived needs, their expectations or hopes of accomplishment, and their understanding of function in relation to one another.

EMOTION

Determination of the meaning intended by the sender of a message requires an awareness of and sensitivity to emotional influences acting on the participants. The meaning is affected by individual differences, attitudes, experiences, and the situation at the moment. An account of one episode reveals a student's awareness of emotions in operation. The student planned to talk with a patient scheduled for a cholecystectomy with the aim of helping in exploration of her feelings about her experience. The student stated that she felt quite anxious and somewhat disappointed on encountering the patient, who responded slowly to the student's "Good evening": "Yes. Good evening". (A straight-faced, somewhat stern but quiet and polite expression). The student recorded that she felt rather uncomfortable and had the feeling that this patient needed to "get something out in the open," and responded accordingly:

Student: You look angry, Mrs. T. You sound angry. What's troubling you?
Patient: I've been here four hours. I can't even get a drink of water. I've asked three times. I hate to ask again. I've asked three nurses what time I'm going to surgery tomorrow—so I can let my sister know before she goes to bed. They all said they would find out. Does it take this long to find out?

The student met these needs and also provided many bits of information desired by the patient in this, her first hospital experience.

The next incident demonstrates one student's lack of awareness of emotional influences in an interchange with a 49-year-old patient who was to have an abdominal hysterectomy:

Student: (After a brief silence). Did your doctor tell you about your surgery and explain it to you?
Patient: Yes, he did.
S.: Do you live here in A.....?
P.: No, I'm from B......
S.: Where is that?
P.: In the eastern part of the state. Where are you from?
S.: I'm from C......
P.: Oh—my daughter will be going to school there next Fall.
S.: What is she going to take?
P.: Medical technology.
S.: Gee, that's nice. She'll be quite a ways from home, won't she?
P.: Yes, but we have relatives there. (Brief silence).
S.: Have you had any other operations?
P.: I've had an appendectomy. I've had a full tooth extraction. And—I've had my children.
S.: So, you are a little bit familiar with what is going to happen.
P.: Yes, all my operations went very well. I can't wait to get this one over with though.
S.: How many children do you have?
P.: Four. Two girls and two boys.
S.: How old are they?

P.: The youngest is 8, the oldest is 18.
S.: Quite a range there.
P.: Yes.
S.: Where is your family now—home, or with relatives?
P.: They are here in A......
S.: They all came for a sort of holiday, huh?

The conversation continued along the same vein.

The student's report of this incident did not include recognition of her own discomfort in her stated effort to "get the patient to talk." Her discomfort can be inferred from her frequent attempts to elicit information, with seemingly no intent to use it for the patient's benefit, also from her evaluative comments (e.g., "Gee, that's nice") and interpretive comment (i.e., "They all came for a sort of holiday").

Nor did the student in the above incident demonstrate awareness of the patient's anxiety. Her conclusion that the patient "was not anxious or apprehensive at all" was invalid. In her report of the incident, she assumed, for example, without validation, that the patient's statement "all my operations went well" indicated lack of anxiety. In addition, the student apparently did not perceive any clue to the patient's feelings in such statements as: "I can't wait to get this one over with."

ATTENTION

Attention to what is being communicated in a situation is largely a function of interest. The degree of attention and interest is largely determined by the first two phases of the listening model—i.e., by participants' emotional states and purposes. These determine whether or not the persons want to hear or do hear what is communicated, as well as whether or not they attend whole-heartedly with only occasional shifts of attention or, instead, attend with innumerable distractions.

As with emotion and purpose, effective listening requires a certain amount of personal responsibility—responsibility for focusing entire attention on the other participant and on pertinent aspects of the environment. In order to give full attention, the listener must exert the effort necessary to suppress his prejudices, biases, preoccupying personal matters and other internal and external distractions. Effort that could be used to give complete attention is sometimes wastefully directed toward giving the impression of attention. Whether or not the listener is sincerely attentive can be gleaned more from his verbal response than from his physical maneuvers, which may or may not be genuine. There is, for example, the person who appears "at attention" by looking another straight in the eye while "listening" and then gives spoken evidence of having been daydreaming.

Following is an example of one of the ways in which emotion, purpose and attention are interrelated. It illustrates a marked shift of the student's focus of attention from expressed concerns of the patient to ideas prompted by a word in the patient's expression.

The patient had related some details about a very recent change of residence from town to farm. She commented on the inconvenience of surgery at this particular time and expressed some doubt as to whether or not the move was beneficial, and then concluded:

Patient: My daughter just loves it out there. I'm so glad we moved.
Student: How old is she?
P.: She's 11. We adopted her, so we love her more than we should.... We spoil her.... I worry about her because this is the first time I have really been away from her.... We just bought her a horse. She's going wild over it. She just loves it.
S.: What kind is it? (The student recorded her own interest in and fondness for horses.)

The remainder of the conversation had to do with the quality and value of horses.

In the early part of this encounter the student had been directing her attention toward gaining knowledge about the patient's concerns, with intent and desire to assist in their exploration. Having received an answer to her question as to the child's age, she shifted her attention abruptly because of feelings and ideas prompted by the word "horse." The change in the focus of her attention interfered with her original purpose. The student presented no evidence of having heard, or of intending to clarify, anything indicating potential concern of the patient; for example, age of the child, feelings of overconcern, overindulgence, and worry regarding separation.

VERBAL RECEPTION

Again, the preceding listening phase (attention) is prerequisite to verbal reception with understanding. Consider the infant who is continuously spoken to long before he can understand and speak.

During this long period it is only with attention to words—attention stimulated by his purposes and related emotional states—that he can eventually hear with understanding and speak with meaning. While a participant is listening, his emotions, purposes and attention are primary determinants of which spoken words he will hear, attach meaning to, and use to formulate into ideas. Conversely these ideas, once formulated, may change the nature and degree of attention from complete concentration to total indifference—or vice versa.

The listener can experience influx of words, but they hold no meaning unless they are familiar, in context, and organized in a sequence which he can comprehend. An unfamiliar foreign word is perceived only as a sound. An English word outside the scope of the listener's vocabulary means little more, although some meaning may be derived from the speaker's tone, timing, inflection and nonverbal behavior. Also, meaning may be derived by "filling in" for the unfamiliar word through context.

Comprehension depends not only on the listener's education, general knowledge, and experience, but also on his current physical and emotional state. Indeed, the listener's emotions, more than his intellect, lend meaning to that which is heard. If a person's physical or emotional state interferes with rational thinking, he may receive words or sentences incompletely, inaccurately, or not at all. Even at best, *total* and completely accurate reception of everything spoken is impossible.

ASSESSMENT

Assessment implies translation and interpretation of ideas expressed in verbal symbols. Implicit in this process is listening between the words and lines for implied or indirectly expressed messages. This impels the effective listener to be cognizant of the parts of speech the speaker chooses, and how, where, when and how often he uses them. These provide clues which help the listener to get a clear, distinct and relevant message. The listener needs also to have a sense of words that are avoided, and of unverbalized sounds. He also listens for meaning in voice quality, tempo and inflection. He can, for example, detect indications and degrees of responsiveness, sincerity, understanding, expectation, fear, anger and other emotional or intellectual states.

The effective listener looks for relationships and discriminates between major ideas and minor details. He needs to be aware of his use of the differential between thought speed and speech speed. Nicholas confirms the fact that most persons talk at a speed of 125 words per minute, but normally think at a speed of about 600 words per minute.[3] The effective listener uses this excess thinking time advantageously for purposes of assessing what he hears—for example, in questioning himself as to what major points the speaker has already made and what point he is about to make. Otherwise the listener's thoughts may go off on frequent tangents until he finally becomes completely inattentive.

Another factor important to assessment is the use of emotionally charged words and phrases. The good listener identifies words that upset him and tries to understand and thereby control their emotional impact. In conversation he avoids those that are likely to have an undesirable effect on the other participant, because such words tend to stop or distort communication.

The listener's assessment of symbols is influenced by his attitude toward the speaker as a person. He may be influenced, for example, by his perception of the speaker's personal appeal, social status, authority, prestige, etc. For example, if he stereotypes the speaker as a "foreigner" and resents foreigners, he may negatively interpret the speaker's positive message. On the other hand, if a certain speaker particularly appeals to him, the listener may either ignore any unpleasant or disagreeable words spoken or distort them in such a way as to maintain his initial attitude toward the speaker. The effective listener is aware of these possibilities of distortion.

Still another factor that influences the listener's assessment and translation of a message involves certain personality traits. For example, the listener who possesses inner security generally displays initiative and flexibility of thinking when the situation indicates the need for change. He therefore assesses and interprets a message much more accurately and completely than the one who, in spite of his intellectual ability, is unsure and anxious. However, despite negative influence of background and experience, it is possible for the latter person—with well-directed interest and effort—to become more adept in the process of interpreting correctly and responding appropriately to what he hears.

RESPONSE

Response is the listening phase that represents the listener's reaction to his translation of a message into language meaningful to him. His response is the result of conscious and unconscious motivations. It may be verbal or nonverbal and may be communicated during, immediately following, or long after his reception of the message.

As in the above described phases in listening, the effective listener—the one who looks for the real meaning that the speaker is trying to get across—assumes personal responsibility for responding to the speaker with adequate and appropriately timed reflection of his understanding of the message. He makes it clear that he is genuinely interested in the speaker and in what he has to say. His external response is the speaker's only way of knowing how well his message was understood and of the need for clarifying or correcting any misunderstanding. Only then is the message complete. This feedback aspect of listening, then, is essential both to understanding the original speaker and to finding out if the speaker understands him.

In the following excerpt from clinical data, the student's inadequate and inappropriate responses made it clear to the patient (a 34-year-old woman who was scheduled for laminectomy and spinal fusion) that the student exhibited no genuine interest in, or attention to, her and what she had to say, and that the student grossly misunderstood her message.

Patient: I'm concerned about my children. They are scattered all over the country while I'm in here.

Student: Are they going to school?

P.: Oh no—one is in S. . . . ., one is in L. . . . with her grandparents, one is in A. . . . here with my sister-in-law and one is home keeping house for her Dad in G. . . . .

S.: That's real nice.

P.: The one at home is nine years old and she wanted to cook for her Dad.

S.: That will be real nice.

P.: He didn't know how it was going to work out. (Nervous laugh).

S.: Perhaps *he* will end up being the housekeeper yet. I'll bet the children will be glad when you get home.

P.: I think the oldest one is affected most. She is 15 years old and has been in the hospital so much of the time. She really knows what the hospital is like. . . . The youngest boy was talking about dividing up my things if I didn't come back—even before I left.

S.: Oh really? (Student noted that patient seemed anxious. Student was surprised at the patient's latter statement).
P.: Yes, it's just my luck to have a bunch of normal growing kids. No wonder I've got back trouble.
S.: Yes, that does sound normal for a little boy.
P.: What year are you in school?

The student recorded her interpretation of this question as the patient's attempt to change focus—possibly because of her interest in nursing. The patient asked several more questions about the student's educational program, including one as to when she would have experience in a certain facility for handicapped children.

Student: We don't go there. I wish we could. I think it would be good experience and very interesting. Have you ever been there?
Patient: Yes, I have—and then I work with handicapped children at home. My oldest daughter is handicapped. I sure enjoy working with those kids. I suppose that's how I hurt my back—packing them around so much.
S.: I'll bet it's real interesting work.
P.: I haven't been able to work for the past couple of months. My back has hurt so badly that I decided to get something done about it before it cripples me. Now I think I should have waited until it is cooler—the cast is going to be real warm.
S.: It sure is warm out these days.
P.: Do you come from a large family?

The ensuing conversation concerned the student's family. It might be assumed that the patient's question, "What year are you in school?" implies wonderment at the student's complete lack of attention and understanding. Perhaps she is "asking" if this can be due to the student's ignorance, immaturity, and lack of experience. Perhaps the patient is also saying, "If you are not truly interested in me, let's talk about you. Perhaps you will then become interested."

The student recorded awareness of anxiety in both self and patient but was not aware of its significance. She noted several times that she was trying to further conversation and to reassure the patient. She recognized that the patient was expressing concern, but was unable to respond in such a way as to help the patient clarify her messages or to validate her own assumptions as to the patient's messages. The extent to which the student's responses were influenced either by anxiety or by lack of knowledge is not discernible from the student's comments about her own responses—or those of the patient. It may be inferred that only the student's anxiety could have caused her to "assess" the scattering of the patient's children as "real nice."

During feedback, when the listener becomes the speaker or message sender, he in turn needs to search for, provide for and elicit feedback from the person to whom he is talking. It is wise in this respect to attempt to anticipate at what point misunderstanding of his own or the other person's message may possibly occur. In the event of a potential misunderstanding it is necessary that the participants verify with one another the correctness of any assumptions each may make concerning the other's message. A student's anticipation of a patient's possible misunderstanding and her subsequent verification of her impression are revealed in the following example:

The student recorded that the patient was being unusually free in expressing her religious beliefs in relation to the progress and outcome of her illness. While speaking, the patient frequently would glance at the student and partially close her left eye. The student recorded the following thoughts: "Does she wonder if I think she is unreasonable and insincere in what she is saying? Does it make any difference to her? She *does* hesitate often. Does she want to know whether or not I understand her views? She obviously wants very much to talk about how her religion helps, but she's not convinced that I understand." This impression was reflected by the student at one point where the patient exhibited the above behavior.

Student: You glance at me rather doubtfully every once in a while.

Patient: Yes. I have been accused of being a fanatic. But I truly believe that with faith in God's help I will be able to face this much better. (This was a clear summarizing statement of the views the patient had been expressing).

The nature of the listener's response, then, can help or hinder a speaker in satisfying his need for expression. It can promote or prevent the creative relationship that is implied in the positive aspects of the designated phases in reflective or critical listening.

SATISFACTION

A speaker's evocation of an understanding and accepting response from a listener is highly conducive to the pleasure and satisfaction of the communicating participants. The understanding and accepting approach of the listener is likely to bring about a similar approach in the speaker.

Such a listening attitude, which conveys the message that the speaker is worth listening to, in itself communicates genuine concern

Listening

for his integrity and gives him a sense of importance, which is always satisfying—even when there is disagreement during communication. The feeling of freedom to express oneself, and having the opportunity to sense more clearly what is going on, can lead to a desire for responsibility and cooperation. Mutual efforts toward the goal of understanding—as well as toward other goals inherent in the situation—may not be easy but are always satisfying. These efforts invariably lead to necessary action toward the goals. Satisfaction is most aptly illustrated in the clinical examples cited on pp.   and

The examples cited, as well as the account that follows, illustrate the "spiraling" development implied by the model presented in this chapter. In the following account it should be noted that the patient and student are operating in the climate created by their purposes and emotions. This climate subsequently influences their attention to, and assessment of, each other's messages. Evident is the successful completion of the final phase of the sequence, i.e., satisfaction associated with their validated responses. Their responses lead once more to a changed psychological climate in which expression is apparently facilitated in terms of understanding and feelings. Again, the ensuing satisfaction affords support for a creative, progressive relationship. In the earlier part of the interaction, the student recorded her own feeling of discomfort when she noted that the patient, who had been admitted for a cesarean section, was obviously upset (sullen expression, speaks rapidly, voice strained, bites lips often). She also noted that the patient's anxiety decreased and her own understanding of the patient became increasingly clear as she helped the distressed woman to clearly, but gradually, reveal the following information:

The patient's recent move from another state had necessitated a change of physicians. Her previous physician had encouraged vaginal delivery, but her present physician told her that she must be delivered by cesarean section. She related that the latter "didn't take me seriously," and that he responded to her objection to a section with: "If you wait long enough, you won't have to have a cesarean section," and that she had been tempted to wait too long. Her first delivery, which she described as miserable, had been vaginal and resulted in coccygeal fractures. Her second had been cesarean section, complicated by a respiratory infection, adverse effects of anesthesia and a twenty-pound weight loss, all of which she said, had resulted in a 14-day hospital stay, during twelve of which she was restricted to bed. The student reflected her impression that this "was a long, uncomfortable seige." The conversation then continued.

Patient: Indeed it was. I've sure dreaded the thought of another broken tailbone—and the thought of ether and of feeling so awful sick for so long, too.... The tailbone was really more miserable than the cesarean section—I guess that's really why I finally decided to come in for the cesarean section. (Pause) When I think of it now—I shouldn't be looking for any trouble this time. I have no cold. And I'm not having ether. (The student noted that she knew from the O.R. schedule that the patient was to have spinal anesthesia). There is no reason to worry about 12 days in bed. (More relaxed facial expression, speaking slowly, smoothly and deliberately.).

Student: There are a number of ways, then, that you expect this cesarean section to be different from your first.

P.: Indeed. Oh—I'm going to have a spinal anesthetic instead of ether. At a card party the other night I heard a lady say that she had an awful backache for weeks after she had a spinal. Until then, I was relieved to know that I would have a spinal instead of ether. I've known several people who had spinals. I never heard them say they had a backache.... I haven't really worried about it, but I've wondered ever since if I'll get a backache.

This point was further discussed and the patient assured of the unlikelihood of occurrence of backache.

In such a progressive relationship, the nurse aims to understand the patient as a unique person and also to be understood. She continuously works toward the satisfaction associated with clear understanding of the patient's purposes and feelings, as well as her own. Her effort in this direction is reflected in her responses, which indicate: (1) awareness of the purposes and feelings involved; (2) willingness to be attentive, and (3) eagerness for confirmation, correction or denial of any impressions, assumptions or inferences on the part of either self or patient. Also conveyed in the nurse's responses is her intent to make maximum use of her knowledge and abilities to learn about the patient, his health problems, and the nature of their concern to him, so that his nursing problems can be dealt with.

This kind of preparation on the part of the nurse is essential to the process of listening with the intent of hearing patients' verbal expressions of need. The ability to explore, identify and take proper action toward meeting expressed needs varies with the educational background, experience and uniqueness of the individual nurse. This applies to any nurse-patient contact in which language, background and the patient's condition permit verbal communication. As Bird and Brandenburg have said, "Without listening there is no communication."[4]

REFERENCES

1. Barbara, D. A.: The Art of Listening. p. 80. Springfield, Ill., Charles C Thomas, 1958.
2. National League for Nursing: Psychiatric Nursing Concepts and Basic Nursing Education. p. 123. Proceedings of the Conference at Boulder, Colorado, June 15-18, 1959. Osmond-Johnson, 1960.
3. Nichols, R.: Listening is a 10-part skill. Nation's Business, July, 1957.
4. Bird, D. E., and Brandenburg, E.: Management Improvement for Hospitals; Improving Communication Through Listening. V. p. 4. Catholic Hosp. Ass. U.S. and Canada, 1959.

BIBLIOGRAPHY

Abdellah, F., Beland, I., Martin, A., and Metheney, R.: Patient-Centered Approaches in Nursing. New York, Macmillan, 1960.

Barbara, D. A.: The Art of Listening. Springfield, Ill., Charles C Thomas, 1958.

Bird, B.: Talking With Patients. Philadelphia, J. B. Lippincott, 1955.

Bird, D. E., and Brandenburg, E.: Management Improvement for Hospitals; Improving Communication Through Listening. V. p. 4. Catholic Hosp. Ass. U.S. and Canada, 1959.

Brown, E. L.: Newer Dimensions of Patient Care, Part 2. New York, Russell Sage Foundation, 1961.

Browne, C. G.: Communication means understanding. *In* Davis, K., and Scott, W. G. (eds.): Readings in Human Relations. pp. 331-336. New York, McGraw-Hill, 1959.

Burton, G.: Personal, Impersonal and Interpersonal Relations; A Guide for Nurses. ed. 2. New York, Spring, 1964.

Cannel, C. F. and Kahn, R. L.: Interviewing: An essential executive function. *In* Davis, K., and Scott, W. G. (eds.): Readings in Human Relations. pp. 336-346. New York, McGraw-Hill, 1959.

Crow, L. D., and Crow, A.: Child Development and Adjustment—A Study of Child Psychology. New York, Macmillan, 1962.

Dean, H. H., and Bryson, K. D.: Effective Communication. ed. 2. Englewood Cliffs, N.J., Prentice-Hall, 1961.

Joint Commission on Mental Illness and Health, Final Report: Action for Mental Health. New York, Science Editions, 1961.

Lesser, M., and Keane, V.: Nurse-Patient Relationships in a Hospital Maternity Service. St. Louis, C. V. Mosby, 1956.

Lindesmith, A. R., and Strauss, A. L.: Social Psychology. ed. 3. New York, Holt, Rinehart & Winston, 1968.

Meyers, M. E.: The effect of types of communication on patients' reactions to stress. Nurs. Res., *13*:126-131, Spring, 1964.

National League for Nursing: Psychiatric Nursing Concepts and Basic Nursing Education. Proceedings of the conference at Boulder, Colorado, June 15-18, 1959. Osmond-Johnson, 1960.

Oliver, R. T.: Conversation. Springfield, Ill., Charles C Thomas, 1961.

Orlando, I. J.: The Dynamic Nurse-Patient Relationship. New York, G. P. Putnam's Sons, 1961.

Pearson, M. M.: Strecker's Fundamentals of Psychiatry. ed. 6. Philadelphia, J. B. Lippincott, 1963.

Peplau, H. E.: Interpersonal Relations in Nursing. New York, G. P. Putnam's Sons, 1952.

Reik, T.: Listening With The Third Ear. New York, Garden City Books, 1951.

Reiter, F., and Kakosh, M. E.: Quality of Nursing Care. A Report of a Field-Study to Establish Criteria. Study conducted at Teacher's College, Columbia University, 1950-54. Available at New York Medical College, New York, no publisher given.

Sullivan, H. S.: The Interpersonal Theory of Psychiatry. New York, W. W. Norton & Co., 1953.

9

Reality Orientation in the Aging Person

Dorothy V. Moses

>   Mrs. M. is 85 years old and has been hospitalized for four weeks. After the death of her husband six years ago she continued to live alone in an apartment, but became progressively more confused and dangerous to herself as she left the gas stove on, burned food, etc. A friend filed a petition for commitment. In talking with Mrs. M., I found myself getting more confused, upset and uncertain as to what to say. Mrs. M. thinks the year is 1889 and that she is in Michigan, and she wants to write a letter to her husband, who is away on a trip. She also wants to show me all her lovely "things."
>   How does one know how much hard reality to face this fragile, lonely, elderly lady with? Does one tell her that her statements are incorrect and that she is in a hospital and doesn't have any belongings and that she can't write letters to dead people? How much can a person stand? How to deal effectively with this type of patient is not found in any textbook but, I guess, has to be learned by experience.
>   I certainly had compassion and interest in this sweet little old lady, who has no family, no home, no money and no belongings. I wanted to help her but felt completely helpless.

The above statements are quoted from a young nursing student's diary. As more and more older people enter our hospital wards and nursing homes, this type of problem will recur with greater frequency. The use of the term "senility" to describe deviations in the mental status of older people has become widely accepted in our culture. It may denote any state from slight confusion to complete disorientation and psychotic behavior. Many people assume mistakenly that the process of becoming senile is a normal concomitant of the aging process.

The term "reality orientation," as used here, refers to the way in which a person views himself in relation to his situation in a particular environment at a specific location in time. The purpose of this chapter is to present information that will foster a better understanding of the older person and his problems of reality orientation. How does the older person view himself in relation to his situation? What are the variables that influence a person's adaptation to the aging process? What is healthy reality orientation in the aged? When and why does senility develop, and how can the nurse help the older patient?

The words "confused" and "disoriented" may be the most common adjectives found on the hospital charts of older patients. They may or may not be a true description of a patient's condition. Often these words merely mean that no one took the time to sit down and really attempt to communicate with him.

DEFINITIONS

Reality testing, according to Hinsie and Campbell's *Psychiatric Dictionary*[1], is an ego function which provides an objective evaluation and judgment of the world outside the ego or self. The functions of perception and memory are essential factors in reality testing. Reality testing further provides a mechanism for handling the external world and the excitation it creates. By judging reality objectively and directing one's actions accordingly, integrity is achieved. Perceptualization is the act or process of representing reality as it appears to the senses rather than to the intellect. Orientation is knowledge of one's temporal, personal and spatial relationships. Orientation is said to be intact when related correctly or successfully to one's surroundings. Equally important to reality perception is reality feedback. By mid-life one has accumulated a storehouse of experience with significant others, and with the world at large, which provides a substantial store of reality feedback, leading to an orientation of the self as helpful or detrimental in the lives of others. This image of the self provides the main source of ego strength and determines to some extent the capacity to cope.

Reality orientation is a continuum throughout the life cycle which constantly changes in relation to intrapsychic needs, biological needs and environmental stimuli. Reality is defined by the society or culture within which one lives. Reality orientation in infancy starts with the pre-theoretical stage, in which reality is that which is presented by the parents. As growth takes place, one soon acquires a body of knowledge that includes a theory of deviance. In our society those with deviant versions of reality are subjected to all kinds of repressive technics by the self appointed custodians of "official reality."

Change or shift in one's perception of reality necessitates consequent changes or adaptations in one's customary life style. The need to make such changes always poses somewhat of a threat and results in varying degrees of anxiety. But no other time of life requires the drastic adaptations that have to be made in old age.

DYNAMICS OF THE AGING PROCESS

Special interest in gerontology as a respectable field for research is rapidly emerging. The last five years have seen a dramatic upsurge in literature focusing on this field. Many of the old myths of aging are being rapidly dispelled. People are beginning to realize that the aged have much to contribute to society and that they *can* enjoy life.

An example of this new attitude toward aging is the American Medical Association's change in the name of its Committee on Geriatrics. The name was first changed to the Committee on Aging, and now it is called the Committee on Living. After seven years of study, this committee has expressed the conviction that "there are no diseases that occur because of the passage of a certain number of years. Most illness and deterioration is environmentally dependent, and these entities can therefore be modified by changing and controlling the environment when possible." The committee further states: "Compulsory retirement is a waste of human resources that this nation can ill afford—it contributes measurably to ill health resulting from lack of work, exercise and responsibility."[2] This new attitude toward a field that was once considered depressing and unrewarding gives considerable hope and challenge.

In viewing the aging process in totality, it can be seen positively as implying growth and attainment of wisdom, or it can be viewed negatively as implying decline and loss. Realistically, both aspects must be considered.

Erik Erikson describes the eighth stage of development as the age of ego integrity, in which the person understands, accepts and loves the life he has lived.[3] He possesses wisdom and is willing to share this wisdom as a detached concern with life itself, even in the face of death. Wisdom maintains and conveys the integrity of experience, in spite of decline of bodily and mental functions. However, society's ability to accept the wisdom of lifelong experience is limited by the rapidity with which basic skills and basic concepts become outmoded. When there is an impatient march into the future and a restless spirit of change, the wisdom of the older generation seems to decrease in value. Society even rejects the wisdom these older people have in the "art of living."

William E. Henry feels that the wisdom and perspective attributed to elders requires a base in leisure, which is not often available in earlier life.[4] Leisure is time at one's command, free from engagement, wherein the individual is able to structure time as he chooses, rather than being commanded by time. With the leisure that is available after retirement, a man can become a true philosopher and perform the useful function of transmitting history and culture.

Among prominent theories of aging, probably Elaine Cumming's and William E. Henry's disengagement theory has attracted more attention and created more controversy than many of the other studies.[5] Briefly, disengagement implies a mutual process in which, as the individual withdraws from society, society also withdraws from the individual. The aging person tends to be less self-assertive and less likely to embrace and challenge life. He has less ego strength available for responding to the environment and responds more to inner stimuli and physical aches and pains.

Critics of this theory claim that this is not a generalized reaction but only one method of coping. Critics further point out that the individual who has always been highly engaged remains so throughout his life. The three important variables that influence engagement are health, mobility, and financial situation. But it remains a fact that the older person must disengage himself from such former ties as his job and his friends and relatives who have died.

Erich Fromm feels that in old age the person is freed from many former anxieties, such as those connected with making a living or pleasing others, and now has an opportunity to be more genuinely himself, to live, and to "feel."[6] He can use his available energy for confronting the philosophical and religious aspects of life. Fromm feels it is wrong to associate "meanness" and "nastiness" with the aging process, when behavior thus labeled may really be the fulfillment of released inhibitions. It just isn't important any more to be "nice" all the time.

Maurice Linden feels that people who are psychologically well-endowed may become even more mentally healthy in old age, because their agressive drives have diminished and been sublimated by the experiences of a lifetime.[7] Some writers see anxiety increased in old age, because of the war between generations, the youth orientation of society, the loss of friends, and the lack of mobility and resilience. Stanley Cath sees the anxiety of older persons as differing both qualitatively and quantitatively from anxiety in earlier life.[8] The aged person is not threatened by instinctual pressure alone (erotic or aggressive), nor by excessive stimulation from without. But rather, he feels a greater threat from emotional exile—or total annihilation—because of the gradual depletion of the inner self, and outer objects, along with decreased capacity to remedy the situation. In time, somatic sources from which energy is derived also undergo progressive attrition.

In order to place the aging process in proper perspective, it is necessary to look at middle age as the period of life in which the reality of aging begins to have its impact. Middle age, frequently called the "prime of life," might better be called the fulcrum of life, at which time introspection starts, and the person suddenly realizes that youth is past and that the future may not be too pleasant. Up to the age of 50, a person usually talks about how old he is, but around 50 the focus often changes to how many years are ahead. In middle age one usually begins to face the reality of approaching death. The youthful visions of immortality gradually disappear. Fantasies of youthful achievements are gone, dreams of fame and glory have faded. A person really starts looking at his life in retrospect, and time assumes a different perspective.

It is the woman who suffers more acutely from this particular phase, when her children have left and a "tired marriage" may become intolerable. Women manifest three to four times as many psychiatric disorders in middle age as men. At this time men are still engrossed in the business of making a living. The commercial market has taken advantage of this problem of middle-aged women, as witnessed by the abundance of products and methods for regaining youth. Overuse of such beauty aids may represent a form of denial of the aging process. Another common adaptation is found in compulsive activity, as represented by the committee and club work engaged in by middle-aged women.

Several writers point to the fact that denial can sometimes be a helpful and useful mechanism. Denial of pieces or parts of reality can be functional. For example, in mild cases of arthritis, the older person who can deny or ignore the presence of pain and keep going may prevent permanent stiffening. In contrast, denial of serious symptoms of cancer can lead to disastrous results. Refusal to recognize an overall decline in one's capacities can have tragic consequences. A prominent judge so completely denied the failure of his physical and mental capacities that he was removed from the bench. Even after this, he continued to maintain his law practice, despite the fact that no clients sought his services. The ultimate result was bankruptcy.

Sociocultural factors may be the most important determinants of reality orientation in the aging process. Margaret Clark and Barbara Gallatin Anderson, in their book *Culture and Aging,* present a most interesting study composed of comprehensive interviews with aged persons from all levels of socioeconomic status.[9] In general, these authors feel that personal adaptation depends upon self-perception, which in itself is shaped by social expectations. The social expectations reflect the value systems of the culture, and these cultural definitions come to be perceived as reality. Many writers point to the lack of a clearly defined role for the aged in our society as a cause of considerable ambiguity and role confusion. With the increase in the number of years of life left after retirement, people now may have as many years in the last period of life as the first, the years before adulthood.

Clark and Anderson have classified the problems of aging as perceived by the subjects in their study into the following seven categories:

1. Change in physical appearance.
2. Partial or total retirement from active, significant duties.
3. Lower energy level.
4. Greater possibility of ill health.
5. Greater possibility of the need for help or dependence on others.
6. Changes in cognitive and intellectual functioning.
7. Greater uncertainty about duration of life.

The seven areas that the subjects in this study identified as problems reflect antitheses of primary values in our society. The fact that these older people viewed these elements as stresses reflects their acceptance of the cultural values.

DEVIATIONS OF REALITY ORIENTATION

Any deviation in reality orientation always deserves careful evaluation and study in order to detect treatable conditions. Among the many physical conditions that can cause temporary reality distortions ("pseudosenility"), nutritional deficiencies and anemia are common. Many older people living alone do not have the energy or financial means to shop for the proper foods. Old people are also very susceptible to food faddism and quack health food promoters. Metabolic or electrolyte disturbances and infections are also frequent causes of mental confusion.

The nurse can play a vital role in early case-finding, in health education and in other preventive measures for older people. Recently, a friend discussed with me his conviction that his mother needed permanent institutionalization because of senility and her refusal to accept aid from any of her children. I was able to convince him that he should take her to an internist for a complete checkup. This examination revealed that she had undetected diabetes. After a week in the hospital and six weeks in a nursing home, her mental confusion completely cleared, and she is back in her own home living independently and happily. This personal experience illustrates how hazardous is the tendency toward the attributing mental deviations seen in older people to irreversible brain changes.

Failing sensory perception has a major impact on the maintenance of reality orientation. Hearing and vision are the two major means of perceiving external stimuli. In regard to visual abilities, a gradual decline may be more significant than a specific eye disease, because gradual loss may not be perceptible to the individual, thus causing him to miss or misinterpret important clues. This points up the importance of increased illumination in the environment.

Pain is another sensory stimulus that may diminish in aging. This means that the nurse must be an alert observer in order to detect signs of illness or injury which may go unnoticed by the patient. I recall vividly an 84-year-old lady who woke one morning with a severe case of jaundice. Examination and surgery revealed a ruptured gallbladder, although she had never complained of any pain, just mild indigestion.

As these other sensory receptors decrease in sensitivity, touch may assume new importance. For example, it is quite common for older people to reach out and attempt to hold on to the person with whom they are speaking. This tendency may also be an attempt to draw the listener closer so that he can be seen better, or an attempt to keep him longer. The effects of severe sensory deprivation on all age groups have been well documented and must be constantly borne in mind when planning care for the aged. At the opposite extreme, too much stimulation, or stimuli that are ambiguous, can be confusing and detrimental to older persons. Faulty interpretation may lead to distortions of reality and the arousal of fears. If these distorted messages from the outside world are interpreted negatively, reality may become intolerable, resulting in increased isolation of thought and affect. The end result may be a spiraling effect with regression into the past, as seen in the case illustration at the beginning of this chapter. Denial of present reality becomes the major defense.

Grief and depression may be said to be the constant companions of old age. The elderly person is very much aware of the inability of his body and mind to respond readily and defensively to stress. He is also very aware of the deaths and disabilities of his peers. Although reality orientation is based mainly on the here and now, past remembrances of who you were and what you did also influence the here and now. In addition, it is important to have a future orientation that contains some openness or hope. The future orientation of the aged, however, must inevitably include death, as death is the ultimate reality of life. A major task of the aging, then, is to resolve the problems of the past, present, and future. These problems are: How to account for past life; how to live in the present with losses; and how to face death.

Because the question of how to face death must not only be dealt with by the older person, but also by those who are caring for him, it cannot be covered adequately in this paper. There is a great deal of good literature becoming available on the subject of death, and nurses need to give attention to this literature. Nurses also need a healthy philosophy of the meaning of life and death for themselves.

Dr. Robert Butler, in a five-year follow-up study of normal aged men, concluded that the best defenses against senility are good health, good humor and a busy life.[10] Most of the men in Dr. Butler's study were married, and the few who were widowed during the study bore their grief successfully. The group characteristically lived independent lives. Though their adaptability often resulted from insight some came from the reverse—a refusal to admit aging changes. Another defense mechanism—counterphobia—led them to excessive activity to demonstrate their continued vigor. Failing eyesight at times was put to good use as a "defensive impairment" that served to exclude what they did not choose to see. All displayed mental flexibility, rather than the stereotyped "rigidity" of old age.

NURSING INTERVENTION

Geriatric nursing can be one of the most challenging and satisfying fields of nursing, provided the nurse has an attitude of interest and concern. But in order for it to be truly rewarding, efforts must be applied not so much to "cure" as to "care."

In terms of "care" for the elderly patient, the nurse frequently becomes the most "significant other" in the older person's life, whether she sees him in his home, in a clinic, or in an institution. The understanding, perceptive nurse who really "cares" and is concerned about her older patients can be the most important factor in creating a therapeutic environment for them. Also, the maintaining of meaningful object relationships may be the most important factor in holding on to reality orientation. One of the major goals in geriatric nursing is the maintenance or elevation of functional capacity, both physical and mental.

Jules Henry, in his book *Culture Against Man*, gives a vivid description of the effects of environment in three different types of institutions upon the behavior of patients.[11] Chapter 10, "Human Obsolescence," describes three hospitals for the aged. One is comfortable and humane; one is inhuman; and the third is somewhere in between. The inhuman institution, besides being dirty and run-down, is staffed by callous personnel who completely dehumanize the patients.

The reality of an aged person's environment must be pleasant enough to be acceptable, otherwise he may choose to combat the intolerable situation with denial and regression. Every institution establishes a culture in terms of definitions of its inmates as special kinds of entities and in terms of its conceptions of inmates' capacities for seeing, hearing and understanding. The staff behaves toward the inmates according to these definitions. When older people are defined as "childlike," they are treated accordingly and talked to as children. When the staff projects such a distorted view of reality on a patient, they create an environment that may be intolerable to him. He may respond by actually regressing into a childlike state—to bring his behavior into accordance with the staff's expectations—or he may shut out the present environment entirely and maintain the illusion that he is still a responsible, functioning adult, such as the head of a household. Many other previously learned coping mechanisms may be resorted to in handling anxiety.

Many patients in institutions for the elderly are suffering from truly irreversible brain damage. However, many of these can be helped to attain a higher level of functioning. But depression and low morale are too often mistaken for evidence of brain damage. I recall an attractive 78-year-old woman who was admitted to the psychiatric service with a diagnosis of chronic brain syndrome. Her repeated response to any comment or question was, "I don't remember." Finally, I asked her if she really wanted to remember. Her immediate response to this inquiry was an emphatic, "Hell, no! Why should I?" Further conversation and work-up by the staff revealed that she was actually suffering from a reactive depression to the death of her husband. The present situation without her husband was unacceptable, and she resorted to complete denial. With short-term psychotherapy and the concern and interest of the staff, she improved enough to be returned to the community.

In making a nursing assessment of older patients, decline and disability are often the easiest factors to isolate. Therefore, we tend to assess pathology instead of abilities. Another common error is that of making our assessment prematurely. For example, sometimes we evaluate the patient immediately upon admission, without recognizing the severe trauma that sudden change in environment creates. The majority of older patients are often brought to institutions against their will. The nurse must use her skill, knowledge and ingenuity so as to determine the patient's positive assets and abilities and plan nursing care accordingly.

Clark and Anderson have identified six components necessary to the "good life" for the aged. These are:

1. Sufficient autonomy to permit continued integrity of self.
2. Agreeable relationships with others, some of whom are willing to provide help when needed.
3. A reasonable amount of personal comfort in body, mind, and living arrangements.
4. Mental stimulation in a nontaxing way.
5. Sufficient mobility to provide variety in surroundings.

6. Enough involvement with life to prevent preoccupation with death.

These six ingredients should be minimal standards for any institution. By looking at these six factors individually, perhaps the implementation will become clearer. The first two statements involve individuality, independence, and freedom of choice and actions. The dependence-independence conflict can become accentuated with aging, owing to the fact that our society, which places a high value on independence, forces its aged population into assuming a dependent role. This is a difficult shift to expect, and the nurse must exercise considerable judgment and tact in determining how much independence is possible for the patient and when help must be offered. Independence and autonomy are necessarily limited by the safety factor. However, we need to examine many of our institutional safety regulations, in order to determine whether or not they are really necessary and whether they allow for individuality. Patients can be helped to maintain a feeling of autonomy if they are permitted to make a few simple choices.

For example, an extremely important method of helping older persons to hold on to reality is to allow them to keep familiar treasures and objects. A pet dog, cat, or a favorite rocking chair, might be the most significant object relationship the older person has. Although much lip service is given to treating patients as individuals, often we blame institutional regulations as inhibitors of needed actions when these regulations are, in fact, made or maintained by us.

Another factor identified by Clark and Anderson in the "good life" is agreeable relationships with others. This need highlights the importance of interpersonal relationships between staff and patients, as well as the desirability of placing patients in congenial arrangements with each other. Some persons need and prefer privacy, while others may need and prefer to share a room with a congenial companion. Institutions for the aged should consider a variety of arrangements in their planning.

The factors of comfort in mind and body, mental stimulation in a nontaxing way, and enough involvement with life to prevent preoccupation with death are interrelated, and they point to the need for occupational and diversional activities in institutions. Here again, if we are really concerned about the individuality of our older patients, it will be recognized that such programs include a wide variety of activities. Moreover, activities must be meaningful, and not just busy work. In one institution, for example, the older men, many of whom were severely disoriented, made wooden toys. Arrangements were carried out for them to personally deliver the completed toys to a children's day nursery. As another example, the government-sponsored Foster Grandparents' programs have had fantastic success in helping both the children and the foster grandparents.

With this emphasis on activities it needs to be stressed that not all disengagement is necessarily bad. There is a fine line between being lonely and enjoying solitude. There are some individuals who like to be alone, or who like to sit on the sidelines and watch. They may derive as much satisfaction from being fringe participants as others would from being actively involved. This is where we need to respect the person's right to make a choice, because the essence of freedom is having a choice.

The last factor in Clark and Anderson's list of needs involves sufficient mobility to provide variety in surroundings. This can be accomplished even in an institution with bedridden patients. Wheelchairs and beds can be placed in different locations. The hazards of prolonged bed rest have been well documented. Every patient should be out of bed for as long as possible every day. Wheelchairs can be placed in the doorway or out in the hall near a main door so that people coming and going cannot avoid some social contact with the person in that wheelchair. Even a patient who is necessarily confined to bed can have the bed moved about within the room so that a variety of views from the window or doorway can be observed. Beds can sometimes be moved into the day room or activity room for social interaction or observation of special activities. The outside world can be kept alive for those who are limited in mobility through television, visitors, and volunteer workers who have time to stop and chat.

Many other technics are helpful in improving the behavior and adjustment of long-term patients. The remotivation therapy that has been supported financially by the Smith, Kline and French Foundation is one method that has proven its value.[12] Another interesting program, called Reality Orientation, has been developed in Veterans' Administration Hospitals.[13] This program focuses on maintaining a controlled environment, with staff attitude of acceptance, concern and expectation. Feelings of calmness, consistency and security are communicated to patients. Emphasis is placed on always calling the patient by name, focusing on where he is and where he is from. Calendars are prominent, and the days are marked off. The patient is directed back to reality-oriented activities.

In Boston there is a Society for Gerontologic Psychiatry, which publishes a semiannual journal. Nurses should be familiar with the research and publications from Duke University done under the supervision of Dr. Ewald Busse, and with the work done at the University of California at San Francisco Medical Center under the supervision of Dr. Alexander Simon. The Group for Advancement of Psychiatry has a special study committee on aging, and the American Psychiatric Association has some publications on aging.

A few psychiatrists have pioneered in demonstrating that old people are receptive to both individual and group psychotherapy. Four leaders in this country who have published extensively are Alvin Goldfarb of New York, Robert N. Butler of Washington D.C., Maurice Linden of Philadelphia, and Jack Weinberg of Chicago. Because it is not likely that there will ever be enough psychiatrists with interest in geriatric therapy, the psychiatric nurse specialist might well be utilized very effectively in conducting both group and individual therapy, particularly in institutional settings for the aged.

PREVENTION

Many studies have shown that good adjustment in later life is closely related to good adjustment in earlier years. The basic human needs do not change appreciably over the years, although their priority may assume different positions throughout life. The factors assuming major importance in satisfactory old age adjustment are, first and most important, those of good health and the ability to overcome physical deficits. Versatility, adaptability, and a multiplicity of sources of gratification are important. This might be summed up as an ability to "roll with the punches." An appreciation of one's own individuality and uniqueness, as well as an ability to appreciate the individuality of others, can be most helpful. Social reality throughout life is based on meaningful relationships with other persons, and this need becomes paramount in aging, as other means of gratification diminish. A confidant, or "significant other" person, is vital to mental health. One must also be able to retain some element of hope. All of these attitudes must be developed early in life.

The nurse can be the key person in early case-finding, in knowing community needs and resources, and in making appropriate referrals. Community tolerance and understanding of aging persons are vital. Multiphasic screening programs to detect and treat physical problems are needed. The needs of the aged are so multiple and so interrelated that a team approach is essential. Adequate income, suitable housing, preretirement preparation, recreation centers, clubs, friendly visiting programs—all can help prevent the loneliness and deprivation so often suffered by the aged. Additional services, such as "Meals on Wheels," home health care programs, homemaker services, and protective services are needed in every community. Emotional withdrawal and apathy are easily reversed in early stages, but tend to become fixed and irreversible if allowed to continue.

A great deal more research into the physiological and psychological processes of aging and into the major diseases that affect the aged person is needed. This country is far behind many other countries in such research, as well as in providing a variety of services for the aged. The recent Federal heart, cancer, and stroke programs are a major step in the right direction.

RECAPITULATION

Although the foregoing discussion has focused primarily on reality orientation, which is psychological, it needs to be emphasized that the aging process is a biological, psychological and sociological phenomenon. We all fail to understand and utilize the assets of the aged. This is a time in life when a person is freed from the roles and norms of earlier life, and when he can be free for self-actualization. Why don't we see more creativity among the aging? There are some outstanding examples, such as Grandma Moses, but what of all the others? The attitudes of society need to be carefully examined and re-evaluated in terms of what we offer our older citizens. We also need to examine our own feelings about growing old and determine how our feelings affect our nursing care of the elderly. Geriatric nursing involves our attitudes, interest, motivation, and concern. Everyone needs to experience gratification and accomplishment in his own life. We have to look at our own reality orientation and set realistic goals in caring for the aged. These goals must be realistic in terms of improving the activities of daily living and improving or maintaining the physical and psychological functioning of our patients. We can achieve a real feeling of accomplishment by preserving the alertness and personality of the older patient. The major psychotherapeutic role that we can perform is that of being an interested listener. We can share the past successes and achievements that are so essential to maintenance of ego integrity. We can allow and encourage the patient to reminisce as much as he wants to, for this serves a very helpful function.

It is always dangerous to generalize about anything, and it is particularly dangerous to generalize about the aged person. The longer a person lives, the more unique he becomes. The sixty-year-old is as different from the seventy-year-old as the eighty-year-old is from the ninety-year-old. Those who live the longest are a very select group. However, a fairly safe generalization is that inherent in the aging process is a loss of functional reserve, which reduces the ability to withstand stress. That this loss of functional reserve is both physical and psychological makes the relationship between the two even more vital. The older patient must be treated as an integrated human being, with the recognition that any physical stress will cause deviations in behavior, just as a psychological stress may manifest itself in physical illness.

The young nursing student needs a great deal of help and support in learning to appreciate the strengths and assets of older patients and in developing communication skills appropriate with this age group. Most important, the young student needs exposure to expert nurse models who demonstrate real interest and concern in older patients.

Both youth and old age may be prolonged periods of dependence. Methods of handling the dependency vary considerably, but many have some common elements. The young child is just discovering reality, while the older person may have seen too much reality and found it unacceptable. The older person may need a few fantasies to maintain ego integrity. We must be careful about taking away supports unless we can offer successful substitutes. We must carefully evaluate the meaning of the patient's fantasies and understand his past experiences and customary life style.

The nurse can provide a true anchor to reality by being consistent and by setting reasonable limits. The older person may outwardly resent firmness and limitations, but secretly be grateful to be treated as an adult. The entire staff must be taught to avoid presumptious judgments. They must assume their role in the therapy of friendship and respect, so that present reality is pleasant and inviting.

REFERENCES

1. Hinsie, L. E., and Campbell, R. J.: Psychiatric Dictionary. pp. 632-633. New York, Oxford University Press, 1960.
2. Quoted in Quarterly Report. Region 9, U. S. Department of Health, Education, and Welfare, Social and Rehabilitation Service, Administration on Aging, October 1967, p. 18.
3. Erikson, E. H.: Childhood and Society. ed. 2. pp. 268-269. New York, W. W. Norton & Co., 1963.
4. Henry, W. E.: Engagement and disengagement: Toward a theory of adult development. *In* Kastenbaum, R. (ed.): Contributions to the Psychobiology of Aging. pp. 19-35. New York, Springer, 1965.
5. Cumming, E., and Henry, W. E.: Growing Old: The Process of Disengagement. pp. 14-16. New York, Basic Books, 1961.
6. Fromm, E.: Psychological problems of aging. Journal of Rehabilitation, *32,* 5:10-12, 51-57, September-October, 1966.
7. Linden, M. E.: The emotional problems of aging. Nurs. Outlook, *12,* 11:47-50, November, 1964.
8. Cath, S. H.: Some dynamics of middle and later years: A study in depletion and restitution. *In* Berezin, M. A., and Cath, S. H. (eds.): Geriatric Psychiatry: Grief, Loss, and Emotional Disorders in the Aging Process. pp. 21-72. New York, International Universities Press, 1967.
9. Clark, M., and Anderson, B. G.: Culture and Aging: An Anthropological Study of Older Americans. Springfield, Ill., Charles C Thomas, 1967.
10. Butler, R. N.: Aspects of survival and adaptation in human aging. Am. J. Psychiat., *123,* 10:1233-1243, April 1967.
11. Henry, J.: Culture Against Man. New York, Vintage Books, 1963.
12. Fong. T. C. C., Rawson, H. E., and Briggle, C. G.: Intensive rehabilitation of the aged. Hosp. Community Psychiat., *18,* 1:39-40, January, 1967.
13. Taulbee, L. R., and Folsom, J. C.: Reality orientation for geriatric patients. Hosp. Community Psychiat., *17,* 5:23-25, May, 1966.

10
Hostility

Sister Mary Martha Kiening

The concept of hostility has been receiving increasing attention in contemporary literature. This is particularly true since the phenomena of aggression and violence, two of its outward expressions, have escalated to the point of becoming major areas of world concern. Hostility is, perhaps, one of the most difficult barriers for the nurse to overcome when she encounters it in her work with others. It is a common human trait, which can operate not only between nurse and patient, but between the nurse and members of the patient's family, among members of the professional team and, not uncommonly, between family members and the patient. In the larger society, it operates within groups to impede the work of the separate groups, and among groups to hamper and impair progress toward desirable social goals. Most importantly, it operates within the individual, often unconsciously, so that he is unaware of the hostile impulses and wishes that form the motives for many of his actions. The perception that an individual has of others can thus be distorted by his own hostile outlook on his life situation.

In its broadest sense, hostility may be seen as a continuum, the manifestations of which range from overly polite behavior to extreme forms which may be externalized in murderous rage or homicide, or internalized as depression or suicide. Most problems that the nurse encounters in her day-to-day contacts with patients, families, and co-workers stem from covert hostility or from the milder types of aggressive behavior that signal its presence. This article attempts to focus on hostility as a symptom or sign of unmet nursing needs, which, then, form the basis of an emergent nursing problem.

188   Hostility

The degree to which the nurse is aware of her own hostile impulses and wishes, and of the behavior patterns she has adopted to cope with them, are crucial factors in determining how effective her nursing intervention will be in dealing with the hostile behavior of a patient. Because hostility is so often an automatic response, this awareness is not easily achieved and, in cases in which the sources of the hostility spring from the very early developmental period, they are probably not recognizable at all.

Webster defines hostility as unfriendliness or animosity. Symonds says that hostility is a "state of enmity and ill will."[1] Saul makes careful distinction between hostility and the closely associated emotions of aggression, anger and hate. According to him, "hostility is the tendency of an organism to do something harmful to another organism or to itself." He goes on to point out that aggression may have a constructive meaning and need not always be hostile, just as hostility may be passively rather than aggressively expressed.[2] Nor can one equate hostility with anger, for anger usually is short-lived and is compatible with love. Hostility may be accompanied by anger and, in human beings, this is often the case. Although Buss lists resentment as one type of hostile behavior,[3] Graham cautions against defining hostility as resentment. According to him, resentment is a "feeling of indignant displeasure" of which hostility is not always a necessary consequence, but hostility is "a feeling of antagonism or enmity implying a wish for aggressive action."[4] For the purposes of this article it may be useful to define hostility as a feeling of antagonism, accompanied by a wish to hurt or humiliate others, which may produce subsequent feelings of inadequacy and self-rejection owing to loss of self-esteem. This feeling may be repressed or dissociated, or it may be expressed in various kinds of covert and overt behavior.

Hostility is thought by many authorities to be the result of frustrated and unfulfilled needs or wishes; according to Horney, repressed hostility is one of the major sources of anxiety.[5] Originally part of a basic, biological mechanism through which the individual adapted to threats, irritations and frustrations, hostility is not a disorder or a disease of itself, but rather one of our necessary human endowments. For primitive man, withdrawing from or destroying a threat to his basic biological integrity may have spelled the difference between extinction or survival. Normal hostility derives from justifiable fear or real danger; irrational hostility originates in anxiety. Hostility becomes a disordered reponse when it is kept alive to generate anxiety, the energy of which is then expended futilely rather than constructively. Such is the case when it is used to strive toward immature goals or when it is substituted for understanding and cooperation in dealing with life problems. The person who becomes the "patient" in a medical system is a person under stress, who attempts to alleviate his anxiety or to deal with his hostile feelings in ways that have previously proved at least partially effective. The regression engendered by illness makes it all the more necessary for him to revert to earlier childhood patterns of response and defense.

It has been suggested that a rudimentary form of hostility may be present even in the fetus, inasmuch as this feeling may be laid down as one of the earlier engrams; if this is the case, it is manifested as early as the 14th week of gestation.[6] Whether or not this is so, it is certain that the early roots of hostility can be discerned soon after birth. A baby will turn its face away from a threatening stimulus or even "attack" it by crude attempts to push it away. Later, the infant uses its powers of locomotion by physically removing itself from the threat. As the child grows older, threats begin to come from the environment as a reaction to something that he has done which brings disapproval from significant others. He may then externalize hostile feelings in the form of angry behavior, such as defiant looks at the reproving or punishing adult. Or, he may project this hostility upon the other person and behave as though the "badness" were in the other person, thus justifying his own anger. Later in his development this overtly hostile behavior may be replaced by shyness, retreat and withdrawal. The three-year-old has already developed the ability to anticipate blame or punishment from an adult and to protect himself by retiring to a safe area. He feels weak and inadequate in the face of a powerful person against whom he cannot openly vent his hostile feelings. These frustrated or unmet needs for status, prestige or power form one of the bases for later hostility in adult life. Janis sees this type of hostility operating in the hospitalized patient in whom parataxic distortions of earlier childhood experience lead him to perceive the nurse as an authority figure, against whom childish, hostile impulses may again be reactivated.[7]

In the very young child, the need to repress hostility stems chiefly from two sources:
  1. Fear of jeopardizing his parental relationships:
      a. He depends on these powerful adults for his very existence.

  b. He fears them in the face of his own weakness and inadequacy.
  c. He desperately needs and craves their love and approval.
2. Reflected self-appraisal:
  a. He rejects the "bad-me", the components of his personality that have previously brought disapproval from significant adults.
  b. This rejection leads to further anxiety and an attempt to disown or dissociate the hostile feelings by projecting them onto others, or by pushing them back out of awareness.

  This is, of course, an over-simplification of a complex dynamism, but it should help to develop an understanding of why certain situations serve to evoke hostility in later adult life. The person who finds it intolerable to acknowledge himself as hostile or angry tends to perceive his world as hostile, unfriendly and dangerous.

  Although social and cultural standards demand that controls and limits be set on aggressive tendencies, healthy self-assertion is a mark of maturity. If the child is constantly required to repress all expression of these tendencies, the impotent anger thus engendered eventually becomes dissociated, but the hostile impulses and wishes remain in the unconscious and generate anxiety and guilt. Horney describes the process as a cycle in which anxiety, when based on a felt threat, provokes reactive hostility which, if repressed, may again create anxiety.[8]

  The disapproval with which our society views the outright expression of anger, particularly in polite social settings, makes it difficult for a person to maintain his right to healthy self-assertion. What is sometimes labelled as "demanding", "uncooperative" or "unreasonable" behavior of a patient may be a normal and even commendable attempt on his part to maintain his dignity as a human being, in a highly institutionalized, impersonal setting. A person whose needs for growth and self-realization are really threatened is acting in a mature way when he takes a stand for himself. The nurse needs to be perceptive in order to assess what is healthy and necessary for this person. She also needs to feel herself reasonably free from bureaucratic and institutional pressures in order to individualize his care. Much has been done in recent years to recognize the fact that the hospitalized child has a need to protest openly and even angrily, but social pressures within the system still operate all too effectively in silencing the adult who feels aggrieved and angry at his unwelcome—and often unforeseen—situation.

Viewed operationally, then, the development of hostility may be described as follows:

1. A person has experienced frustration, loss of self-esteem or unmet needs for status, prestige or love in the past.
2. A situation occurs in which he holds certain expectations of self or others.
3. Expectations are not met.
4. The person feels inadequate, hurt or humiliated.
5. He experiences anxiety in the form of hostility.
6. He may then act in one of three ways:
    a. repress the hostility and withdraw.
    b. disown the feeling and over-react by being extremely polite and compliant.
    c. engage in some type of overtly hostile behavior, either verbal or nonverbal.

The influence of hostility on the cause and progress of illness has long been recognized. In ancient times, imbalance of the bile or choleric humor was believed to produce certain bodily diseases. Washington Irving's classic character, Rip Van Winkle, came home to learn that his shrewish wife had finally "burst a blood vessel in a fit of anger." In more recent times, Dunbar,[9] Alexander,[10] and others have focused on the role that hostility plays, not only in many psychosomatic conditions, but to some extent in most or all disturbances of physiology. Although earlier theories concerning hostility as a specific cause of various psychosomatic illnesses have not always been borne out by the available data, a number of studies do lend some credence to this belief. Kaplan and his associates see a relationship between hostility and hypertension, but advance the possibility that expressed hostility may be caused by elevation of blood pressure rather than vice versa.[11] Alexander notes that "persons suffering from rheumatoid arthritis have difficulty in handling their aggressive, hostile impulses."[12] Hirt sees "much of the hostility felt by asthmatic patients as directly related to their dependency needs."[13] Schoenberg reported a study in which overall results seemed to substantiate his hypothesis that "hostility is a significant factor in the etiology of neurodermatitis."[14] Weiner and his associates, in an attempt to link hostility to peptic ulcer, found that the majority of patients in his study who were hypersecretors of gastric enzymes seemed to have had as the source of their anxiety, "hostile impulses that they felt must not be revealed or directly expressed."[15] Even pain can, in some instances, be traced to guilt feelings about aggressive impulses. Engel maintains that some individuals feel guilty about expressing aggression and that they may actually experience pain as a result.[16]

More pertinent for the nurse, perhaps, is the literature that deals with situations in which there seems to be a fairly high potential for hostility. Bowlby's studies have led to a greater awareness of the hospitalized child's need to express his grief and frustration by angry outbursts and tears.[17] What is not so universally recognized, however, is the fact that most adults experience some degree of hostility during a period of enforced illness and hospitalization. The initial reaction to any illness is anxiety, which may be expressed as hostility. The dependency feelings that accompany acceptance of the illness may lead to feelings of hostility if this is the pattern that the patient usually follows in his attempt to cope with stress. The period of convalescence may be prolonged if the patient has repressed his resentful, hostile feelings toward medical personnel during his period of accepted illness.

Referring to preoperative cancer patients, Henderson says that hostility is common. Although the patient sees the surgeon as the injuring agent, he may fear retaliation and so displace his hostility onto nurses, social workers or family members.[18] The now classic work of Janis demonstrates that "absence of fear before operation appears to bear a marked relation to subsequent reactions of anger and resentment during the postoperative period."[19] Leake notes that the tendency to focus frustration on others may lead to serious problems in the care of the chronically ill. It may be particularly damaging to relationships between the patient and his family. As the patient becomes more aware that some of his basic emotional needs cannot be satisfied, he may become quite disturbed. Persons closest to him, such as devoted family members, may then become the objects of his jealousy and displaced hostility. Early recognition of this danger and frank discussion with him of the realities of the situation lead to greater self-understanding for the patient. Attempts to assist him in reaching a balanced satisfaction through appropriate and satisfying activities within his capacities and limitations help prevent this unhealthy focusing of frustration onto others.[20]

Regardless of the type of illness for which the person seeks medical help, the circumstances surrounding the event are usually sufficient in themselves to call forth a high degree of anxiety and/or hostility. He is placed in much the same situation as he was when early childhood experiences first evoked a hostile response. He is again weak and inadequate in a world of powerful authority figures upon whom he must depend to ward off danger or threat; he is painfully aware of his dependent status; his needs for love and approval are intensified by stress; and his very self-identity is threatened by the alien, impersonal world of the hospital. The highly organized routines through which his medical care is delivered serve only to augment the ego-alien stimuli. Maslow observes that being "rubricized" denies the person's individuality or pays no attention to his personhood. The person resents being casually classified, and deprived of his uniqueness and difference from all others. Anger then serves to protect this identity.[21]

Not all people are alike in their ability to feel or express anger. Likewise, it is seldom possible to assess the degree of hostility present by the directness or the intensity of its expression. Behavior indicative of hostility varies considerably with the individual. Even the ways in which the person acts out his hostility may differ according to the circumstances in which he finds himself and the degree of stress that he is undergoing. Nor is it always possible to detect who is really the focus of the patient's hostility, for the tendency to displace this feeling on those less threatening and less able to retaliate is a common one.

Unless the nurse is working in a psychiatric setting, she rarely encounters the violently aggressive behavior that signals that the person has temporarily lost control. If this should occur, it must be dealt with as a psychiatric emergency. This aspect of nursing has been ably handled by Lange.[22]

Covert expressions of hostility may be frequent, but are not always easily identified. A patient may be silent because he is resentful, withdrawing from a perceived threat, or seething with anger to such a degree that he dare not trust himself to speak. He may be depressed, a sign of the hostility that is turned inward upon the self. A perceptive nurse picks up many nonverbal cues indicating that the patient may feel hostile; facial expression and bodily posture often betray inner turmoil. She may wonder why the patient is so placating and obsequious, or why he finds it necessary to adopt so ingratiating an attitude toward those who care for him. She can only surmise as to what the patient is trying to communicate, unless he himself can say what it is that he is feeling. She cannot act directly upon her assumptions or hunches until she has validated them with the patient. What the nurse perceives as dangerous, threatening or discomforting may not be felt in this way by him at all. Often, the basic cause of his hostility cannot be identified, nor is such "depth psychotherapy" either appropriate or necessary in order to deal with a presenting problem. If the nurse can help the patient identify what it is in the here-and-now situation that seems to threaten him, she can help him deal with the problem at hand and resolve his hostility, or at least prevent it from interfering with his needed care. In cases in which a real personality problem exists, psychiatric consultation should be sought, so that professional psychotherapy can be instituted if it should be indicated.

Overt expressions of hostility may take the form of sarcastic, abusive or rude remarks. Freud tells us that a hostile joke is one way to satisfy an instinct by circumventing an obstacle that stands in the way of this satisfaction.[23] The person may be argumentative, demanding, verbally attacking or threatening. Rejection and fault-finding are other indications of a hostile attitude. Such behavior is usually motivated by fear and a distorted perception of a threat to the self or the self-image. The hostility thus generated is then displaced onto another object which in some way symbolized the danger.

Resentful silence or deliberate avoidance needs to be dealt with gently but directly before any meaningful communication or therapeutic nursing intervention can take place. The nurse may tell the patient that she observed his silence or avoidance, and she may inquire if something has happened. Recognition of the fact that he appears troubled will convey the nurse's concern and willingness to help. Regardless of whether this brings only further silence or an angry outburst, the nurse must be prepared to accept the patient as he is and to continue to meet his nursing needs in every way she possibly can.

Accepting the patient does not in any way imply that the nurse should abdicate her responsibility to set reasonable limits or controls, should this become necessary. Occasionally, the free expression of hostile feelings may excite the patient instead of relieving the tension. The subsequent feeling of guilt then tends to be projected onto the nurse in the form of hostility, because he sees her as responsible for his behavior to some degree. Some patients, especially those with strong authoritarian traits, respond to limit-setting much more readily than they do to discussion and ventilation. Their anxiety is lessened when they feel that the "danger-control persons" show no signs of weakness, but seem to be really in control and can be depended upon to help them preserve their self-respect. Only a sound understanding of the dynamics of human behavior, derived both from theory and clinical experience, will enable the nurse to make the discriminating judgments necessary in deciding upon the most helpful approach for any given individual. The following clinical examples illustrate a variety of approaches, most of which seemed to be of some help in reducing the patient's anxiety and enabling him to begin to cope with his situation in a more constructive manner.

One of the most difficult of all situations for the nurse to face and to deal with occurs when overt hostility, which she had in no way anticipated, is focused directly upon her. When the hostility is anticipated, some thought and planning can be given to dealing with the problem. However, when such open hostility and verbal abuse are unexpectedly encountered, the nurse is placed in a very difficult position as she tries to deal with her own anxiety and the patient's evident antagonism and rejection. The following incident exemplifies such a situation:

The A family had been scheduled for a routine clinic appointment, but failed to keep it. A nursing student who had been working with the family visited the home to ascertain the reason for the missed appointment. Greatly to her surprise, she was received with unmistakable signs of hostility. At first, they refused to open the door and, when they did, they blocked the entrance to her. When she gained reluctant permission to enter, both family members placed their legs up on the available chairs in such a way that she was prevented from being seated. The mother accused the nurse in loud, angry tones, stating that she had not contacted the clinic to clarify the patient's appointment as she had said she would. The father spoke to the mother in loud tones saying (about the nurse) "She is no help . . . you see you don't depend on her." Both expressed a wish to have the nurse discontinue her services to the family. The nurse attempted to calm both parties and to encourage description in sequential order of the wife's missed appointment and her understanding of the arrangements. Both patients resisted these attempts and continued to express their hostile feelings. At this point, the nurse realized the futility of attempting to discuss the matter and permitted them to verbalize their hostile feelings. Upon leaving, she stated she would contact them at a later date.

After conferring with the mental health consultant, the nurse wrote a letter to the family, explaining the misunderstanding and saying she would call them the following week. It was decided that a letter would be the best approach at this time, because it would give them something concrete to refer to and would also give them time to prepare for the visit. When the nurse telephoned the home to confirm the appointment, the mother was still taciturn and monosyllabic. However, when she did make the visit, both clients were very friendly and open, even to the point of prolonging the visit beyond the scheduled hour.

In retrospect, it can be said that the nurse used the only approach open to her at the time of the initial visit: she accepted the persons as individuals by permitting them to talk without retaliation and counter-hostility. Possibly the most important factor in re-establishing working relationships was the nurse's concern for the welfare of her clients. She demonstrated by her actions that she considered them important and would proceed with any nursing intervention they needed if they would permit it. Her letter not only presented whatever factual information was necessary to clear up the misconception, but again acknowledged their importance as people who had a right to an explanation.

Hostile relationships among patients can pose a ward problem that, once it is identified, calls for a creative and consistent approach on the part of the nursing team. An attempt must be made to reduce hostility-provoking stimuli and to provide a measure of acceptance and security for these patients. The following is an example of overt hostility which was, nevertheless, indirectly expressed:

Two elderly ladies occupied beds next to each other in a four-bed ward in a general hospital. One carefully kept her curtains drawn all day, thus creating for herself an area of isolation which could not be disturbed without vociferous protest. Because each took a considerable amount of nursing time, they were usually assigned for care to two different nurses who worked simultaneously. During the time each was receiving morning care, one of the patients kept up a running line of comments about the "old lady in the next bed. She's really not all there, you know." . . . "She doesn't like anyone." . . . "She's pretty sick, do you think she'll make it?" Meanwhile, the other patient was remarking to her nurse about that "mean old woman in that bed over there." The problem was discussed at a team conference. It was noted that each of the participants in the "feud" could communicate with the other only indirectly. By using the nurses as deflectors of a sort they were able to establish at least a negative relationship with each other. Because direct confrontation might have proved too traumatic and resulted in a need to save face by still further strengthening of defenses, it was decided to try an indirect approach, which would provide opportunity for the two patients to speak with each other directly while both nurses were present, to facilitate the process and to provide a feeling of security.

The following morning, both patients were taken in wheelchairs to the lounge area by their respective nurses. They were formally introduced to each other and both nurses sat down to engage them in friendly conversation. This became a daily event and, as they began to know each other better, nursing personnel were able to gradually withdraw. The two ladies found a number of common interests and began to enjoy each other's company, even within the ward situation.

One might conjecture at length on the basic motives for the original hostility. As it was, for some reason, each of these patients had felt in some way threatened by the other. When the misperceptions began to be cleared and they had additional first-hand information about each other, the hostility between them seemed to be resolved. Acceptance of their need to communicate through a third person and working from this knowledge was the approach chosen by this particular nursing staff. Other alternatives might have been tried, but the basic principle from which nursing intervention was derived is that of recognizing the hostile behavior, accepting the patient's need to deal with a perceived threat, and trying in some way to reduce the threat by clarifying the misperceptions from which it seems to emanate. When the unknown became the known, the fear had no further foundation in reality.

Most patients find it difficult to express anger or hostility toward authority figures, particularly if they themselves are authoritarian personalities. If the patient has invested the nurse with an authority role, she may need to be even more perceptive in recognizing distress signals that appear in the guise of hostility. She may find, too, that the patient needs considerable encouragement before he can trust her enough to voice what it is that is distressing him. One such incident is recounted below:

A highly successful professional man had been hospitalized and placed on bed rest. A new nursing supervisor was struck by the apparently hostile feeling of the nursing staff toward this patient. He was described as "impossible," "with a chip on his shoulder" and "sarcastic." When the supervisor entered his room, she found a very unhappy, taciturn man in the bed; his wife sat quietly by with a worried expression. The nurse introduced herself and the patient remarked sarcastically:

Patient: "Oh, so they sent the supervisor."
Nurse: "I've been trying to get acquainted with the patients. How is everything with you, Mr. B?"
P.: (sarcastically) Oh, everything is just fine."

N.: "That's not the impression I get, Mr. B. Something seems to be troubling you."

P.: "Oh, no, nothing at all. There's no use going into all that! Just forget about me. I guess I'll be o.k."

N.: "You don't sound very convincing to me, Mr. B. Is there something I can do to help?"

Here, the patient began to pour out, in an angry and aggrieved tone all the frustrations he had been brooding over for the past few days. At this point, his wife placed her hand on his arm, admonishing him not to complain. The nurse continued to encourage him to describe and clarify. Some of his protests were legitimate struggles against complete helplessness and dependency. Added to this was the stress of apparently trying to live up to his wife's expectations of what a good patient should be and do. After a nursing conference, adjustments were made in the plan of care, thus individualizing it more. Time was also set aside during which he could talk about the things that were disturbing him, and an effort was made to respect his needs and preferences as much as possible. By the time he was discharged the following week, his anxious, hostile behavior had abated, and a better understanding was beginning to develop between him and the nursing staff.

The initial reluctance to speak displayed by this patient in the presence of an authority figure was overcome by the encouragement and acceptance that the nurse conveyed. Empathy and sensitivity are especially important in a situation of this kind. Pushing a patient into revealing what he is not yet ready to discuss can be harmful and it may result in intensification of the anxiety that caused the problem in the first place. He needs time to learn how far he can trust, and it may take more than one visit before he feels free enough to speak about what is troubling him. The nurse can inquire directly what the problem seems to be, but the patient must be ready before a productive working through can take place. In the example just cited, mutual withdrawal of the patient and the nursing staff from each other had become progressively more pronounced and would have continued, had the intervention not been direct and prompt. This patient was behaving in a way that was alienating and rejecting the very people on whom he most depended for help at this time.

The following incident illustrates what can occur when the nurse is unaware that her actions are not only one cause of the patient's hostility, but that they actually serve to reinforce the hostile, resentful behavior adopted by him in an almost last-ditch fight, in order to defend his self-image and to punish those who seem to deprive him of the esteem and approval he so sorely needs.

Mrs. L. occupied the first bed next to the door in a five-bed ward. Mrs. K, the patient next to her, was a very sweet, compliant person, with many friends and visitors, and well liked by everyone except her next-bed neighbor, Mrs. L. This neighbor's rude remarks to Mrs. K. frequently reduced her to tears, yet she never fought back. Students assigned to Mrs. K were indignant with Mrs. L for her seemingly unjust attacks on Mrs. K., but were at a loss to know how to deal with Mrs. L's hostile behavior. In an effort to comfort Mrs. K., they redoubled their efforts to give her tender, loving care and withdrew still more from Mrs. L. The problem was discussed with the psychiatric consultant, and the students were helped to see what a vicious cycle had unwittingly been set in motion. As Mrs. L. saw herself more rejected, her anxiety rose, and, with it, the need to defend herself in the only way she knew; hostility and verbal attack. As a first approach, it was suggested that each nurse who passed her bed would acknowledge Mrs. L. by a friendly, "Good-morning, Mrs. L," being careful to use her name, or by a smile or nod of recognition. An attempt was made by Mrs. L's nurse to spend time with her daily, talking with her in a friendly, relaxed way. The staff were also helped to recognize the psychological harm being done Mrs. K by the reinforcement of her neurotic, compliant behavior and her attempt to control the situation by playing the martyr. Through their strong positive response, they were providing effective feedback, which encouraged this behavior still more. As the plan went into effect, Mrs. L's sarcastic, biting remarks became less frequent, and nursing personnel were agreeably surprised to find her a friendly, humorous person, who now dealt with them on a much more mature level.

Covert hostility, of which the hostile person himself is not aware, may be unwittingly translated into behavior that is perceived by the other person as hostile. The following is an interesting example of how the nurse's own unconscious may have betrayed her into an automatic, hostile response:

Mrs. X. had undergone extensive surgery for a radical mastectomy. While the nurse was assisting the physician for the first postoperative dressing, the patient started to look down at the unsightly incision. Quickly but gently, the nurse placed her hand on the patient's cheek, turning her head to prevent her from seeing the wound. The patient accepted this submissively, without comment. Several weeks after she had been discharged from the hospital, the patient met the nurse during one of her return visits for a check-up. She remarked to the nurse: "Do you remember the day you slapped me? I'd never have believed you would slap me, but you did." Surprised at this misinterpretation of what had been meant as a kindly gesture, the nurse protested that she had not slapped her. No amount of explanation, however, would convince this lady that it had not been a slap. Not a very hard one, of course, but still a slap.

One might, as a first reaction, say that the patient's own hostility caused her to project these feelings onto the nurse and thus see the nurse as hostile. However, as the nurse began to look at herself more honestly, she asked herself a number of questions: Why did she react so automatically to the patient's gesture? What would have happened had she permitted the patient to look at the wound? Was she being over-protective? If so, perhaps this reactivated the patient's childhood feelings about an overprotective parent. Or, to be still more honest, perhaps the nurse saw her own self-image as the good nurse or the "good mother," threatened by some imaginary harm to the patient for which she might be responsible. If this were really the case, the hand that she placed on the patient's cheek might not have been as gentle as she liked to think. The answers probably lie somewhere in between, for the complex dynamism of human behavior usually does not admit of any simple explanation. It does point up, however, the fact that hostility can be unconscious, and that it may be a reciprocal process of which neither of the persons involved is fully aware.

Each person who exhibits hostile behavior has his own unique background and reasons for behaving the way he does. If the hostility results from the illness or from some existing situation, it usually subsides as the person becomes better or the situation improves. If the hostility is deep-seated and part of the person's life-long pattern of defense, it will require professional psychotherapy. In either case, the nurse must be able to recognize the cues that signal hostility. Her first action should always be to look at herself and her own feelings. Just as a patient may misperceive or distort a situation, the nurse, who also belongs to the same human race, may have her own childhood experiences and images reactivated by something in a situation.

It is not always easy to distinguish between hostility (which is motivated by the wish to hurt or to humiliate) and healthy self-assertion, which is part of the normal human process of the exercise of individual rights. One of the marks of emotional maturity is a healthy striving toward self-actualization. This implies the ability to perceive reality correctly in relation to one's own life situation and to assume personal responsibility for one's own actions. This self-assertion, which is part of the growth process, may be difficult to exercise within the structure of our highly efficient automated health systems. Persons who do assert themselves with justifiable reason, refusing to surrender their independence, may fail to conform to what is expected of the patient. The staff may criticize him accordingly.

The nurse who has learned to recognize her own feelings and to bring them under conscious control is usually able to respond in a professional and disciplined manner to the patient's hostile expression of his underlying fears. Her response reflects acceptance and understanding; usually the attack is not so much against her personally as it is a reaction to the whole frustrating situation as the patient sees it. She needs to keep in mind, however, that there may be times when she finds herself under a real emotional strain in trying to cope with a particularly trying patient whose hostility seems to be chronic and who is beginning to wear down her own emotional reserves. This is an occupational hazard for which she needs counsel and support from those professionally qualified to help her. The nursing supervisor, mental health consultant or other qualified person should be available to her, in order to lend whatever assistance and support she needs at this time to carry out therapeutic nursing intervention. If she is able to demonstrate sincere concern for the patient and his welfare, she helps him meet and resolve the crisis; once the anxiety is allayed, he can begin to stabilize and to use the proferred assistance in constructive ways. She can only do this if she herself feels relatively comfortable in this anxiety-laden situation.

An understanding of the dynamic bases of hostility—and the behavioral processes which hostility activates—is essential for the competent nursing practitioner. When the nurse perceives behavior that seems to indicate hostility, she needs to check out her observations with someone else in the situation whenever possible. The first necessary step in effective nursing intervention is for her to validate her assumptions with the patient, assist him in the description and clarification of what it is that he is experiencing and the possible reasons behind these feelings. To be aware of her own reactions, to accept the patient without giving either approval or disapproval, and to avoid value judgments will sometimes be difficult for her, but these are the essential ingredients of therapeutic nursing. Skill in detecting the patient's unspoken wish for limit setting, and the ability to control without being punitive or retaliating, demand maturity and professional acumen. Most important of all is the effort the nurse exerts to ameliorate the circumstances causing the hostility and to enable the patient to maintain his pride and self-respect. Working in this way, she truly assists him to grow in self-understanding and to achieve optimal health and self-actualization.

REFERENCES

1. Symonds, P.: The Dynamics of Human Adjustment. p. 82. New York, Appleton-Century-Crofts, 1946.
2. Saul, L.: The Hostile Mind. p. 3. New York, Random House, 1956.
3. Buss, A., and Durkee, A.: An inventory for assessing different kinds of hostility. J. Consult. Psychol., *21*, 4:343, 1957.
4. Graham, D., and Wolf, S.: Pathogenesis of Urticaria, J. A. M. A., *143*:1399, 1950.
5. Horney, K.: The neurotic personality of our time. *In* Collected Works of Karen Horney, Vol. I, p. 63. New York, W. W. Norton & Co., 1937.
6. Cushing, J. G., and Cushing M. M.: A concept of the genesis of hostility. Bulletin of the Menninger Clinic. p. 98. 13, 1949.
7. Janis, I. L.: Psychological Stress. p. 169. London, John Wiley & Sons, 1958.
8. Horney, K.: The neurotic personality of our time. *In* Collected Works of Karen Horney, Vol. I. p. 74. New York, W. W. Norton & Co., 1937.
9. Dunbar, F.: Emotions and Bodily Changes. ed. 4. New York, Columbia University Press, 1954.
10. Alexander, F.: Psychosomatic Medicine. New York, W. W. Norton & Co., 1950.
11. Kaplan, S., Gottschalk, L., Maggliocco, G., Rohowit, D., and Ross, D.: Hostility in verbal productions and hypnotic dreams of hypertensive patients. Psychosom. Med., *23*, 4:321, 1961.
12. Alexander, F., French, T., and Pollock, G.: Psychosomatic Specificity, Vol. I. p. 12. Chicago, University of Chicago Press, 1968.
13. Hirt, M. L.: Psychological and Allergic Aspects of Asthma. p. 200. Springfield, Ill., Charles C Thomas, 1965.
14. Schoenberg, B., and Carr, A.: An investigation of criteria for brief psychotherapy of neurodermatitis. Psychosom. Med., *25*:262, 1963.
15. Weiner, H., Reiser, M., Thaler, M., and Mirsky, I. A.: Etiology of duodenal ulcer; Relation of specific psychological characteristics to rate of gastric secretion. *In* Palmer, J., and Goldstein, M. (eds.): Perspectives in Psychopathology. p. 121. New York, Oxford University Press, 1966.

16. Engel, G.: Psychogenic pain and the pain-prone patient. Am. J. Med., *26*:899, 1959.
17. Bowlby, J.: Child Care and the Growth of Love. Baltimore, Penguin Books, 1953.
18. Henderson, I., and Henderson, J.: Psychological care of patients with catastrophic illness. Canad. Nurse, *61,* 11:901, 1965.
19. Janis, I. L.: Psychological Stress. p. 217. London, John Wiley & Sons, 1958.
20. Leake, C.: Prevention of the focusing of frustration in chronic illness. *In* Harrower, M. (ed.): Medical and Psychological Teamwork in the Care of the Chronically Ill. Springfield, Ill., Charles C Thomas, 1955.
21. Maslow, A. H.: Toward a Psychology of Being. p. 119. Princeton, Van Nostrand, 1962.
22. Lange, S.: The violent patient. *In* American Nurses Association: A.N.A. Clinical Sessions, San Francisco, 1966. New York, Appleton-Century-Crofts, 1967.
23. Freud, S.: Jokes and Their Relation to the Unconscious. p. 101. Trans. by James Strachey. New York, W. W. Norton & Co., 1961.

BIBLIOGRAPHY

Alexander, F.: Psychosomatic Medicine. New York, W. W. Norton & Co., 1950.

Alexander, F., French, T., and Pollock, G.: Psychosomatic Specificity, Vol. 1. Chicago, University of Chicago Press, 1968.

Berkowitz, L.: Aggression: A Social Psychological Analysis. New York, McGraw-Hill, 1962.

Bowlby, J.: Child Care and the Growth of Love. Baltimore, Penguin Books, 1953.

Buss, A., and Durkee, A.: An inventory for assessing different kinds of hostility. J. Consult. Psychol., *21*, 4:343, 1957.

Clack, J.: Nursing intervention into the aggressive behavior of patients. *In* Burd, S., and Marshall, M. (eds.): Some Clinical Approaches to Psychiatric Nursing. New York, Macmillan, 1963.

Cushing, J. G. N., and Cushing, M. M.: A concept of the genesis of hostility. Bulletin of the Menninger Clinic. 13. pp. 94-100. 1949.

Dumas, R. G., Anderson, B. J., and Leonard, R.: The importance of the expressive function in nursing for pre-operative preparation. *In* Skipper, J. K., and Leonard, R. (eds.): Social Interaction and Patient Care. Philadelphia, J. B. Lippincott, 1965.

Educational Design, Inc.: Understanding Hostility. Programmed Instruction. Am. J. Nurs., *67*, 10:2131-2150, October, 1967.

Engel, G. L.: Psychogenic pain and the pain-prone patient. Am. J. Med., *26*:899-918, 1959.

Freud, S.: Jokes and their Relation to the Unconscious. Trans. by James Strachey. New York, W. W. Norton & Co., 1961.

Graham, D., and Wolf, S.: Pathogenesis of urticaria. J. Am. Med. Ass., *143*:1396-1402, 1950.

Henderson, I., and Henderson, J.: Psychological care of patients with catastrophic illness. Canad. Nurse, *61*, 11:899-902, 1965.

Hirt, M. L.: Psychological and Allergic Aspects of Asthma. Springfield, Ill., Charles C Thomas, 1965.

Horney, K.: The neurotic personality of our time. *In* Collected Works of Karen Horney, Vol. I. New York, W. W. Norton & Co., 1937.

Janis, I. L.: Psychological Stress. London, John Wiley & Sons, 1958.

Kaplan, S., Gottschalk, L., Maggliocco, B., Rohowit, D., and Ross, D.: Hostility in verbal productions and hypnotic dreams of hypertensive patients. Psychosom. Med., *23*, 4:311-321, 1961.

Lange, S.: The violent patient. *In* American Nurses' Association: A.N.A. Clinical Sessions, San Francisco, 1966. New York, Appleton-Century-Crofts, 1967.

Leake, C.: Prevention of the focusing of frustration in chronic illness. *In* Harrower, M. (ed.): Medical and Psychological Teamwork in the Care of the Chronically Ill. Springfield, Ill., Charles C Thomas, 1955.

Maslow, A. H.: Toward a Psychology of Being. Princeton, Van Nostrand, 1962.

Magraw, R.: Hostility as a symptom, sign and signal in medical care. Hosp. Med., *2*:105-111, 1966.

Oscarson, S.: Hostile behavior in a maternity patient. *In* American Nurses' Association: A.N.A. Clinical Sessions, San Francisco, 1966. New York, Appleton-Century-Crofts, 1967.

Peplau, H. E.: Interpersonal Relations in Nursing. New York, G. P. Putnam's Sons, 1952.

Schoenberg, B., and Carr, A.: An investigation of criteria for brief psychotherapy of neurodermatitis. Psychosom. Med., *25*:253-263, 1963.

Saul, L.: The Hostile Mind. New York, Random House, 1956.

Symonds, P.: The Dynamics of Human Adjustment. New York, Appleton-Century-Crofts, 1946.

Weiner, H., Reiser, M., Thales, M., and Mirsky, A.: Etiology of duodenal ulcer; Relation of specific psychological characteristics to rate of gastric secretion. *In* Palmer, J., and Goldstein, M. (eds.): Perspectives of Psychopathology. New York, Oxford University Press, 1966.

Weiss, F., Zuger, B., Thompson, D., Landman, L., and Joost, M.: Dynamics of hostility, a panel. Am. J. Psychoanal., *19*, 1:4-27, 1959.

11

Ambivalence

Rose Kemp

Nursing students and practicing nurses constantly face and deal with a maze of concepts relating to human behavior. Nurses must decide which is the primary motivation for the patient's behavior. One behavior characteristic that clouds understanding between patient and nurse, and sometimes blocks positive action toward recovering health, is ambivalence. Ambivalence may be described as the presence within one person of opposing emotions, attitudes, ideas or wishes toward the same object or situation.

The concept of ambivalence evolved out of psychoanalytic theory, and it has acquired a well recognized place in psychiatric literature. Today, both lay and professional people use the term to describe a variety of situations.

The concept of ambivalence usually is introduced to students during their psychiatric nursing experience, and it generally is associated with severe mental illness. However, ambivalence can best be understood by relating it to the development of the child, its manifestations in the normal adult, and the problems it poses in everyday nursing situations.

Because ambivalence in all degrees is one of the main threats to interpersonal relationships, a sound grasp of all its aspects—normal and abnormal—should increase the nurse's effectiveness with patients and colleagues.

A review of most of the literature about ambivalence written since the late 1920's discloses that the meaning of the term has changed, gradually and almost imperceptibly. The word now has a number of connotations.

Eugen Bleuler used the term to describe a phenomenon in which pleasant and unpleasant feelings simultaneously accompany the same experience. He stated that ambivalence is characteristic of the child and of the unconscious. The overt appearance of ambivalence in the adult, Bleuler says, implies the presence of definite psychopathology. He saw ambivalence as a primary symptom of schizophrenia and manic-depressive psychoses, and he used the term extensively in relation to these psychiatric diseases.[1]

Sigmund Freud and others adapted the term ambivalence to fit their theories of psychic life and extended its use to the neuroses. Throughout his writings, Freud continued to elaborate the concept. Because contemporary authors quote from different periods of Freud's writings, they introduce subtle differences into the definition of ambivalence.

One major variation among the definitions of ambivalence hinges on the question of movement. Does an ambivalent person oscillate between two feelings, or is he locked in a static position, immobilized by the presence of two opposite feelings?

This question arises because ambivalence frequently is used to describe the simultaneous existence of love and hate toward the same object, without regard to how this state affects behavior. One definition implies that ambivalence is the simultaneous pressure of opposed tendencies, particularly love and hate, toward the same person.[2] This definition suggests a tension between two feelings which is so strong that it might conceivably lead to a paralysis of feeling. In contrast, phrases such as "co-existence of antithetic emotions" and "simultaneous attraction to and repulsion from an object" imply the possibility of movement between two points.[3,4]

A recent article proposes that to regard ambivalence as oscillation enhances the dynamic aspect of the concept because it allows for a shift of feeling into both polar positions. This shift, in turn, allows for variation of feeling along a continuum.[5] At different times, it is possible for the adult to experience either oscillation or stasis between two feelings. Two authorities point out that the paralyzing inability to focus on either of two feelings indicates a disorganized ego, whereas alternation between love and hate reflects a more highly organized ego.[6]

Freud used the concept of ambivalence to express the polarity of psychic life. The content of psychic life has been categorized into biologic, intellectual, and psychologic polarities. For example, there are numerous biologic opposites, such as wakefulness and sleep or the basic division of living things into male and female. These fundamental opposites are necessary to each other.

Some authors attribute intellectual polarity to our ability to grasp one side of a meaning only in relation to the other. Expressions such as "on the other hand" and "conversely" illustrate this point. By this reasoning, ideas and feelings are not independent, but linked together in pairs.

The polarities of opposites pervade all of psychology: active-passive, conscious-unconscious, pleasure-displeasure, independent-dependent, urge to rebel-urge to conform.[7] Students of nursing encounter the idea of polarities throughout the curriculum in biology, philosophy, psychology and other courses.

The governing of psychic life by polarities would seem to be a concept in itself, but one that is quite similar to ambivalence. However, the presence of polar opposites does not necessarily imply ambivalence. For instance, an individual may have, simultaneously, an urge to disrupt order and an urge to conform. Through his mode of adjustment, he may find suitable outlets for each of these urges. He may join various organizations, participate in "sit-ins," and so forth and, at the same time, wear conventional clothes and decorate his office conventionally. A different phenomenon might occur if both these urges—to rebel and to conform—were to come into play around a single factor, such as deciding whether to move into a residential area with many restrictions.

Ambivalence has been interpreted in two distinct ways, the psychoanalytic and the clinical. According to Tarachow's "Studies In Ambivalence," the psychoanalytic concept of ambivalence refers to the problem of fusing love and hate.[8] The child's task is to merge his separate feelings of love and hate into a more mature attitude that embraces both feelings. The young child and some mentally ill persons cannot fuse or integrate love and hate. Their hate is not tempered by love.

The clinical concept of ambivalence, as differentiated by Tarachow, simply refers to the conscious evidence of indecision or the presence of opposites.[9] Both uses of the concept will be discussed and illustrated later.

Whether the term "ambivalence" is used in the psychoanalytic or the clinical manner, the experience of ambivalence is purely subjective. Because ambivalence is a feeling, one can only infer its presence by observing another person's behavior or by experiencing ambivalence oneself. This engenders some confusion about the concept.

First, the fact that ambivalence is a feeling leads to a discussion of drives or needs. Feelings are often considered to be interchangeable with instinctual drives.[10] Rapaport states that feelings are released and are indicators of unconscious impulses or wishes.[11] For example, the feeling of anger can be released through the aggressive drive. However, aggression does not necessarily express anger. The aggressive drive can find outlets in sports or in other self-assertive, non-angry actions.

The writer will not attempt to differentiate between feelings and drives inasmuch as the literature refers to ambivalence of both. The reader should have in mind that unconscious drives, feelings and the behavior that results from them are all interrelated.

An individual can love one person and hate another and express each of these feelings appropriately toward the person to whom it is directed. If, however, the love and hate are directed toward the same person, all degrees of ambivalent behavior may be seen—from teasing and practical joking to the classic sadistic-masochistic forms of behavior.

A final source of confusion lies in the similarities and differences between ambivalence and conflict. One author points out that ambivalence has been used to describe all contradictory feelings, including the conflict between aggression and submission, male and female, and other opposites. The fact that conflict and ambivalence are used interchangeably and that no clear distinction is made between the two terms raises many questions for a reader of the psychiatric literature.

Sorting out the similarities between ambivalence and conflict is like deciding whether the chicken or the egg comes first.

Both ambivalence and conflict may extend from the emotional level into other areas such as thinking and acting. Conflict, however, covers a wider range than ambivalence. In conflict, two or more contradictory feelings clash. This battle may occur between intrapersonal or interpersonal forces. Compromise solutions or defenses are used to resolve the conflict. Frequently, ambivalence is thought of as a result of conflict. At other times ambivalent feelings are seen to be the cause of conflict, which then leads to defensive behavior. In children, in the mentally ill, and in mild forms in adults, ambivalence may occur *without* precipitating conflict. The mature person may or may not be aware of his ambivalence because one side of the ambivalence usually is unconscious in adults.

The following examples illustrate how ambivalence and conflict differ. A husband might feel ambivalent about his wife's working. On the one hand, he appreciates the extra money she earns. On the other, he misses the housewifely comforts she is unable to provide because of the demands of the job on her time. The husband's feelings are both negative and positive, but they do not necessarily stem from deep conflict, such as a threat to his masculinity. However, when a man is offered a substantial promotion but feels undecided about accepting the position, his indecision may reflect ambivalence or a deeper conflict. To him, acceptance of the new position may mean that he is being aggressive. This may clash with his need to submit and to avoid competitive situations. If the conflict is severe, it may lead to anxiety and be solved by a compromise. One solution might be for him to develop a somatic symptom that could help him avoid the higher position.

HOW AMBIVALENCE DEVELOPS

The growth of the child's ego, his relationships to others and the development of ambivalence are interrelated. It is generally agreed that ambivalence is a fundamental characteristic of the child's emotional life, but opinions vary as to how and when ambivalence originates.

Fenichel says that it is meaningless to talk about ambivalence before the child has a concept of objects.[12] Most authorities accept this statement and believe that ambivalence is not part of man's original, innate equipment but develops with the child's growing awareness of others.

Ambivalence is a reaction to deprivation and frustration of basic needs. This inevitable frustration calls forth the child's aggression toward his love object, his mother, and gives rise to the beginning of ambivalence. The child's mixed feelings of good and bad toward his early object relations make him split the figure of the mother into psychic representations of the good object and bad object.[13] This duality persists and colors all relationships to some degree.

Ambivalence begins in the later part of the oral period and is well established in the two-year-old. The toilet training period offers even

212   Ambivalence

more opportunities for the child to experience opposing feelings toward people and situations.

Until he begins to operate on a fairly realistic basis, his ambivalent feelings can exist for a long time without causing conflict. For example, a child on her first day at camp may write, "Dear Mommie, I hate you, Love, Mary."[14] As the child's ego develops, however, and his ability to form relationships expands, he becomes aware of his opposing feelings. This provokes conflict because the feelings are difficult to reconcile. But, as hatred gradually is tempered by love, the opposing feelings fuse into a stable, more mature attitude.

Ambivalence is largely resolved during the family triangle period. The child usually relates to more people during this period and this enables him to displace his feelings. The child has a right to his feelings and needs the freedom to express them. If both negative and positive feelings are available, they can be fused, displaced, and dealt with. In contrast, the child with few warm relationships, who perhaps has only one major object to relate to, has greater difficulty with his feelings. One side of his ambivalence may be repressed and, therefore, not available for use in forming other ego defenses.

In the older child, various ego defenses concerned with impulse control become more stabilized. Engle mentions the ego defense of undoing. Here "something positive is done which actually or magically is the opposite of the forbidden impulse, and in a sense negates it ... ambivalence in such behavior as undoing is obvious. Certain oaths, vows, rituals, and superstitions of children and adults incorporate this principle, such as the child's game, 'don't step on a crack or you will break your mother's back'."[15]

Reaction formation is another way in which to deal with ambivalence. In this process an acceptable feeling or behavior remains conscious, and its opposite exists unconsciously. Reaction formation, which can become a part of character formation, is the avenue by way of which the obsessive-compulsive personality takes shape.

Several writers, in describing other ways in which ambivalence affects behavior, discuss the reciprocal nature of ambivalence between parent and child, and the ways in which parents reinforce ambivalence in children. The term "double bind" is proposed for the relationship of a child to a mother who is both accepting and rejecting, who expects and demands the child's affectionate response, but refuses or avoids it when it is offered. This *continual ambivalence* of the mother creates a persistent confusion in the child. He cannot build a dependable expectation of his mother's attitude, feelings, and treatment, nor can he resolve the ambiguities of language by which he tries to relate himself to the world of people and symbols.[16] This extreme situation explains why ambivalence may remain to trouble the adult, and sometimes even may cause him to become mentally ill.

Ambivalence plagues adults in other, milder forms. Doubt is thought to be an expression of the ambivalence conflict. "Do I love or do I hate?" is transferred to the thinking process and raises doubt. Pity is another ambivalent feeling, in that the elements of hostility and contempt toward the suffering person are masked by the feeling of sympathy.[17]

Persistent jealousy, too, is rooted in deep ambivalence. This is not the occasional jealousy that corresponds to the intensity of the love feeling.[18]

One can say that ambivalence is a feeling or subjective state which is a universal characteristic of man. Ambivalence can be experienced as a paralysis of two feelings or as an oscillation between two feelings. It influences other areas of the personality, such as thinking and action. In the adult, ambivalence causes one or both opposing feelings to be relegated to the unconscious.

The development of ambivalence includes the following steps:

1. As the child distinguishes himself from his environment, he sees his mother, the external source of comfort and discomfort, as a separate object.

2. The child realizes that the mother provides both good feelings and bad.

3. The child forms an internal image of both a good and bad mother and a good and bad self.

4. Experiences such as weaning, toilet training, and limitations of activity provide added opportunities for opposing feelings toward parent, people, and situations.

5. Opportunities to feel and express negative and positive feelings toward parents of the same sex arise in the family triangle period.

6. Opportunities for displacement of the negative feelings arise as the child matures and encounters an increasing number of objects.

7. Growth of ego makes opposing feelings intolerable to a child so that he either fuses the opposing feelings or relegates them (usually only the negative feelings) to the unconscious.

8. Behavior such as doubt, indecision, and conflicting feelings or simultaneous opposite attitudes indicate residual ambivalence.

AMBIVALENCE IN ADULTS

According to most writers, all relationships are inherently ambivalent because it is impossible for the needs of two persons always to be confluent. The concept of normalcy, in the sense of the ideal, if present in the mature adult, would make him free of ambivalence in his relationships. However, normalcy, in the sense of the average, implies the recognition that ambivalence persists throughout life to some degree.

The traditional relationship between mother-in-law and son-in-law illustrates that adult relationships are still colored by ambivalence. This relationship is considered to include both affectionate and hostile impulses. Another common idea is that women and girls tend to be more ambivalent than men and boys. Helene Deutsch holds that ambivalence in the adolescent girl acts as a positive force for maturation in that the girl's hateful feelings help free her from the mother.[19]

In one research study on ambivalence, the investigators tried to measure ambivalence and discover predictable factors that influence fusion of opposing feelings. The criteria for ambivalence were indecision, doubt, conflicting feelings, or simultaneous opposite attitudes. The sample was composed of psychiatric patients. Results of this study suggested that the group that rated high in ambivalence came from smaller families, had fewer older siblings, and fewer opportunities for warm, long lasting relationships than did the group rated low in ambivalence.[20] So far as is known, this type of study has not been extended to a general population.

The lack of research on ambivalence probably indicates that the important characteristics and consequences of ambivalence are conceptualized under a different framework. Such important theorists as Horney, Sullivan, and Fromm do not even mention ambivalence. Perhaps they conceptualize it in other ways.

How the adult deals with ambivalence is discussed by Tarachow in detail. He uses ambivalence to mean two opposites which have not been fused. For example, when aggression is not modified by love, the aggression is left unresolved in the unconscious. It is the ego, then, that must contain the aggression. Tarachow points out that we all need periodic relief from the burdens of ego functions, especially synthesis and fusion of ambivalent tendencies. Comedy, art, and other creative acts help adults to re-experience the paradoxes of childishness and rebellion alongside maturity. In Tarachow's view, ambivalence is a state of the instincts, ambiguity is a state of the ego, and comedy is the adaptive process by which we deal with these.

Wit and comedy are special technics that enable one to express both sides of ambivalence at the same time. The very popularity of the comedian rests on the fact that we harbor immaturities and ambivalence. The comedian rescues our ambivalence by letting us enjoy a momentary revival of our repressed feelings. Laughter occurs when the aggressive side of the situation has been made tolerable. The healthy person can release his aggression through a joke. Tarachow believes the normal adult, the educated adult, and the repressed adult all have made four sacrifices in common: ambiguity, ambivalence, inconsistency, and fun.[21]

Tarachow quotes another author to make the point that neither the completely cruel man nor the completely moral man can laugh, but the ambivalent man can.[22]

Art, Tarachow says, is a more mature resolution of ambivalence than comedy. For example, the Mona Lisa has continuous appeal because it strikes deep chords of ambivalent and ambiguous responses, whereas posters are clear and concise. Posters restrict. They exhort us to be adult. They direct us not to litter or set fires, but their appeal is short-lived because the other side of the ambivalence soon demands expression.[23]

There are many common examples of adults dealing with ambivalence. The drug addict refers to his drug as "crap" and says he is "clean" when he is not taking drugs. The poster of a beautiful model is soon altered by the addition of sideburns and a moustache. Women suspect at times that fashion designers bear subtle and hidden anger against them because fashions occasionally seem almost ugly.

Many persons speculate that ambivalence affects society as a whole. There is some agreement that irrational thinking and emotional responses develop most frequently in regard to political figures. The source of such disturbed thinking in an adult can be found in the way the child originally coped with ambivalence. Splitting an object into a fantastically good and a fantastically bad person leads, in religion, to the concept of God and the devil. Splitting the object into good and bad, in less extreme forms, results in an exaggerated notion of the good qualities of one's own party, class or group in contrast to the exaggerated bad qualities of the other.

The more mature person can perceive both the good and bad aspects of his religion, political party, or social group. As this critical ability is thought to increase with learning, extreme ambivalence probably decreases in the more educated societies.

NURSING IMPLICATIONS

The literature yields very little information about nursing intervention based on the concept of ambivalence. However, some ideas presented in this paper seem pertinent to the understanding of the importance of ambivalence in nursing situations. It is helpful if nurses can anticipate and identify circumstances in which children and adults may become ambivalent.

Children naturally feel two ways about parents, teachers, nurses, and others who have authority over them. The following example shows how a nurse helped one parent recognize and cope with her child's ambivalence.

> The mother told the nurse that she was worried about Rita, who had just entered first grade, because Rita had come home from school saying, "I hate my teacher. I won't go back." Wanting Rita to make a good start, the mother asked the nurse if she should go to school and iron things out.
> The nurse replied, "Kids do that, don't they. One minute they love you, the next minute they don't. They get mixed up in their feelings just like we do. Allowing Rita to voice her strong feelings was a good way to handle the situation. I think you have already taken care of it."

Children need opportunities to voice both their negative and positive feelings. Adults can assist them with this if they are able to acknowledge their own feelings comfortably. The following calm, uncritical statements to children about their ambivalent feelings are supportive because they convey that even mixed-up feelings are understandable.

> You have two thoughts on the subject—you would like to go to school, but you also want to stay home.
> You seem to have two feelings about your brother—you love him, but you also resent him.
> You seem to feel mixed up—you love your mother, but you're angry because she's left you in the hospital.[24]

Compare these nonjudgmental reflections of ambivalence with the following situation:

During her psychiatric nursing experience, a student reviewed a list of patients with a staff nurse in order to select one patient to work with more closely. After much hesitation by the student and considerable discussion of the pros and cons, the staff nurse said, "Boy, are you confused! One minute you are willing to work with a patient, the next you're not. Make up your mind for once!"

The adult may feel quite ambivalent without allowing this feeling to block appropriate action. The nurse should anticipate such a response in many situations—when a family faces the need to institutionalize a retarded child, when a young mother faces assumption of the complete care of her premature infant, when a family is trying to decide whether grandparents should be placed in a nursing home, when a man is confronted with the possibility that his cancer may be controlled if he has an ileostomy, or when a woman has to decide whether to have an abortion.

Adults, too, need to express both sides of their feelings. At times, the adult may be unable to figure out why he feels so mixed up. Sometimes, just the verbalization of opposing feelings can enable a person to find a more mature approach to a difficult problem.

It is well known that teasing masks ambivalent feelings, as anyone who has been playfully pinched can testify. Nurses should realize that much seemingly good-natured joking and teasing is a release for ambivalent feelings toward hospitalization, the doctor, and themselves.

It is difficult to be the target of ambivalent feelings, and young nurses find this extremely hard to handle. One student described her experience with an older patient this way:

> Miss Q. always asks for me. She tells the others I can help her best, but when I go to help her she is so critical. Like, just as I am about to do something for her she will ask me for it in an irritable manner. If I offer to help her get up before she requests it, she says I'm trying to make a cripple out of her. If I don't offer, she whines and says, "can't you see I need help." I'm damned if I do and damned if I don't with her. I guess I pity her.

This student was close to recognizing her own ambivalent feelings about the patient. Having been allowed to voice them, she may have been freed to recognize other factors, such as regression, that were operating. Inasmuch as regression is common among hospitalized patients, one can speculate that Miss Q. had regressed so that her mixed feelings about being dependent were now conscious. She could tolerate incongruities in her behavior to a greater degree, and thus she gave many confusing messages to the student, "You're making me a cripple—can't you see I need help?" Ambivalence, some theorists say, is one of the first signs of regression. In the adult, regression permits ambivalence to exist without the conflict it usually generates.[25]

The nurse should understand that indecision and contradictory behavior may indicate ambivalence. When she encourages him to explore the contradictions, the patient may be freer to help himself, as this incident illustrates:

Miss Smith was assigned to Mr. Benton, who was recovering from a myocardial infarct suffered several days previously. Miss Smith was concerned because, although she had carefully gone over the restrictions of complete bedrest, Mr. Benton continued to do more for himself then he should. After she found him getting back into bed a second time, the conversation went like this:

Nurse: You know, I've noticed that this is the second time you've been out of bed and I'm wondering what you make of this.

Patient: Oh, is it? Well, I guess you're right.

N.: It's just that it seems so contradictory, since I overheard you telling your wife you understood you must stay in bed.

P.: I guess it does seem funny . . . even to me.

N.: Not so funny. You must feel both ways at times, like you want to cooperate and yet you can't see the sense in it.

P.: That's right. I don't see how getting up can hurt me.

The nurse went on to explore Mr. Benton's behavior. He was able to talk about his fear and anxiety over his illness, and he began to approach his present condition more realistically.

Frequently, it comforts patients to realize that they don't just hate someone, but also love him, unconsciously. A nurse applied this knowledge in the following situation:

The Green family had been using the visiting nursing service for years. One of Mrs. Green's recurrent themes during almost every visit was her mother's mistreatment of her and anger toward her. Mrs. Green claimed that she hated her mother and gave endless examples of her reasons. After assessing the problem carefully, the nurse started this conversation:

Nurse: Mrs. Green, you've told me your mother moved to Denver after you did, and that when you moved to another part of town she moved into your neighborhood.

Patient: That's true. She did it just to bother me. She's even lived right behind me for months.

N.: It seems strange to me that anybody should go to all that trouble just to pester someone. What do you make of that idea?

P.: Well . . . You just don't know my mother.

N.: I think you're right. I wonder if either of us knows what she feels? She sure keeps in touch with you. I find it hard to believe she doesn't like you. She just might not realize how to show it.

P.: Well—well (less emphatically), she sure doesn't. She never has. She's always treated me this way.

N.: It makes you unsure of how you feel about her?

P.: No! I *am* sure—or pretty sure.

N.: You say you don't like her, but I have noticed we talk about her all the time. I always know when you are worried about her health.

P.: You think I care about her?

N.: Yes, I do.

P.: (cries) Well, I sometimes do.

N.: Mrs. Green, we often can be angry and love someone at the same time, only we usually aren't aware of our anger. With you and your mother, it's the other way around.

P.: I have thought about that. We're just backward and can't show our love. That's what my husband says.

In this situation, bringing the patient's positive feelings into the open seemed to enable her to make a more realistic response.

Occasionally it is best to allow ambivalent behavior to resolve itself. Simple awareness of opposing feelings is enough. The following is a case in point:

> A mother arrived to pick up her son from school, and found him struggling with himself. As she watched, he backed down the steps of a high slide, walked to the front of the slide, and looked up. Presently he remounted the steps only to back down after he had viewed, and probably speculated on, the trip down from his high perch. The mother felt unsure about what to do. She wanted very badly to reassure him, to help in some way, but she did not move or call to him. At this point, the boy climbed the steps with determination, banging each foot down as he made the trip, sat down, hurriedly gave a push, and was off. This was a victory for both parent and child. The mother immediately joined her son and shared his triumph.

So, too, knowing when not to help is as important as knowing when to help. However, the nurse may experience contradictory feelings in helping a patient to face a disability and then to master it.

The following situation is an illustration of this frequent occurrence in nursing:

A 17-year-old girl patient and a school nurse seemed to share the same goal, improving the girl's personal hygiene and grooming. The girl seemed more confident as she attended to her appearance more consistently. The question of diet came up because she was quite overweight. They discussed this and made joint plans. After a few weeks, it was obvious that the girl could not follow through, but she insisted she was interested and asked the nurse to repeat all the diet instructions. The nurse was firm with her but the following week the girl again looked very unkempt. She expressed her dilemma this way. "Oh! I want to lose weight, but I can't, I am just stuck." At this point, the nurse decided to abandon the diet discussion. The nurse recognized that the girl's ambivalence indicated a deep conflict, because she became increasingly anxious as she moved closer to one side of her ambivalence.

What action can the nurse take in such a situation? She can seek consultation, refer the patient, or lead the conversation into other areas which may indirectly bear on the problem and point the way to its resolution.

Another characteristic of the highly ambivalent person is his tendency to separate his ideas of people into sharply delineated pictures of them as good objects or as bad objects. Because of his ambivalence, he shifts from one to the other easily. He becomes hyperalert for indications that the external object is changing from a good person to a bad one. He keeps careful score on the behavior of others and is quite changeable in his response to them.

The public health nurse had visited a Mrs. Hall weekly for over three months. Recently, she had been able to persuade Mrs. Hall to accept medical help. The patient responded well and was full of praise for her nurse. This step taken, Mrs. Hall began to seek help with the problems of her teen-age daughter.

At this point, the nurse was ill and Mrs. Hall was not notified that her weekly visit would be omitted. At the next visit, Mrs. Hall was polite, remote, and stubbornly silent. The nurse spent two or three visits working through this stalemate. In appraising this development, the nurse realized that in the past she had been careful to include Mrs. Hall in planning her care, to arrange Red Cross transportation, to visit punctually, and to return Mrs. Hall's telephone calls promptly. Together the nurse and patient explored what had happened. They concluded that the meticulous planning had meant to the patient that the nurse cared about her and was a "good nurse." Mrs. Hall's reaction to the nurse's one slip, forgetting to call about a postponed visit, revealed how sensitive Mrs. Hall was and how well she kept score.

This experience was used to further the working relationship. Unfortunately, this is frequently not done. Much of the interaction between patient and nurse becomes clouded through unintentional mistakes. This confusion probably accounts for many of our failures in relating to each other.

Ambivalence in Mrs. Hall's case was a persistent characteristic. With some persons, ambivalence is a sporadic response. In such instances, the nurse may intervene, not to deal with the ambivalence itself, but to help the person move in the right direction. For example, most instructors have had a student request an appointment and then change it or fail to appear. When the student finally arrives at the office, she stands literally in the middle of the doorway, one foot in, one foot out, until the instructor asks her, very firmly, to be seated. The instructor does not reflect the student's behavior back to her, but adds weight to one side of the ambivalence by her direct manner. Often this technic is all that is needed to help another person choose the action he wants to take.

These illustrations pertain to a few nursing situations. Readers can apply much of the knowledge about ambivalence to many other areas of nursing.

To practice nursing therapeutically, one must always remember that "a sophisticated view of human reality takes account of the possibility that where there is love, there is also some hate; where there is admiration, there is also envy; where there is devotion, there is also hostility; where there is success, there is also apprehension . . . (and) that all feelings are legitimate: the positive, the negative, and the ambivalent."[26]

REFERENCES

1. Bleuler, E.: Dementia Precox; The Group of Schizophrenias. Trans. by Joseph Zinkin. pp. 53-55. New York, International Universities Press, 1966.
2. Symonds, P.: The Dynamics of Human Adjustment. p. 93. New York, Appleton-Century-Crofts, 1946.
3. Hinsie, L. E., and Campbell, R.: Psychiatric Dictionary. ed. 3. pp. 30-31. New York, Oxford University Press, 1960.
4. Webster's Seventh New Collegiate Dictionary. p. 28. Springfield, Mass., G. & C. Merriam, 1963.
5. Grauber, D., and Miller, J.: On ambivalence. Psychiat. Quart., *31*:458-464, 1957.
6. Redlich, F. C., and Freedman, D. L.: The Theory and Practice of Psychiatry. p. 816. New York, Basic Books, 1966.
7. Jaspers, K.: General Psychopathology. p. 342. Chicago, University of Chicago Press, English Translation, 1963.
8. Tarachow, S., Freedman, S., and Korin, H.: Studies in ambivalence. J. Hillside Hosp., 7:67-97, 1958.
9. *Ibid.*, p. 69.
10. Novey, S.: A clinical view of affect theory in psycho-analysis. Int. J. Psychoanal., *40*:95, 1959.
11. Rapaport, D.: On the psychoanalytic theory of affects. Int. J. Psychoanal., *34*:178, 1953.
12. Fenichel, O.: The Psychoanalytic Theory of Neurosis. p. 64. New York, W. W. Norton & Co., 1945.
13. Engle, G.: Psychological Development in Health and Disease. pp. 54, 123. Philadelphia, W. B. Saunders, 1962.
14. Tarachow, S.: Ambiguities and human imperfections. J. Am. Psychoanal. Ass., *13*:90, 1965.
15. Engle, *op. cit.*, p. 134.
16. Bateson, G., Jackson, D., Haley, J., and Weakland, J.: Toward a theory of schizophrenia. Behav. Sci., *1*:27-32, 1956.
17. Engle, *op. cit.*, p. 185.
18. Fenichel, *op. cit.*, p. 512.
19. Deutsch, H.: Neuroses and Character Types; Clinical Psychoanalytic Studies. p. 142. New York, International Universities Press, 1965.
20. Tarachow, S.: Studies in ambivalence, *op. cit.*, pp. 67-97.

21. Tarachow, Ambiguities and human imperfection, *op. cit.*, pp. 85-101.
22. *Ibid.*, p. 93.
23. *Ibid.*, pp. 95-98.
24. Ginott, H.: Between Parent and Child. p. 33. New York, Macmillan, 1965.
25. Graubert and Miller, *op. cit.*, p. 463.
26. Ginott, *op. cit.*, p. 34.

BIBLIOGRAPHY

Balint, M.: Problems of Human Pleasure and Behavior. New York, Liverright, 1957.
Bateson, G., Jackson, D. C., Haley, J., and Weakland, J.: Toward a theory of schizophrenia. Behav. Sci., *1*:27-32, 1956.
Bergler, E.: Three tributaries to the development of ambivalence. Psychoanal. Quart., *17*:143-151, 1948.
Bleuler, E.: Dementia Precox; The Group of Schizophrenias. Trans. by Joseph Zinkin. New York, International Universities Press, 1950.
Deutsch, H.: Neuroses and Character Types; Clinical Psychoanalytic Studies. New York, International Universities Press, 1965.
____ : The Psychology of Women; A Psychoanalytic Interpretation. New York, Grune & Stratton, 1944.
Engle, G.: Psychological Development in Health and Disease. Philadelphia, W. B. Saunders, 1962.
Fairbain, W. R.: An Object-Relations Theory of the Personality. New York, Basic Books, 1952.
Farber, L.: The Ways of the Will. New York, Basic Books, 1966.
Fenichel, O.: The Psychoanalytic Theory of Neuroses. New York, W. W. Norton & Co., 1945.
Freud, S.: Totem and Taboo. New York, W. W. Norton & Co., 1952. 1952.
Ginott, H. G.: Between Parent and Child. New York, Macmillan, 1965.
Gould, J., and Kolb, W. L.: A Dictionary of the Social Sciences. New York, The Free Press, 1964.
Graubert, D. N., and Miller, J.: On ambivalence. Psychiat. Quart., *31*:458-464, 1957.
Hinsie, L. E., and Campbell, R. J.: Psychiatry Dictionary. New York, Oxford University Press, 1960.
Jaspers, K. I.: General Psychopathology. Chicago, University of Chicago Press, English Translation, 1963.
Jourard, S.: Personal Adjustment; An Approach Through the Study of Healthy Personality. New York, Macmillan, 1958.
Menninger, K.: Love Against Hate. New York, Harcourt, Brace & World, 1942.

Munroe, R. L.: Schools of Psychoanalytic Thought. New York, Dryden Press, 1955.
Novey, S.: A clinical view of affect theory in psycho-analysis. Int. J. Psycoanal., *40*:94-104, 1959.
Rapaport, D.: On the psychoanalytic theory of affects. Int. J. Psychoanal., *34*:177-198, 1953.
Redlich, F. C., and Freedman, D. L.: The Theory and Practice of Psychiatry. New York, Basic Books, 1966.
Symonds, P.: Dynamics of Psychotherapy. New York, Grune & Stratton, 1957.
——: The Dynamics of Human Adjustment. New York, Appleton-Century-Crofts, 1946.
——: The Ego and the Self. New York, Appleton-Century-Crofts, 1951.
Tarachow, S.: Ambiguities and human imperfections. J. Am. Psychoanal. Ass., *13*:85-101, 1965.
Tarachow, S., Freedman, S., and Korin, H.: Studies in ambivalence. J. Hillside Hosp., *7*:67-97, 1958.
Webster's Seventh New Collegiate Dictionary. Springfield, Mass., G. & C. Merriam, 1963.

12

Transactional Analysis and Nursing

Silvia Lange

Communication and interpersonal relations are two vital concomitants of the nursing process. The basic nursing unit consists of two persons, the patient and the nurse; in this interpersonal relationship the two individuals bring their past experiences and expectations to the present situation and attempt to find ways to express, understand, and act on them.

As nursing has accepted the responsibility of giving comprehensive care, the profession is faced with the problem of understanding human behavior and using this understanding for therapeutic results. Sanford stated:

> If medical care is to be truly comprehensive, and truly humane, there cannot be treatment of mere cases or mere symptoms. There must be treatment of people—whole people, complicated people, weak and strong and courageous and frightened and cantankerously individual and mousily conformist people.... It is the nurse who must carry the therapeutic light in this very human side of medical care. It is the human skills—skills based on both knowledge and on personal attributes—which give the nurse a highly unique therapeutic function, the true significance of which has very probably not yet been fully appreciated.[1]

The body of knowledge about human behavior has expanded explosively in this century. Many schools of nursing have utilized concepts from psychiatry, psychology, sociology, and anthropology toward better understanding of patients, colleagues, and the nursing situation. Writings of men such as Freud, Sullivan, Erikson, Rogers, Maslow, Reusch, and Skinner have presented theories and findings in the areas of psychodynamics, psychopathology, communication, and behavioral change, all of which have become increasingly useful in nursing.

In the 1950's Eric Berne introduced a theoretical framework and a treatment approach called transactional analysis.[2] Transactional analysis is a study of the communication process—the ongoing exchanges (transactions), verbal and nonverbal, between people. This particular approach gained acceptance among professional psychotherapists who received training in transactional analysis seminars. It has been found that transactional analysis is applicable in settings other than traditional mental health services. Workers in probation, education, marital counseling, prisons, welfare agencies, medicine, and nursing have applied its concepts.

The tremendous popular success of Berne's book, "Games People Play," verified the interest of the general public in understanding more about human behavior.[3] In this book the basic concepts of transactional analysis are expressed in terms that are easily understood; the jargon is deceptively simple at times.

The purpose of this paper is to relate transactional analysis to nursing, in order to understand better the communication network in nursing situations. Transactional analysis provides the nurse with conceptual guidelines to plan and carry out more effective intervention. The following concepts of Berne, which have significance for nursing, will be discussed: recognition hunger, time structure, ego states, transactional analysis proper, and script.

RECOGNITION HUNGER

Recognition hunger refers to the need for attention and acknowledgment from other people—a response Berne calls "stroking." Recognition hunger develops from an earlier, primitive need for sensory stimulation. The infant's need for stimulation is generally met by holding, feeding, caressing, jiggling, patting, and diapering. In order for a child to develop properly, physically and emotionally, he needs this contact. As he gradually develops the capacity to use action and verbal language, he shifts from his sensory needs to recognition needs. To tell a six-month-old baby that you love him, you must hold and pet him. You can blow a kiss to a two-year-old. With an adult, you can sit across the room and signal with your eyes, or you can write in a letter your feelings of love and compassion.

Stroking can be as casual as greeting someone on the street. But think how disconcerting it is if your greeting is ignored! Stroking can also be a tangible thing, such as a paycheck or a raise in position.

(Criticism, punishment, and notoriety are also forms of strokes because at least one is being noticed and reacted to.)

Along with the need for recognition, there remains a need for continual sensory input to maintain psychosocial equilibrium. Controlled experiments in sensory deprivation confirm this as well as the anxiety, discomfort, and distorted perceptions of reality which have been experienced by patients in isolation, extensive body casts, and respirators.

People vary in their need for "strokes." Some people need a great many to keep going; others get along with very few. Illness generally disrupts the usual means of obtaining recognition and gratification. Anxiety, preoccupation with the body, and egocentricity increase the need for strokes. The "demanding" patient is generally signaling in desperate ways that he *needs* attention. If the nurse anticipates the requests of such a patient and spends time with him rather than ignoring or grudgingly answering his light, the frequency and extent of his demands will generally decrease.

Physical care, given in the form of a bedbath or a backrub, may provide a sense of being cared for, because it revives earlier relationships with the pleasure of being physically stroked. Spending time with a person is also a form of stroking. A patient who has definite ideas in regard to the person who gives him nursing care—a registered nurse, a nursing student, or an aide—may be expressing his need for selective stroking. If the team leader takes the time to establish her concern for the well-being of the patient, she will be better able to interpret the nursing team concept to him.

Recognition hunger is related to learning theory. Basically, what is learned is that which is reinforced by strokes. To the growing child, any reaction at all from the parents is better than indifference. If he is not able to receive recognition of positive behavior, he will get attention by undesirable means—temper tantrums, failing in school, or getting sick. Patterns of achieving recognition through positive or negative behavior become part of each person's personality. More subtle in adult patients, these patterns are easily observable on pediatric wards. Children use all sorts of behavior to cope with the fears and threats of illness and separation from parents. Difficulties over eating, sleeping, medication, and general behavior may be unwittingly reinforced by the nursing staff if they stroke the children through attention for negative behavior.

The nurse must evaluate her own needs for recognition and stroking. To whom does she look for her major sources of satisfaction, appreciation, and gratification? Sometimes, staff members become unhappy and disgruntled because a patient seems unappreciative—"You can't do anything to please her," "She never says thanks," and "He won't *let* you help him." When feelings like these predominate, the staff generally begins to withdraw from the unrewarding, puzzling patient, who is left with his own pattern (often lifelong) of unsatisfactory interpersonal relations. Periodic evaluation and supervision can meet the nurse's need for recognition, as will acknowledgment of her worth by the medical staff.

TIME STRUCTURE

Time structure refers to ways in which time can be spent. According to Berne, there are six possible ways, each with a special meaning assigned it: withdrawal, rituals, activities, pastimes, games, and intimacy. To a large extent, the way one gains recognition depends on how he structures his time.

When a person becomes ill and shifts into another setting, such as the hospital, his usual patterns of time structure shift. Hospital routines that structure time for the whole unit may interfere markedly with an individual's choice. The nurse, after identifying the particular ways in which a patient is structuring his time, can help him to find more effective and satisfying means if this is indicated.

1. *Withdrawal* Withdrawal refers to solitary behavior, with or without the presence of other people. A person may withdraw into preoccupation or fantasy, ignoring others. In withdrawal, a person retreats to privacy, isolation, or sleep. He may be actively involved in doing something by himself, but more often he turns his energies and interests inward. This is a common experience for patients who are too physically ill to structure their time any other way. As they fantasize about their physical condition, impending surgery, or an uncertain future, they may become increasingly anxious and depressed.

People who use alcohol and drugs to excess may be using these means to withdraw from painful reality and uncomfortable relationships with other people. Some mental illnesses, particularly certain types of schizophrenic and depressive reactions, are characterized by profound withdrawal, to the point of muteness and stupor.

A certain amount of withdrawal accompanies physical malfunction and is useful in allowing the patient to regress, to let others care for him, and to facilitate rest and recovery. If a person is not able to withdraw into sleep, he becomes progressively disorganized and distressed. When withdrawal extends beyond the helpful state, the nurse can help the patient to shift into one of the five remaining ways to structure time. Withdrawal cuts one off from other people; recognition is therefore denied.

2. *Rituals* A ritual is a socially programmed, stereotyped, predictable exchange of transactions. It is routine, relatively automatic, and safe. A ritual serves a purpose, in that it decreases continual decision-making in situations that occur frequently. There is little commitment to the other person involved, but there is some pleasure derived from the feeling of being in step. The greeting ritual—"Hi." ... "Hi. How are you?" ... "Fine. How are you?" ... "Fine ... well, goodbye." ... "Goodbye."—acknowledges the presence of each party. Manners, social events, holidays, many religious events, and customs are rituals.

Rituals can be useful, but they can also interfere with the most effective way of doing things unless they are continually evaluated. All institutions have routines to accomplish frequently performed tasks. The purpose of the procedure book is to standardize routines for greater efficiency. Nurses must remain flexible and cognizant of the need to alter routines and rituals in line with patients' needs. Such things as taking TPR's, passing bedpans, and the morning bath should take into consideration the patient for whom the ritual is being done.

Most patients, like most people, have developed their personal rituals. A patient may be described as showing obsessive-compulsive behavior because he insists on having his bedstand in a certain order, or on having his morning care done in a particular way. Deviation from his ritualistic ways results in more anxiety. With this person, it is generally helpful if one allows him to control his environment as much as possible, by giving him the opportunity to direct his own care when able.

The human tendency to establish rituals may be utilized in helping patients learn to give their own treatments, such as insulin or colostomy care. A person who is so disorganized that he has no routines or rituals, such as a getting-up-in-the-morning ritual, needs to be helped to establish this means of structuring time. Certain routines of the hospital should be explained to the patient so that he knows what to expect next, and is therefore less anxious.

3. *Activities* Activities, in Berne's meaning of the term, are generally synonymous with work and productivity, whether at a job, at home, or in hobbies and recreation. An activity has to do with external reality and can be recognized by a completed project, a paycheck, a tangible accomplishment. Activities usually result in important satisfaction of interpersonal, as well as financial, needs, with consequent feelings of accomplishment, self-worth, respectability, and mastery. However, activities can be a way of structuring time which may help to avoid association with others. An example is the businessman who works late and brings his paperwork home to avoid intimacy with his family.

Illness interferes with a person's ability to work and may necessitate major changes in his usual patterns of being productive. Even when such changes have to be made, a person may feel anxious, useless, and insignificant because he is not working. A mother may feel guilty over temporarily abandoning her family chores. For some patients, it is more helpful to allow them to maintain some of their job and family responsibilities even when quite ill, so that they can reduce anxiety. It is also helpful to convey to many patients the idea that the process of getting well is their major activity at this time.

4. *Pastimes* The term pastimes here refers to the matrix of superficial, social exchange—to the socializing behavior, verbal and nonverbal, that conveys the message to people that they are recognized and reacted to. Pastimes can take the form of social conversation or chitchat, recreation, and entertainment. The expression "killing time" fits into this category, and the cocktail party is an arena for pastiming. Pastiming may be a way to get through the day, to get to know others better in a nonthreatening, noncommittal way, and "on a larger scale, until bed-time, until vacation-time, until school starts, until the cure is forthcoming, until some form of charisma, rescue, or death arrives."[4]

After the crisis of acute illness is over, the patient is left with a great deal of time to be passed. Nurses are challenged to provide a therapeutic environment in which this can be done most effectively and satisfactorily. Encouragement of patients to socialize, provision of an environment in which recreation can take place, and referral of patients to occupational therapy are often appropriate.

Generally, the conversation that a nurse has with a patient should be more than social chitchat, unless she has decided that it is helpful to the patient to develop more skill in pastiming. When a nurse pastimes a great deal in her exchanges with a patient, it is generally because she is uncomfortable, unaware, or unable to talk with the patient about his concerns and needs. Like withdrawal, rituals, and activities, pastimes may help to keep people apart.

5. *Games* The concept of games is a cornerstone of transactional analysis. Berne defined a game as:

> .... an ongoing series of complimentary ulterior transactions progressing to a well-defined, predictable outcome.... a recurring set of transactions, often repetitious, superficially plausible, with a concealed motivation; or, more colloquially, a series of moves with a snare, or "gimmick."[5]

Because many people are afraid of intimacy, and because the other means of structuring time are not satisfying enough, they settle for games—interpersonal games. Although games may bring compromise, misery, disappointment, or ultimate disaster, they do provide some human relatedness.

Games are a means of getting recognition from others while avoiding intimacy and responsibility. When a person becomes a patient, he brings his characteristic games with him. He may find himself in a treatment situation through such games as Alcoholic, Addict, and Look How Hard I Tried (often part of psychosomatic illness). Other games common in treatment situations are: Ain't It Awful; Gee, You're Wonderful, Doctor; How Do You Get Out of Here?; If It Weren't for Him. These colloquial names suggest the theme of the game; the reader is encouraged to read about them in detail in the book, "Games People Play."[6]

As the nurse becomes more familiar with game theory and the ongoing patterns of the patient and his family, she becomes much more aware of the games he plays, and of the degree of their destructiveness. Proper referral to psychiatric services may be helpful to a person who wants to make changes in his modes of interacting with others. The nurse can also become more aware of the interpersonal games that she plays with patients, co-workers, and the medical staff.[7] Although games serve a useful function, there are more effective and direct ways to communicate. The game of I Was Only Trying to Help is often played in clinical settings, as well as Let's You and Him Fight.

6. *Intimacy* Intimacy is a gamefree exchange of open, honest feelings. It has to do with love, trust, vulnerability. It is made possible in the absence of fear and exploitation. In our culture intimacy is rare and also is frightening. Therefore, people use the other ways of structuring time to ward off the risk and anxiety of being vulnerable.

One of the greatest challenges in nursing is the opportunity to participate in the intimacy of a person's response to life and death. To enter into the moment of open human need by just being there as another human being is an awesome responsibility. The held hand, the concerned smile, the willingness to listen to the hurt, anger, and fear that a patient may be experiencing all comprise moments of treasured intimacy. In addition to participating herself in this intimacy, the nurse should be aware of the patient's need for intimacy with his family. She structures the environment so that privacy is available during visiting hours, and during terminal illness and at the time of death. She should also be aware that patterns of intimacy—emotional and sexual—may be disturbed by illness, a poor prognosis, and treatment procedures, especially surgery. Alert to these possibilities, she is better able to help the patient express his problems and come to a solution.

The nurse can use the concept of time structure to evaluate the present behavior of the patient, to determine whether to encourage him to structure his time differently, and to do pre-discharge planning. She can evaluate her own behavior in terms of the balance among withdrawal, rituals, activities, pastimes, games, and intimacy as she structures her time in her professional and personal life.

EGO STATES

Another concept from transactional analysis that is useful in understanding human behavior is that of structural analysis of the personality. Structural analysis is the identification of the specific ego state in operation (see Fig. 12-1). Ego states refer to the three observable patterns of thinking, feeling, and behaving that are part of everyone's personality. These parts are called the Parent, Adult, and Child and are considered to be present in all people, regardless of chronological age. The Child is present at birth; the Parent begins at birth; the Adult develops in early infancy. In discussing the work of Penfield, Harris concluded that the brain functions as a high-fidelity tape recorder that stores up all the material of which a person is consciously aware.[8] The memory and associated feelings are available for replay at any time, and an ego state is "produced by the playback of recorded data of events in the past, involving real people, real times, real places, real decisions, and real feelings."[9]

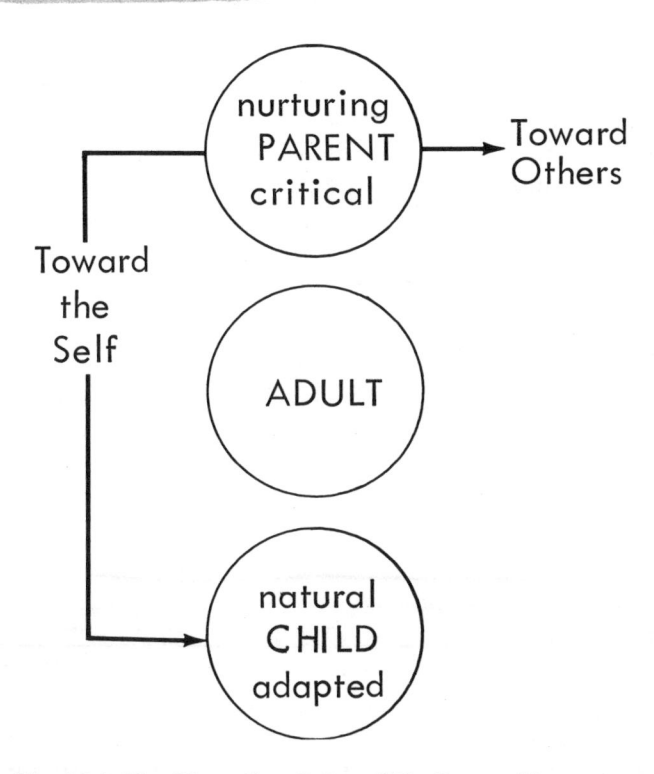

Fig. 12-1. The Three Ego States of the Personality.

Ego states are often rapidly shifted and can be identified by such things as gestures, posture, voice tone, choice of words, and subjective feelings.

The Parent ego state reflects the ideas, feelings, and behavior of one's own parents, particularly as expressed during the first eight years of life. It can be identified when behavior includes the language, intonation, attitudes, posture, and mannerisms of one or both parents.

In the Parent are recorded all the admonitions and rules and laws that the child heard from his parents and saw in their living. They range all the way from the earliest parental communications, interpreted nonverbally through tone of voice, facial expression, cuddling, or noncuddling, to the more elaborate verbal rules and regulations espoused by the parents as the little person became able to understand words. In this set of recordings are the thousands of "no's" directed at the toddler, the repeated "don'ts" that bombarded him, the looks of pain and horror in Mother's face when his clumsiness brought shame on the family in the form of Aunt Ethel's broken antique vase.[10]

The Parent ego state is necessary when the time to raise children comes. It also makes many automatic responses concerning ethics, manners, and the way things "should" be done. The Parent ego state refers to both these aspects of the personality—the nurturing, sympathetic, reassuring, caring part, and the critical, opinionated, prejudiced, and judgmental parts. The Parent ego state can be recognized by such words as "should," "ought," "right" and "wrong." The Ten Commandments reflect a cultural Parent, as do many laws of the land.

For many a woman, it is the nurturing part of her Parent that is attracted to nursing—the desire to care for and to be of help to others. In the process of nursing education, the student acquires knowledge and information (in her Adult) to accomplish this purpose on more than a sympathetic, intuitive level—she develops "an educated heart."

The statement that the nurse should not be judgmental means in TA (transactional analysis) terms that she shouldn't let her own critical Parent pass open judgment on how the patient chooses to live his life. Even if her own background, morals, and religious beliefs are much different from those of the patient, she can respect his individuality and dignity.

The critical aspects of the Parent also can be directed toward oneself. When a person condemns himself as being inadequate, or a failure, or a coward, it is in response to earlier recordings from his parent. This is a common experience among people who are depressed. A competent nurse who is continually dissatisfied with her performance despite reassurance from others may be demonstrating this part of the Parent ego state.

Clues to the Parent include pursed lips, the pointing index finger (as in accusations), hands on hips, tongue clucking, and patting on the head. Most evaluative words are Parent—stupid, lazy, good-for-nothing, ridiculous, good, bad, shocking, cute, poor dear, and sonny.[11]

The Adult ego state also refers to that part of the personality which is the computer and data processer. It deals with facts and verifiable information. The Adult begins to develop at roughly 10 months of age; about this time the infant begins to find out for himself what the world is all about, as he explores and tests. He separates himself from his mother and tries out cause and effect.

The Adult ego state operates on what works, what is most efficient, and what will solve the problem. An important function of the Adult is to make decisions based on the computation of information from the Parent, the Child, and previous data in the Adult. It examines data from the Parent to decide if it is still applicable today. It examines data from the Child to determine if feelings and actions are appropriate to the present or are left over from the past.

The key vocabulary of the Adult is who, what, when, where, why, and how. Fact words, such as how much, possible, probable, and objective, indicate that the Adult is in gear. Physical clues to Adult include an attitude of listening straightforwardly.

When people become physically and emotionally ill, they often retreat from the use of their Adult ego state and surrender decision-making and problem-solving to the medical and nursing staff, and to their families. For a period of time this may be helpful and vital to recovery, but the goal for successful treatment is for the person to resume executive control over his life. When a person is extremely anxious, his Adult is generally decommissioned. Information about treatments, surgery, or routines can be misinterpreted. In denial of illness, the person will not allow his Adult to process the data accurately.

The Child ego state is that part of the personality which is a carryover from chronological childhood. These recordings represent the way the child saw, heard, felt, and understood in the world around him. Powerful emotions reside in the Child, and these can be in reaction to past reality or to present situations. Many times a person finds himself feeling and reacting as he did when he was a child, with frustration, rejection, despair, and rage. Within the Child are also the qualities of creativity, excitement, sensual and sexual enjoyment, curiosity, and spontaneity. This is the zest of a person, and is called the natural Child.

There is another part of the Child ego state—the adapted Child. This is the manner in which the child learned to get along with his parents. Adaptation (or adjustment) includes lifelong patterns of withdrawal, anger, and fear; getting sick; or being overly submissive, helpless, or whining. When people become sick, it is common knowledge that they function with their adapted Child ego state. Other people either go along with or reject this behavior.

Clues to Child ego states include many nonverbal expressions—tears, pouting, quivering lip, high-pitched whining tones, teasing, giggling, coyness, boisterousness, temper tantrums, and blushing. "I can't" and "I won't" are clues to the Child, along with "I dunno," "I guess" (or hope and wish). Behavior that is labeled "acting out"—delinquency, alcoholism, drug addiction, violence, and deviant sexual behavior—comes from the adapted Child.

Structural analysis, the identification of ego states, provides a useful framework for viewing behavior in the nursing setting. Under the stress of illness, the behavior of the patient and his family often indicates that the executive control has shifted from the Adult ego state to either the Parent or the Child ego state. A certain amount of regression is common in all illnesses and may precipitate the need for more nurturing. The Child ego state is more clearly seen. Many times the patient is quite aware of this shift, and because of his own critical Parent ego state, he stands in judgment of himself. He may apologize profusely for "being a baby." This is often seen in men who cry out in pain or despair and then are deeply ashamed of their lack of control.

Patients often relate to staff as if the latter were parents or similar authority figures. This is related to early parenting, cultural expectations, similarity of present hospitalization and treatments to childhood experiences, and the behavior of some doctors and nurses. The term "mother surrogate" has been used to describe the specific nurturing activities that nurses perform. Feeding, bathing, soothing, reassuring, protecting, and encouraging are all nurturing Parent actions. Modern concepts of nursing include the expectation that the patient is a partner in his care—that he will use his Adult in exercising responsibility and decisions regarding his life and care.

The nurse uses her Adult ego state to determine the patient's needs. She decides whether he needs her to nurture him or whether she should refrain from direct help. She can view with objectivity behavior that represents the Child ego state—demandingness, flirtatiousness, withdrawal, hypochondriasis, and manipulation—and try to understand how this meets the needs of the patient at this present time. She refrains from labeling this behavior as child*ish* or immature. Working from this basis, she can help the patient to develop more satisfying and more satisfactory ways of achieving recognition.

TRANSACTIONAL ANALYSIS PROPER

In addition to this whole system being labeled as transactional analysis, one particular aspect of it is known as transactional analysis proper. This refers to the analysis of a single transaction by use of the transactional diagram. It refers to the identification of the ego states in the two or more individuals involved in terms of the stimulus by one person and the response by the other. The response becomes the stimulus for another set of transactions.

When the stimulus and response on the diagram make parallel lines, the transaction is considered to be complementary and can go on indefinitely. These transactions can be Parent-Parent, Adult-Adult, Child-Child, Parent-Child, Child-Parent, etc.

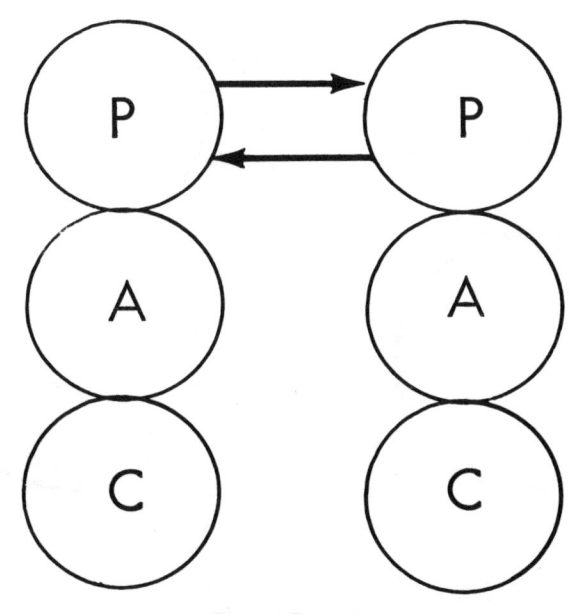

Parent-Parent

Stimulus: The cost for hospitalization is outrageous these days!
Response: And you don't get the good old bedside nurse, either!
Stimulus: Doctor, I told her it was for her own good, but she wouldn't listen to reason and take the medicine.
Response: I'll give her a good talking to.

Fig. 12-2. Parent-Parent transaction.

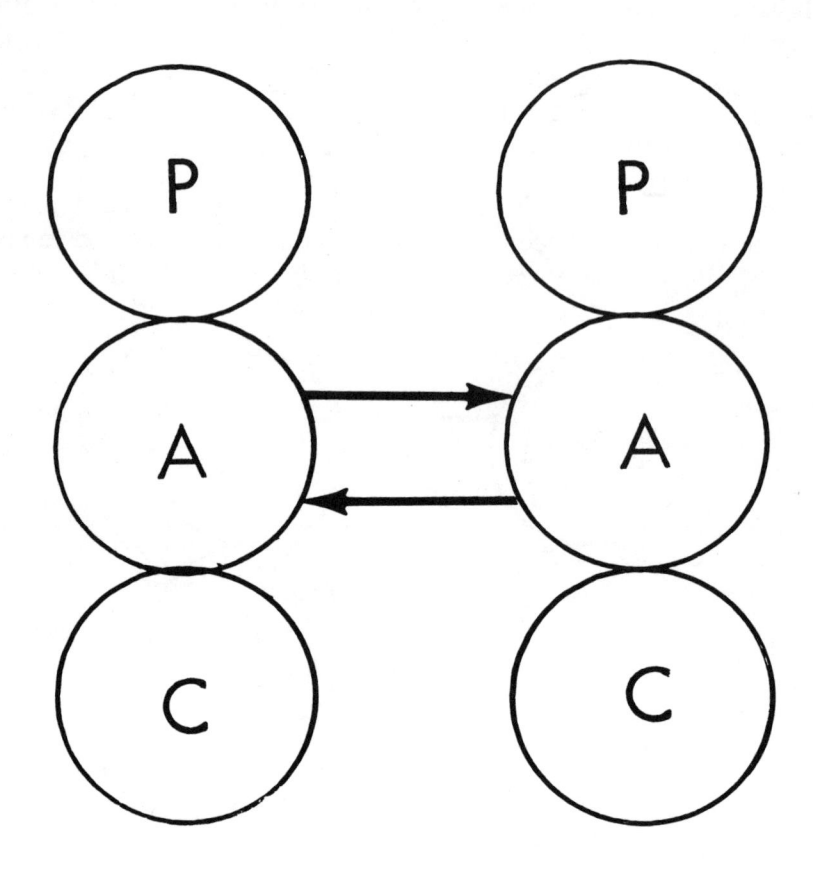

Adult-Adult

Stimulus: What time am I scheduled for surgery?
Response: 8:30 am. Do you have any other questions about it?
Stimulus: I'm not able to sleep.
Response: What seems to be keeping you awake?

Fig. 12-3. Adult-Adult transaction.

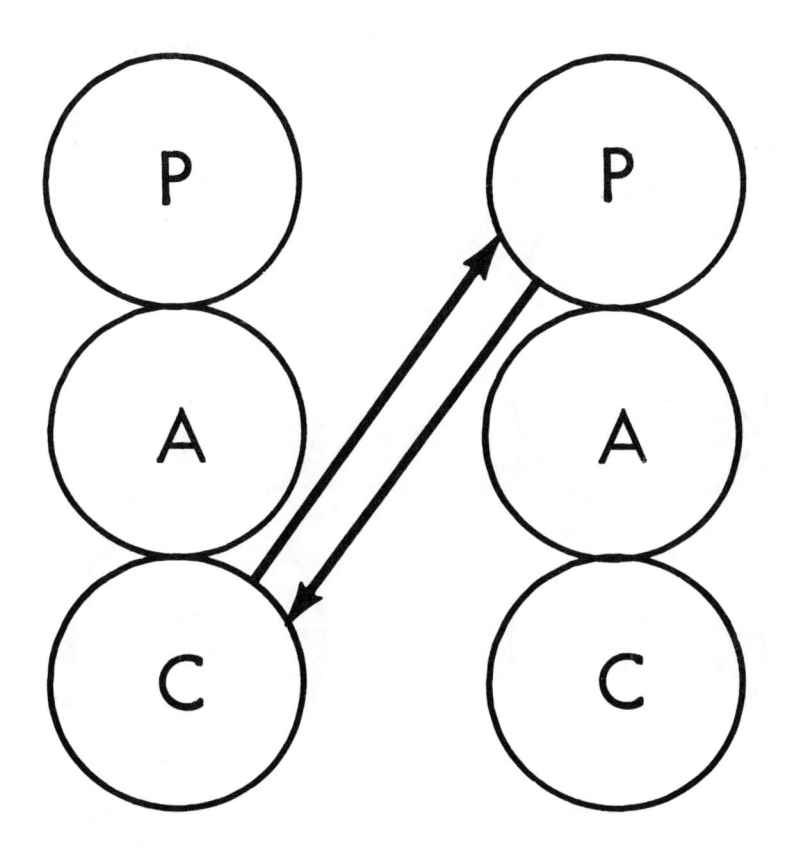

Child-Parent

Stimulus: Nurse, please help me. It hurst so much.
Response: Hold on. I'll get your medication.

Fig. 12-4. Child-Parent transaction.

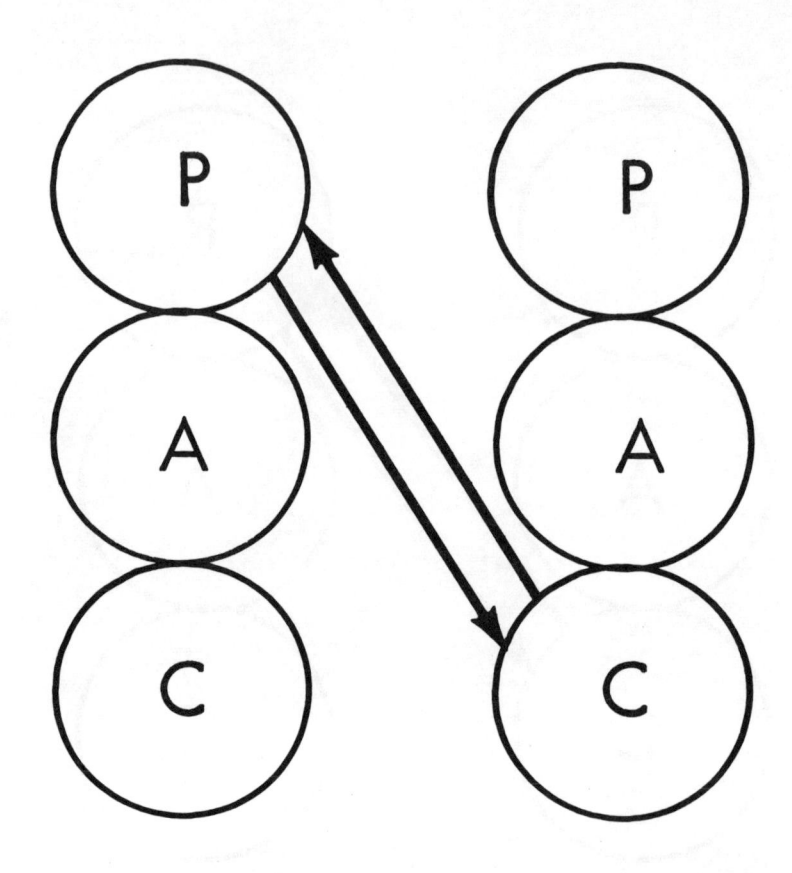

Parent-Child

Stimulus: What are you doing up? You know you're supposed to be on bedrest!
Response: You're always picking on me!

Fig. 12-5. Parent-Child transaction.

In the above examples, the communication could go on indefinitely as long as the ego states do not shift. Communication shifts or stops when the transactional lines cross. This occurs when the stimulus is directed toward one specific ego state but the response originates in another. At this point the communication shifts from the specific subject to the relationship of the two people involved.

Nurse   Patient

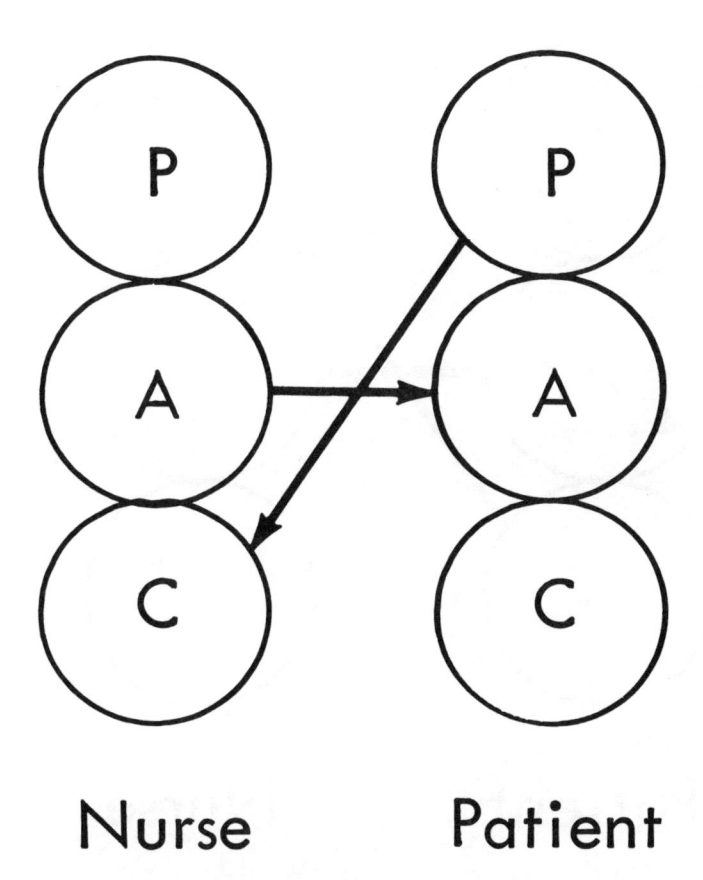

Crossed Transaction

Stimulus: I can help you with your morning care now.
Response: It's about time.

Fig. 12-6. Crossed transaction: Nurse gives information with her Adult, and Patient responds with criticism from Parent.

Now the situation shifts from one in which a bath will be given to one in which the nurse has to defend her time schedule and the patient expresses his feelings of neglect.

Patient ## Nurse

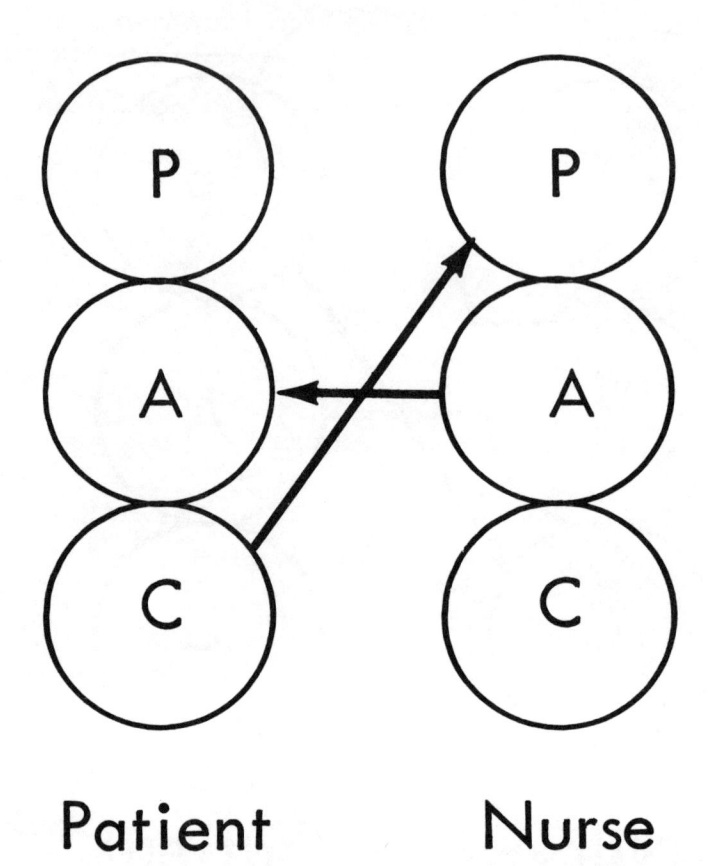

Crossed Transaction

Stimulus: I'm signing out of this hospital and you can't stop me!
Response: I'd like to know what is upsetting you.

Fig. 12-7. Crossed transaction: Patient addresses his angry, rebellious Child to the Nurse's Parent. She replies with information-seeking Adult.

The patient can no longer be the rebellious, angry Child as the nurse has responded with her Adult to problem-solve.

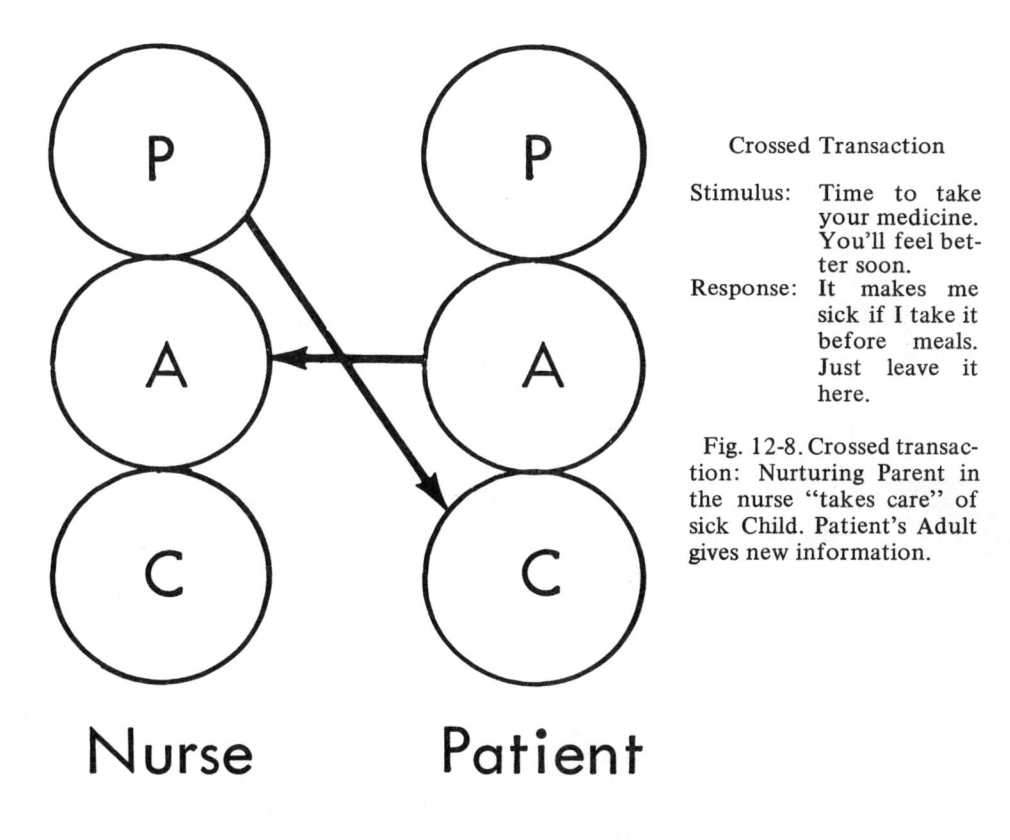

Transactional Analysis Proper 245

Crossed Transaction

Stimulus: Time to take your medicine. You'll feel better soon.
Response: It makes me sick if I take it before meals. Just leave it here.

Fig. 12-8. Crossed transaction: Nurturing Parent in the nurse "takes care" of sick Child. Patient's Adult gives new information.

Nurse   **Patient**

Now they must dicker about the hospital policy concerning leaving medicine at the bedside. The nurse should try to identify the clash in ego states when communication breaks down.

A general guideline for the nurse is this: she should use Adult to evaluate the needs of the patient and the reality of the nursing situation, recognize her own Parent and Child, decide when expressions of these are appropriate, and make deliberate nursing actions based on as much information as she can get.

Harris summarized that a strong Adult is built in the following ways:

    1. Learn to recognize your Child, its vulnerabilities, its fears, its principal methods of expressing these feelings.

    2. Learn to recognize your Parent, its admonitions, injunctions, fixed positions, and principal ways of expressing these admonitions, injunctions, and positions.

3. Be sensitive to the Child in others, talk to that Child, stroke that child, protect that Child, and appreciate its need for creative expression as well as the NOT OK burden it carries about.

4. Count to ten, if necessary, in order to give the Adult time to process the data coming into the computer, to sort out Parent and Child from reality.

5. When in doubt, leave it out. You can't be attacked for what you didn't say.

6. Work out a system of values. You can't make decisions without an ethical framework.[12]

To increase her level of self-awareness and effectiveness, the nurse may evaluate her own ego states in relation to patients and co-workers.

"I felt so sorry for her when she begged me not to make her deep breathe and cough. But I knew she had to, so I insisted." The nurse used her Adult ego state to overcome her nurturing Parent ego stage in response to the patient's frightened, hurt adapted Child.

When a patient developed a pressure sore and the doctor criticized the nursing care, the head nurse burst into tears. He apologized profusely for upsetting her, but privately decided to send his patients to another floor whenever possible. Later, the nurse recognized her pattern of being over-sensitive to critical Parents and avoiding or lessening criticism by crying in a Child ego state. She used her Adult ego state to determine how the pressure sores came about and to initiate proper treatment. She consciously used her critical Parent to supervise her staff, which had become lax.

A nurse's aide had been continually calling in sick or coming in late to work. The nurse felt very angry and critical toward her because of the burden she placed on the rest of the staff. She felt like losing her temper, but after recognizing this as her critical Parent ego state, which would probably just hook the aide's Child, she sat down for a conference. Instead of continuing her rebellious Child behavior, the aide discussed the problems at home. Together, they talked Adult to Adult and decided on reasonal expectations and limitations.

Mr. Smith is considered by all the staff as a "problem patient." He is uncooperàtive, surly, and resistive to care. He rejects attempts to nurse him and then complains to the supervisor that he is being neglected. At a staff conference, feelings of anger, despair, frustration, indignation, and hopelessness are expressed. That staff, having been hooked by his Child ego state behavior, had responded with either reciprocal Child or critical Parent ego states. They decided to shift to either Adult or nurturing Parent ego states in treating him and discussed specific means of accomplishing this.

Ego states can be consciously altered when a person becomes aware that the way he is reacting and responding to other people is not accomplishing what he wants. In meeting the needs of the patient, the nurse should be aware of her own, as well as the patient's, ego state. She alters her behavior accordingly. This is one of the expectations for the professional nurse and is part of what is meant by the therapeutic use of the self.

SCRIPT

Nurses usually are genuinely interested in the people who become their patients. They may come to know them very well or may have only a fleeting glimpse of understanding. They often wonder what happened to a person before, during, and after an experience of illness and how the parts of the human puzzle fit together.

The concept of "script" is useful in viewing a person's life. In TA terms, a script is a life-plan, generally operating on an unconscious level. Based on decisions made early in life, when not all the information was available or accurate and judgmental powers were unformed, a script limits a person to a narrow path in life, which may be constructive or tragic in outcome. Repetitive patterns suggest script behavior. Life patterns, which include suicide, alcoholism, drug addiction, crime, homicide, mental illness, obesity, and recurrent physical illnesses (especially if they are preventable and treatable), are all parts of tragic scripts.

A 25-year-old woman realized that she was following a tragic script by "eating myself to death." She weighed over three hundred pounds and had recently had a severe coronary. Seeking love and affection, she became pregnant, which necessitated a therapeutic abortion for both physical and psychiatric reasons. She saw her slogan as "Underloved and Overfed."

Nurses may not be able to identify script behavior in patients who spend short periods of time in the hospital. Illness and hospitalization may play significant parts in a person's script. Even the delivery of a normal, healthy baby is full of possibilities in terms of how the family balance will be readjusted with ramifications for all family members. Longer-term patients, such as those seen by the nurse in public health, rehabilitation, and psychiatric settings, generally show definite script patterns. How a person faces death is related to his script.

Script is formed in early childhood and is based on the messages, verbal and nonverbal, that children get from their parents. Viewpoints related to worth, lovableness, sex, work, responsibility, dependency, authority and countless other aspects of everyday life fit into a pattern by which one views oneself and acts accordingly as a winner or a loser in life. Tragic scripts are based on such decisions as "I will never trust anyone," "I can never think for myself," "I'll never amount to anything," "I'm doomed to die young." and "The only way I can get attention is to be sick." One of the problems in meeting the emotional needs of children who are hospitalized for extended periods of time is to try to prevent destructive script decisions. Separation from mother for a very young child may result in the decision, "I will never trust women again." Treatment for very painful conditions such as burns may result in a lifelong pattern with the theme of "People will always hurt you."

Another aspect of script analysis has to do with a person's basic position toward himself and others. "OK" refers to a feeling of worthwhileness, competency, intelligence, attractiveness, and lovability. "Not OK" denotes the feeling of lack of these qualities. The four basic positions are:

1. I'm OK—You're OK
2. I'm not OK—You are OK
3. I'm OK—You're not OK
4. I'm not OK—You're not OK

It is speculated that the infant originally feels "I'm OK—You're OK" as his early needs are met through adequate mothering. If he is fed, snuggled, and kept warm by a relatively anxiety-free mother, he experiences good feelings which result in basic trust. Through adverse, repeated actions in the first few years of life, he may shift to one of the other positions. The optimistic view is that a shift back to the original position can be made through other life experiences.

Harris maintained that all children shift to the I'm Not OK—You Are OK when they realize their relative smallness, powerlessness, and inadequacy as compared with their parents and the world.[13] This position is called the depressive position, in which feelings of inferiority, inadequacy, and worthlessness predominate.

The position I'm OK—You're Not OK is called the paranoid or criminal position, in which the individual distrusts others and is suspicious of their motives and actions. This person's slogan is "Look out for Number One because no one else will."

The fourth position of I'm Not OK—You're Not OK represents an attitude of despair, isolation, and futility. Suicide or a life of hopeless withdrawal may result from this position. A person may shift into this position as the result of a traumatic injury or an illness such as paraplegia or stroke.

One of the applications of this knowledge of script and position is in health counseling with parents. As the nurse talks with families in a variety of health settings, she can share her knowledge of growth and development incorporating the concepts of stroking, script formation, and transmission of parental attitudes.

It is also helpful for the nurse to screen her own responses on the I'm OK—You're OK grid in relation to the patients she cares for. The expression "accepting the patient" refers to seeing him as really OK despite socially stigmatized conditions such as drug addiction, mental illness, alcoholism, abortion, old age, and poverty. A problem in treating the terminally ill or dying patient is that the staff may adopt a Not-OK position toward him and withdraw in defeat and discouragement.

REFERENCES

1. Sanford, F. H.: The behavioral sciences and research in nursing. Nurs. Res., *6*:56, October, 1957.
2. Berne, E.: Ego states in psychotherapy. Am. J. Psychother., *11*:297, April, 1957; Transactional analysis: A new and effective method of group therapy. Am. J. Psychother., *12*:735, October, 1958; Transactional Analysis in Psychotherapy. New York, Grove Press, 1961; Principles of Group Treatment. New York, Oxford University Press, 1966; Transactional Analysis Bulletin, 1-present. International Transactional Association, Carmel, California.
3. Berne, E.: Games People Play: The Psychology of Human Relationships. New York, Grove Press, 1964.
4. Berne, E.: Transactional Analysis in Psychotherapy, p. 98.
5. Berne, E.: Games People Play, p. 48.
6. *Ibid.*
7. Stein, L. I.: The doctor-nurse game. Am. J. Nurs., *68*:101-105, January, 1968.
8. Harris, T. A.: I'm OK–You're OK: A Practical Guide to Transactional Analysis. pp. 4-11. New York, Harper & Row, 1967.
9. *Ibid.,* p. 18.
10. *Ibid.,* p. 20.
11. *Ibid.,* pp. 66-67.
12. *Ibid.,* pp. 95-96.
13. *Ibid.,* p. 37.

13

Privacy

Dorothy Bloch

Uppermost in the mind of the person who is entering a hospital for medical or surgical treatment may well be thoughts regarding his recovery. What a shock it is for him to discover suddenly that in the admission process he is confronted with questions, routines, and actions by others that seem to threaten his very being. Questions ranging from "Do you want a private room?" and "Will your expenses be paid by insurance or welfare?" to "Do you have false teeth?" and "Have you had a bowel movement today?" may be asked of this newly admitted patient within the first hour of his walking into the hospital. For the individual who is not accustomed to sharing this type of information with strangers or even members of his family, these questions may serve to invade his private thoughts, feelings, and behavior.

During the past few years increasing discussion and debate have taken place within our society concerning the concept of privacy. Newspapers, television programs and popular magazines have made the American public aware of the many ways in which one's privacy may be invaded. Familiar examples are the multitude of ingenious devices used to record conversations and the psychological tools and tests used to measure personality traits as a screening maneuver. Although nurses do at times refer to the patient's need for privacy, only occasional mention is found in the nursing literature on the concept of privacy and its application to nursing care. Thus, it appears that there is a growing necessity to explore the concept of privacy and how the patient's need for privacy is supported, encouraged, met or inhibited in the provision of health services and especially nursing.

DEFINITIONS AND CONCEPTS

In order to approach the study of privacy from within an established frame of reference, it is important to establish a definition that can be used as a basis for continuing discussion. Perusal of the literature to establish an acceptable definition of the term has resulted in several possibilities. The title of a book by Ernst and Schwartz suggests one simple definition, *Privacy-The Right to be Let Alone*.[1] Another definition by Bates is "a person's feeling that others should be excluded from something which is of concern to him and also a recognition that others have a right to do this."[2] Westin, in his comprehensive book on the importance of privacy as an essential in a free society, defines privacy as "the claim of individuals, groups, or institutions to determine for themselves when, how, and to what extent information about them is communicated to others."[3] From this basic definition Westin elaborates on the relation of the individual to a social group, stating that privacy is the temporary and voluntary withdrawal of an individual by physical or psychological measures.[4]

From these several interpretations a composite statement on privacy would include the following aspects:

1. the individual's right to exclude others from certain knowledge about himself;
2. the awareness by a person that others have the same privilege as he desires for himself;
3. the factors of time, place, manner and amount of information, which may all be aspects to be considered; and
4. the exclusion of oneself from others; this may be voluntary, temporary and achieved by physical and/or psychological means.

To derive the meaning of privacy that will be utilized in this paper, other terms were necessarily reviewed for their relationship and similarity to or differences from privacy. Among these were such terms as secrecy, confidentiality, and solitude. Sociological concepts such as social distance and avoidance were also considered.

After these initial steps involving the development of pertinent aspects of privacy and the identification of related concepts, the behavioral science literature was surveyed for material on privacy. The sources which will be reviewed in this paper were those few citations which developed the concept in some depth, contrasted to the numerous brief references to privacy made in many books and articles. As stated previously, privacy has been brought to the attention of the American public through a variety of popular publications. These are identified in the reference list for the reader's interest, but they will not be reviewed.[5]

The definitions stated in this paper refer in most instances to the individual, but one definition does allude to groups and institutions as well. However, the literature reviewed will be in the context of the individual, with only a few references to groups and societies.

Among the questions which may be raised in a study of privacy are those regarding its importance, functions and universality. How necessary is privacy? Do all people need privacy? To what extent is it important? What factors influence an individual's or group's need for privacy? What situations contribute to a change in the degree of privacy? Is there a balance to be achieved between privacy and participation?

Functions of Privacy

To explain further some of these basic questions, the functions which privacy serves can be delineated. Four of these functions, as identified by Westin, will serve as the basis for this discussion.[6]

The first function, *personal autonomy*, relates to the beliefs regarding the uniqueness of man and his basic dignity and worth as an individual. The development and maintenance of individuality have been related to the need for autonomy. Some behavioral scientists have described interpersonal relationships in terms of zones, regions or circles of privacy leading to the core or inner self. The inner portion contains those secrets, thoughts and beliefs which are not shared with anyone except in situations of extreme stress when the person must share for essential emotional relief. In this model there are concentric rings to denote the decreasing degree of privacy from the inner to the outer layer, which is casual communication, observable to all.

Goffman, a leading sociologist, has described ways in which people present themselves to others with the aim of controlling the impression the others receive of them. An aspect of this would be the region where the performance takes place. The "back region" thus becomes the term for the area which is out of bounds to the audience; and "backstage" behavior is the regressive, intimate behavior not presented to the audience.[7]

254   Privacy

The potential threats imposed upon one's autonomy and thus one's privacy are those situations which seek to enter the inner core and learn the secrets. Also threatening is any attempt to move a person into one's "back region."

Emotional release is the second function identified by Westin. Because modern society imposes stresses and strains on man, man needs opportunities for privacy in order to find emotional release. Several authors have noted the special need to obtain relief from tension brought about by the multiplicity of roles played by a person. Another aspect of this function is that of the "safety-valve" effect, which is used to relieve emotional pressure. Examples are seen in the situations where people express anger, tension or anxiety at some authority in the privacy of their home, office or intimate circle of friends. A further form of emotional release is observed when privacy makes possible minor noncompliance with social norms or social etiquette. Exceeding the speed limit, padding the expense account, belching or swearing may all be instances of nonconforming behavior permitted by privacy. Of special importance to the health professionals are the releases in bodily and sexual functions and in emotional expression at times of loss or sorrow. These are further examples of expressions usually condoned only in private.

The third function, *self-evaluation,* describes the process whereby man is able to integrate his experiences and gain some meaningful perspective. Assessment of data and consideration of choices are best handled in private. Closely related are creative thinking and moral inventory-taking.

Limited and protected communication is the fourth function of privacy. The first of the two aspects of this function is the opportunity for sharing confidences because of the social norms establishing privileged communication for certain groups, such as physicians, ministers and counselors. The second aspect serves to set boundaries or distances in interpersonal relationships, such as student-teacher and parent-child relationships.

Degrees of Privacy

Another perspective from which to view individual privacy is through the delineation of four basic states or degrees.[8] *Solitude,* the term used for the first state, describes the individual's separation from the group. While physical stimuli such as sound and heat and psychological intrusions may occur, solitude is the most complete state of individual privacy.

The second state, *intimacy,* refers to the individual's acting as part of a small unit that exercises seclusion. Examples of these units are families or a husband-and-wife dyad. The importance of intimate relationships to meet the basic needs for human contact has been described by Sullivan.[9]

Anonymity, the third state, is characterized by the individual in a public place such as on a bus or at a zoo who is free from being personally identified and supervised. He is not forced to observe rules of behavior that would exist were he known. Anonymity can be preserved with strangers and in the publication of ideas without their originator's identification.

Creation of psychological barriers against invasion of privacy is the most subtle kind of privacy. This fourth state, which occurs in all interpersonal relationships, is the choice made by an individual to limit his communication with others. The balance which ensues as people withhold information, and the respect or disregard afforded by others, are achieved by this state of privacy.

Variables Influencing Privacy

The number of variables which influence the development and expression of privacy is evident as the concept of privacy is explored. Two of these variables will be presented as examples of the multitude of factors which can be considered in examining one's state of privacy.

Cultural. Studies of culture and subcultural groups by anthropologists have increased the understanding of the importance of the cultural values and norms upon individual behavior. Lee, from her study of different cultures, points out the variations in how privacy is maintained. She mentions the notion of having one's own bedroom as a concept previously related to having enough fresh air, but now receiving sanction as a matter of one's mental health. The Tikopia people of Polynesia, for example, find privacy to be intolerable in maintaining their value of the self's continuity with its society.[10] Lee compares this attitude toward privacy with American values on private cars, bedrooms, bathrooms, offices, and secretaries—all of them based upon the value of individualism with self-dependence and individual rights and integrity.[11]

Political systems. A question might be asked concerning the relationship of the political system to the concept of privacy. The differences between the totalitarian state and the democratic system can demonstrate this relationship. In the totalitarian state a high degree of secrecy is afforded the governing body, while disclosure and surveillance is the rule for all other individuals and groups. Because of the loyalty to the state demanded in this society, the person's privacy, autonomy and individualism are attacked as being "immoral" and "antisocial." While eventually a totalitarian state may relax somewhat and thus afford more privacy to institutions such as the church and the arts, the balance favoring disclosure and surveillance is necessary for the functioning of the system.[12]

By contrast, the democratic state favors publicity and open hearings and investigations of the government as a means of control. At the same time, privacy is encouraged for individuals and groups. Democratic societies support the idea that individuals should have interest areas apart from the political system; therefore, these interests are encouraged. Strong family systems, personal retreats, religious choice and variety of groups are all values important in democratic theory. Thus, the balanced state of privacy maintained in a democracy is one in which individual and group needs are protected by privacy, yet governmental groups are usually open to investigation and disclosure. An exception to the disclosure of governmental offices is the high degree of secrecy afforded to the security systems, such as the military and the Federal Bureau of Investigation.[13]

Universals

Following a discussion of forces which may influence the development and maintenance of privacy, it is important to look also at the universality of privacy. Although most people tend to think of privacy as strictly a human desire, some interesting studies of animal behavior have increased the knowledge about privacy and seclusion as necessary components of all animal life.

Privacy of space. As stated in the definition, physical or psychological measures can be used to promote privacy. Hall has done some interesting work on the physical aspects of privacy. In *The Hidden Dimension,* for instance, he presents his concept of proxemics, the term he coined for the theories related to man's use of space.[14] From his description of territoriality and spacing mechanisms as utilized by animals, he developed similar ideas related to man's perception of space. Thus, according to Hall, man also uses rules of personal, intimate and social distance in his interpersonal relationships. Physical senses or animal senses such as smell, taste or touch are employed by man in his defining of boundaries of privacy.

Human needs. While norms regarding privacy do vary among cultures and societies, within each there are social norms to insure individual and group privacy. Within an individual's daily interactions with others, in small groups such as families as well as in larger communities, privacy is maintained.[15]

Individual. The process of an individual's relating to others is marked by periods in which privacy is sought at some times and participation with others at another. The individual sets limits to maintain a degree of distance at certain crucial times when protection is needed. Murphy points out that social distance may be more important in the person's most intimate relationships than in casual contacts.[16]

Family. Primitive and modern societies as well as nuclear and extended family households all maintain rules regarding entry, communication patterns and psychological privacy. For example, when the household is crowded and little physical privacy is provided, psychological measures such as soft voices and restrained emotions may insure privacy.[17]

Groups. In group relationships also, privacy may be observed as a need met through the customs which prescribe privacy for certain rituals. Rites of passage and sacred ceremonies are examples of these secret events.[18]

Counterforces to Privacy

In addition to factors operating to promote privacy, there are also forces which act against the maintenance of privacy. There is some indication that the tendency to invade the privacy of others may be a universal behavior. The trait of curiosity has been observed to begin in very young children. This desire to gain knowledge about others continues to develop throughout life. Gossip, as a means of obtaining and communicating private information, is common among many people. Tales such as the one about Pandora's box or the story of Lot's wife serve to support the presence of this trait.

Along with this individual behavior is the group behavior of observation and surveillance by authorities to enforce the rules of the society. Socially accepted means are established that invade an individual's privacy in order to insure rights of individuals and groups.[19]

Balanced View of Privacy

Since this paper is focused on privacy, primary focus has been given to its desirability to the individual. However, in a balanced view of privacy, the equally important needs for companionship, sharing and socialization must also be recognized. This balance of privacy and disclosure is achieved by man's changing experiences and opportunities as he moves through the states of privacy or finds satisfaction in interpersonal relationships with others. Privacy is not proposed as an ultimate state or even a state to be achieved solely as an end in itself. Privacy is a way of achieving individual goals and adapting to the stimuli of interactions and the environment.

Man seeks privacy when he needs it. However, too much or too little privacy can be inappropriate and cause an imbalance. The values of group participation have been recognized by many theorists in group dynamics and group therapy. The importance of group work and actions, as well as the benefits for the individual member, are among the advantages of group membership. On the other hand, the study of social isolation and sensory deprivation has added to the knowledge about the effects of this extreme degree of solitude. When an individual is isolated from others, emotional deterioration occurs similar to that produced by sensory deprivation.[20] Thus, the individual must strive for the continuous adjustment between these counteracting needs of privacy and compansionship.[21]

NURSING IMPLICATIONS

What knowledge of privacy is necessary in nursing intervention aimed at providing privacy for patients? What situations are especially pertinent as examples of the need for nurses to preserve privacy?

In the following discussion, examples of nursing situations are used to illustrate the concept of privacy and its relationship to nursing. Although the uniqueness of the clinical specialties of nursing is recognized, the reader should be able to make the application to other clinical situations which are not used as examples.

Privacy for Patients

To introduce the relationship of privacy to nursing care, nursing situations will illustrate the four functions reviewed earlier in this paper. The needs for personal autonomy, emotional release, self-evaluation, and limited and protected communication are seen frequently by nurses as they interact with patients in a variety of nursing activities.

The importance of considering the patient's autonomy has often been suggested as an essential aspect of nursing care. Individualized or patient-centered care has been a popular expression in nursing for a number of years. Along with this have gone some of the psychological theories utilized in nursing which support the view of various layers or rings denoting the degrees of confidentiality of one's personality, including thoughts, desires, beliefs. As they are developing interviewing skills, nurses have often been cautioned not to probe or ask penetrating questions that require the patient to reveal more than he desires. Sensitivity on the part of the nurse would help her to respect the individual's right to privacy, and at the same time to interview therapeutically. Providing privacy in regard to the setting might be the approach when certain difficult topics are discussed or when the patient indicates a desire to exclude other patients from the information he is willing to share with the nurse. In addition, are there any tools for measuring the layers to determine what information a person is willing to share?

The process of admission to a hospital may be an example of a situation in which nurses have a responsibility to insure privacy for the patient and his family as a way of respecting the worth and dignity of the individual. Consider also the unwed mother who needs to keep to herself the knowledge that she has not been married. Exposing her marital situation to other patients might be an invasion of privacy and threat to her autonomy as an individual. As an example,

A young woman was admitted to an obstetrical service for the delivery of her child. Following the birth, she was placed in a six-bed ward. A nurse observed her crying when the babies were brought out to the mothers from the nursery. In talking with this patient, the nurse learned that the woman, an unwed mother, had relinquished her child for adoption. At this time when other mothers were having contact with their new babies, she was reminded that she was giving her baby to another person. Also, the others became aware of this woman's situation, which may have been one which she wanted to exclude from other's knowledge. In conversation with the nurse, she revealed that she would have preferred to be in a room alone and not allow her single status to be known. She also indicated that seeing the babies of the other women and the mother-child relationships which she was forced to witness were very difficult situations for her.

Were there alternatives that might have been provided as a means of protecting this patient's privacy? Indeed, in certain situations maintaining privacy might be a very difficult task; however, preparation of the patient for this type of room assignment, if a private room was not available, was a possible approach to alleviating the situation.

In community health nursing, a nurse's entering a family's home at unannounced times could also be viewed as an invasion of privacy. Consider the family whose eating habits, clothing, child care practices, furniture, orderliness and cleanliness of the house and yard, relationships with neighbors, and many other manifestations of personal values can all be revealed by a visit to the home.

A question has often been raised in psychiatric nursing related to the use of therapeutic community concepts and especially the techniques of reality confrontation. A patient who has recently experienced a traumatic event may be encouraged to discuss this openly in a group situation with both other patients and staff. How does the group decide how much to allow or encourage the patient to reveal? There is a possibility that the patient will need assistance to protect his privacy so that he does not later feel "undressed" by the group. On the other hand, the nurse who assumes that the patient will want and need privacy may find that this isn't what he desires. Careful assessment and exploration of the patient's goals will need to be made to avoid false assumptions.

The second function served by privacy, emotional release, is undoubtedly a familiar one in nursing. It has been taken for granted that illness or threat of illness produces stress in the individual. If states of privacy provide people with the opportunity to blow off steam or obtain emotional release, this need would seem to be necessary for those experiencing the multiple stresses of illness. For example:

> A new mother has just been visited by the pediatrician following an examination of the infant. A nurse walking by the room hears the mother crying and saying, "I just can't believe it. I don't want to think of anything being wrong with the baby."

Since the mother is in a four-bed ward, the nurse might consider how she can intervene at this time of stress to provide for privacy so that the disappointed mother can obtain emotional release more comfortably. Or could the state of privacy have been provided before the woman was told of the baby's diagnosis? Physical solitude is one way of excluding others; however, in the absence of this possibility, psychological privacy can be used through a soft voice, slow speech, and well-chosen words. Consideration needs to be given to means of providing both physical and psychological privacy in the health agencies where nurses are with patients and families. The patient's need for emotional support is frequently included in nursing care plans as an accepted goal. While the value of another person's listening and caring is important, at times an individual may need privacy first or at subsequent intervals to gain more from the person providing the emotional support. In this situation also, the desire for a balance between privacy and interaction with others has to be considered for effective nursing care.

For the emotional expression usually found following death, families may need an opportunity to be alone with the deceased prior to being interrupted or involved by the personnel. They should be permitted the release of their tensions, anger, guilt, or sadness through the provision of privacy. Other families may prefer to talk with personnel immediately, then secure moments of privacy with the deceased to be followed again by a desire to talk with the staff. Providing a room where a family can be alone as desired will enable the family to express their emotions in private as they choose, without having to fit themselves into any routinized pattern of behavior.

Nurses deal with people who are frequently in need of assistance in relation to bodily functions. Within the American culture especially, privacy for the body and its functions such as elimination, sleeping arrangements and sexual activities has been accepted. Patients should be provided with at least the privacy measures of screens, curtains around the bed, or a closed door. And when the door is closed, is the patient's privacy respected by the nurse's knocking on the door prior to entering? Or does she enter without asking for permission?

The third function, self-evaluation, can be viewed as a frequently occurring need as the person's illness, altered body image, pain, and other symptoms are integrated and become meaningful to him. Provision for privacy can allow for and encourage this reintegration. A patient having just been told of a terminal illness may need some time to be alone in which he can review the situation, study the possible alternatives of treatment available, and make some decisions. This desire for privacy does not preclude the nurse's being a helpful person in the problem-solving process but, as has been stated earlier, the balance between privacy and companionship is the desired optimum, with neither privacy nor participation ends in themselves. Again, the nurse will necessarily need to determine which is wanted and needed by the patient.

Limited and protected communication, the fourth function of privacy, is familiar within health situations where certain information is privileged due to the norms and boundaries of that relationship. A decision sometimes posed to nurses is that of the patient who says, "I'd like to tell you, but don't tell anyone else." The nurse will not only need to assess the situation to determine if this is indeed a legitimate request for privacy or if the patient is asking another question, such as, "How much do you share with others?" or "Do you care enough about me to tell the others I'm in trouble or suicidal, so you'll help me?"

Privacy for Nurses

So far we have been talking about the patient and his needs for privacy. However, the nurse's own privacy deserves some attention. As has been stated in many philosophies of nursing, the nurse should be aware of her own behavior, values, norms and expectations. This general statement would encompass privacy as well, with the need for the nurse to be aware of her values regarding privacy. In what situations does she require privacy? How does she obtain a satisfactory balance between privacy and participation?

Although the intent of the paper is to focus on nursing, brief mention should be made of the situation in which the nurse's privacy may be the issue because of threats coming from within the nursing experiences. Nurses, too, may be threatened by probing questions asked of them by patients and other staff, or they may feel unable to express in public the emotional responses they experience when a patient goes home or dies or is mutilated. Many of us will remember the nurse's running to the linen closet to seek refuge and privacy for her emotional releases. The "back regions" discussed by Goffman may be the nursing office, the linen room, treatment room or staff lounge where personnel have their private places where emotions can be expressed. The staff dining room can be an alternative place where nurses find privacy from patients if there is no other situation available. Some luncheon conversations would seem to support the idea of need for emotional release.

Knowledge Needed by the Nurse

What sort of knowledge does the nurse need as a basis for intervention aimed at privacy? If the model used to describe nursing process involves the steps of assessment, validation, intervention and evaluation, the nurse may follow this process in utilizing her knowledge for meeting more effectively the patient's needs for privacy. An example is:

A nurse enters a male patient's room and initiates a discussion with the patient about the previous evening. She asks him how he slept and whether he was comfortable. Suddenly the patient says, "Leave me alone. I just want to be left alone."

Based upon this small amount of data, the nurse must make some assessment of the situation and plan and initiate a nursing action. Possible interpretations are that the patient is testing the nurse, he is asking the nurse to stay, or he is expressing his need for privacy.

Before the nurse can consider the possibility of any patient's need for privacy, she must have some awareness of the functions privacy can serve for an individual. She also needs to know some of the variables which influence one's views about privacy. Consider the differences between a woman accustomed to living in a small nuclear family who is now hospitalized in a room with several other patients, and a woman from a large extended family who is now relatively isolated in a single or double room.

Other variables which might be significant and worthy of consideration are related to cultural background, social class, age, or religion. These and other factors may all influence a person's individual needs for privacy. Knowledge of growth and development would suggest to the nurse that a five-year-old boy may much more readily share personal information about himself and his family than a fifteen-year-old boy who is turning toward his peers as his confidants rather than adult authorities, such as the nurse. With these two boys, what differences need to be provided for privacy during visiting hours or telephone calls?

As the nurse establishes a relationship with a patient, she is able to gain knowledge about that person's individual means of expressing the need for privacy. Verbal and non-verbal behavior becomes apparent and certain facial expressions or bodily gestures can be the patient's way of asking to be let alone. For example, a patient turning his face toward the wall during a conversation could be asking to be left alone. Also, because privacy may be needed for emotional release, symptoms of stress may be clues to the need for privacy. When a patient starts to cry, is this a clue that he wishes to be left alone, or does the patient wish to talk about his stress?

As suggested earlier, the nurse's awareness of her own needs for privacy will be another knowledge useful for her successful intervention. Recognition of her tendency to isolate herself or, on the other hand, to reveal her inner thoughts to others will assist her in becoming aware that other people may have similar or different needs relative to privacy.

The nurse's understanding of privacy should also include the concept of the desired balance between privacy and participation. An unvalidated assumption that a particular person needs privacy could lead to the nurse's isolating that person. Therefore, the degree of privacy provided needs to be carefully determined and evaluated to prevent privacy's becoming an end in itself.

SPECULATIONS

This exploratory discussion of privacy and its relevance to nursing raises many questions and ideas. Additional speculation might lead to new knowledge of privacy and further guidelines for the nurse.

In considering the application of privacy to all age groups, one question that emerges is: how does privacy and its meaning develop in children? Are there differences in the expressions of privacy in girls compared with boys? The influences of child-rearing practices upon the continuation or extinction of privacy might be studied in this culture as well as in other cultures.

Along with age, sex, and culture as variables, social class is another factor to be explored as an influence upon privacy. Within the health profession, there may be a tendency to invade the privacy of people in those classes below us, with a hesitation to invade the privacy of those in higher classes. Indications are that at the present time, the lower social-economic groups are being deluged with all kinds of professional workers to study health, social, economic, and educational needs. Do these surveys always consider the privacy of those who are studied? Is the lack of studies about similar needs of the higher social classes due to concern about respecting their privacy?

A question which is related to the nursing process is how the need for privacy may vary as the nurse and patient progress through the stages of the relationship. Also, how is this similar to or different from the group process and its influence upon privacy?

While the intent of this discussion has been essentially to focus upon the importance of privacy, additional studies might be done on the effects of varying degrees of privacy. The possibility of too much privacy has been indicated in patients who have experienced long periods of isolation or seclusion. The knowledge gained by studies of sensory deprivation might be reviewed for its possible relationship to too much privacy. When there is too little privacy, what kinds of behavior are observed? Sensory overload data are a part of this phenomenon, and additional information could be gathered about "people overload" as seen in situations where individuals are kept together in groups with little or no opportunities for being alone.

Study of individual variables would also be useful in our understanding of privacy in order to meet the needs of patients. For example, is the use of a patient's first name an indication to him that his privacy is being invaded? Or, is touching a person an invasion of his privacy? Within each clinical specialty numerous examples occur which can be identified and studied by clinical nursing specialists.

Nursing care will be enhanced as research on the nursing process continues. It is hoped that additional studies on the concept of privacy and its relation to the health-illness continuum, and especially to the practice of nursing, will be done in the future.

REFERENCES

1. Ernst, M. L., and Schwartz, A. U.: Privacy—The Right to be Let Alone. New York, Macmillan, 1962.
2. Bates, A. P.: Privacy—A useful concept. Social Forces, 42:429-434, May, 1964.
3. Westin, A. F.: Privacy and Freedom. p. 7. New York, Atheneum, 1967.
4. *Ibid.*
5. Brenton, M.: The Privacy Invaders. New York, Coward-McCann, 1964; In defense of privacy. Time, 88:38-39, July 15, 1966; Packard, V.: Seven steps to greater personal freedom. Reader's Digest, 88:123-127, April, 1966; The Naked Society. New York, David McKay, 1964; Solarz, A. K.: Privacy at home.... Yours, mine, ours. Family Circle, 71:32, 33, 102, 104, 106, July, 1967; Westin, A. F.: Privacy. McCall's, 45:58, 118, February, 1968; Young, L. R.: A child's right to privacy. McCall's, 43:57, 59, 163, March, 1966; and Life Among the Giants. New York, McGraw-Hill, 1966.
6. Westin, A. F., *op. cit.,* pp. 32-39.
7. Goffman, E.: The Presentation of Self in Everyday Life. pp. 106-140. New York, Doubleday Anchor Books, 1959.
8. Westin, A. F., *op. cit.,* pp. 31-32.
9. Sullivan, H. S.: The Interpersonal Theory of Psychiatry. pp. 290-291. New York, W. W. Norton & Co., 1953.
10. Lee, D.: Freedom and Culture. p. 31. Prentice-Hall, Spectrum Books, 1959.
11. *Ibid.,* pp. 74-75.
12. Westin, A. F., *op. cit.,* pp. 23-24.
13. *Ibid.,* pp. 24-26.
14. Hall, E. T.: The Hidden Dimension. New York, Doubleday, 1966.
15. Westin, A. F., *op. cit.,* p. 13.
16. Murphy, R. F.: Social distance and the veil. American Anthropologist, 66:1259, December, 1964.
17. Westin, A. F., *op. cit.,* pp. 16-17.
18. *Ibid.,* pp. 17-18.
19. *Ibid.,* p. 20.

20. Schultz, D. P.: Sensory Restriction—Effects on Behavior. pp. 164-167. New York, Academic Press, 1965.
21. Westin, A. F., *op. cit.*, pp. 39-42.

14

Inquiry

Florence McDonald

INTRODUCTION

We are at a point in educational history when the subject of undergraduate education needs fresh thought and serious reconsideration. Knowledge produced at an explosive rate presents a dual challenge to American education at all levels. Education must first encourage and sustain qualities of intellectual curiosity and personal commitment among the young students of today. Secondly, it must provide them with the knowledge, the skills, the habits of mind that will enable them to create the kind of society and world they envision. This dual challenge must be met regardless of the specialized field of learning the individual student chooses to pursue. The growing sense of social responsibility for human welfare is creating new and expanding demands for health services and, concurrently, new requirements for the health sciences. Within a social context that is beginning to assume revolutionary character, nursing education is in a period of transition. This state of transition poses a fundamental question: how does nursing as a discipline fit into the structure of higher learning and professional education? The validity of the basic assumption that nursing is a learned profession must be demonstrated within the college or university community that supports the undergraduate curriculum in nursing.

This paper will reflect the belief that the college or university must provide an atmosphere conducive to education of the whole person by making it possible to continue the parallel study of the humanistic disciplines with the emerging science of nursing. The student must have the opportunity to enter into a "community" of scholars, both with faculty and peers; a kind of "community" that values learning for its own sake and makes it possible for the student to develop open-minded intellectual curiosity about what are presently accepted as the necessary knowledge, principles, concepts and methods of nursing. The atmosphere must permit the student to view nursing practice within the larger context of the health sciences. This "community" must make it possible for both the student and the teacher to enter into the process of discovery of what is taught and how it might be taught in the future.

This paper will endeavor to present the concept of inquiry as a cognative process that must be developed as one kind of unifying continuum within the nursing curriculum. This process of inquiry should emerge as a disciplined intellectual approach which becomes a habit of mind, a mental posture for the learner. Sequentially, the attempt is made to explain the what, the why, and the how of inquiry as a process, an intellectual tool, that enhances the integration potential in curriculum development and implementation in nursing. The bits and pieces of application of the concept of inquiry that are presented herein will focus on the learner—the student today—the agent of change tomorrow.

WHAT IS INQUIRY?

The business of Definition is part
of the business of discovery.[1]

Chapter Three of the King James version of the Book of Genesis begins with the immortal story of Eve and the serpent. This story reports what is probably mankind's first research adventure, mankind's first yielding to his inherent curiosity. Man, endowed with a superior brain, incessantly asks questions about himself and his environment. Man asks not only *what* but also *how, where, when* and above all else, *why*. By nature he investigates extensively, persistently. An inquiring mind is a healthy mind.

Webster defines inquiry as "a seeking for information by asking questions; the search for truth, information or knowledge; an investigation; research."[2] It is, then, a process.

The question is the key to most educative activity. Just asking questions does not ensure learning; rather, it is the character of the question, the time, the manner of asking and the content which result in self-discovered learning.

Every student must be encouraged to ask questions beginning with, "What is the nature of nursing?" By asking and dealing directly with this kind of question and others, the student can set intellectual tasks that are related to developing a clearer perspective of herself. (Cross-application: concept of awareness of self)

Search: Human beings persist in seeking out answers to their never-ending questions. In search one seeks a tangible object or person. One engages largely in physical activities. A simple example:

> The narcotic keys are missing. The student who used them last is questioned; she looks for them in the usual places; she retraces her steps where she had them; she then looks in her uniform pocket and finds the missing keys.

Investigation: This word comes from the Latin infinitive investigare which means to track, to trace out. Usage has made it synonymous with research.

Research: In research one may seek tangible objects, but more often one seeks intangible facts or concepts. Finding these kinds of answers chiefly requires intellectual activity. Research has one characteristic in common with search, namely, persistent attention and action directed toward finding that which one seeks; however, it differs from search in dealing more extensively with intangibles and in requiring much more complex intellectual activities.

The development of this paper on inquiry as a behavioral concept essential for integration within a program in professional nursing represents a research activity.

Inquiry: This term goes back to the Latin infinitive quaerere, to ask. It is the most general term applicable to search regardless of the means used (questioning, interviewing, observing, experimenting, investigating) or the end in view. The word "inquiry" is a synonym for either search or research and, depending upon the context in which it is used, implies the more complex intellectual processes that distinguish search from research.

The examples of application that are cited throughout this paper represent the concept of inquiry in operation.

Process: Parker and Rubin explain process to encompass all of the random, or ordered, operations which can be associated with knowledge and with human activities.

> When embellishments are stripped away, the fact is that we know little about the way people learn. We know that they learn in different ways and at different gaits. It is for this reason, in part, that we argue for a concep-

tualization of process as the life-blood of content and for a point of view which holds that they cannot be a dichotomy.³

Synonyms for the word "research": During recent years the word "research" with its prestigious, almost magical overtones has become so exceedingly popular that it has all but supplanted the two older generally synonymous terms—investigation and inquiry. These three terms can be used interchangeably; however, for the purposes of this paper, "inquiry" is preferred because it connotes an intellectual process that is fundamental to all levels of education, provides for the scope of processes essential to a learned discipline, can be a thing or a process conjointly or separately.

THE WHY OF INQUIRY

The concept of inquiry is basic to all learning. It is the process through which all of learning takes place. The development of an attitude of critical inquiry as a disciplined intellectual approach is a vital component of many education and nursing practices. The process of inquiry is a pivotal concept in relation to individual mental health; and in the implementation of this process, the concept of communication becomes an inseparable part.

The student is to give a bath to a 35-year-old woman who has a "fractured back." The doctor has written an order that the patient is not to be moved in any way for any reason. The patient's anxiety about herself is probably matched by the anxiety of the student as she prepares to give the bath. At this point the doctor arrives, talks with the patient briefly, reminds the student that the patient must not be moved in any way and leaves the room. The patient then asks the student for the bedpan. The student recognizes the paradox of this total situation. After some thought, she excuses herself, goes out to the chart room and asks the doctor if he would please return to the patient's bedside with her. She explains to him that she is inexperienced and would he be kind enough to show her how she can maintain his order for immobility and still care for the basic needs of the patient. The doctor acknowledges the problem, helps to clarify the situation with the student and the patient and thanks the student for teaching him a long overdue lesson in patient management. (Cross-application: concepts of trust, relationship control, and role change)

As the student pursues learning in structured patterns as well as independently, she will develop appropriate forthrightness, the habit of inquisitiveness and will derive stimulation and satisfaction from the process of exploring what she is doing at any given time. To achieve this kind and quality of learning, there must be some reason or specific objective for whatever situation the student is in the process of assessing.

The student prepares a clinical profile of an appropriate syndrome for presentation to an interdisciplinary group of peers and staff. She interviews the patient before the total group. Her process of assessment must be guided in such a way that the learning objective is accomplished, yet at the same time the patient's right to privacy is respected and maintained. (Cross-application: concepts of privacy, listening, empathy)

It becomes increasingly apparent that the concept of inquiry has cross-application to most all behavioral concepts and can best be derived within a social system where questioning is encouraged throughout the total learning experience, where ideas are respected and creativity is valued. This spirit of inquiry, emerging as a knowledgeable, perceptive approach, will enable the student to identify, understand, and deal with such affective elements in learning as the self-reactions of shame, fear, grief, and humor. (Cross-application: concepts of shame, humor, grief)

The student must be provided with the opportunity to develop a philosophy of critical inquiry and an appreciation for the experimental point of view toward learning. The ability to use knowledge and past experience, to maintain motivation until a difficult task is completed or a baffling problem is solved, to gain confidence in herself as a self-actuating creative person, to learn how to fill gaps in knowledge or to call on experts when necessary—all of this is of fundamental importance to the student who is learning how to organize and give competent nursing care.

The student will recognize learning as a developmental task of life and discover that she has the power to learn and to learn how to learn. The assumption has been set forth that self-esteem is an important element in individual mental health. A further assumption is "that self-esteem is partially dependent on the inclusion of a sense of power within [one's] self-concept, that an effective . . . mentally healthy person must be able to perceive himself as at least minimally powerful, capable of influencing his environment to his own benefit, [and for others,] and . . . that this sense of minimal power has to be based on the actual experience of, and the exercise of, power."[4] This sense of power as a quality of experiential learning for the student is achieved, in part, through the process of discovery in new areas of learning. Carl Rogers observes:

274 Inquiry

> ... that anything which can be taught to another is relatively inconsequential, that is, it will have little significant influence on his behavior. The only kind of learning which significantly influences behavior is self-discovered or self-appropriated learning, truth that has been personally appropriated and assimilated in experience.[5]

Inquiry as a learning strategy has only recently emerged as a significant concept in nursing literature, acceptable and respectable in education for nursing. Through the development of the method of inquiry as a process of learning, knowledge can be acquired and employed not merely as a composite of information but as an ongoing system that supports continual learning. The nurse can function only at the level of basic knowledge and understanding that she brings to the reality of the working situation.

The entire curriculum must be developed in a pattern that will provide for sequential experiences and opportunities that will activate these intellectual processes—inquiry, analysis, synthesis and independent creativity. The student, sustained by the motivation that comes through discovery, learns from the triad of knowledge, experience and assessment technics.

THE HOW OF INQUIRY

Nursing is a service to someone, by someone. It is always an interpersonal relationship, a reciprocal interaction process for the reason that it comes into being because of its concern with people either directly or indirectly. Thus nursing education uses experience as a method of education and assumes the obligation to make this education effective. Nursing situations being experiences in time and place, are always in a state of change. In both quality and quantity the concept of inquiry has the potential to enhance the effectiveness of experiential learning. Experiential learning is an essential segment of the nursing education continuum that enables the learner to test and clarify knowledge, technics, concepts and understanding against a variety of real life situations. This process provides for constant refinement of perceptions and appropriate use of self. Herein, the application of the concept of inquiry as learning methodology is limited to the teaching-learning process and to the development of a core theme of independent study in a curriculum.

The Teaching-Learning Process: The critical path in the development of a spirit of inquiry and a rational attitude toward the concept and process of inquiry as a basic approach to learning lies in the teaching-learning context. Ideally, the teaching-learning process is a partnership with the teacher serving as a role model appropriate to the particular learning situation. This teaching-learning sequence becomes a tutorial or preceptorial relationship wherein the teacher demonstrates her functional knowledge and understanding of the art and science of nursing to the student and vice-versa. The teacher and the student form a partnership in which the participants learn and practice cooperation through the deliberate and meaningful practice of cooperation. Learning becomes an evolving, dynamic process of change for both the teacher and the student. (Cross-application: Concepts of team plan, interpersonal relations, ambivalence)

Teaching-Learning Sequence—
    Teacher to self: "What do I want the student to learn?"
    Teacher to student: "What do you want to learn?"

The teaching act has four dimensions:

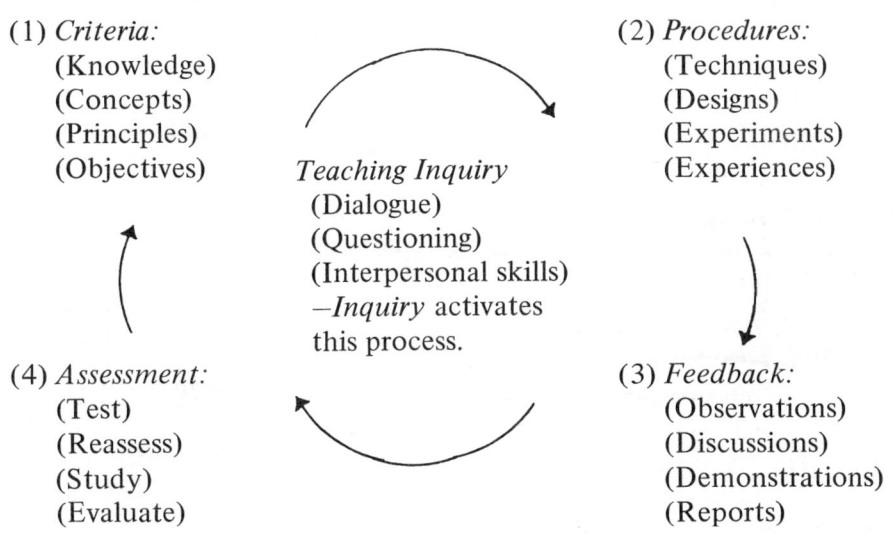

(1) *Criteria:*
  (Knowledge)
  (Concepts)
  (Principles)
  (Objectives)

(2) *Procedures:*
  (Techniques)
  (Designs)
  (Experiments)
  (Experiences)

Teaching Inquiry
  (Dialogue)
  (Questioning)
  (Interpersonal skills)
  —*Inquiry* activates this process.

(4) *Assessment:*
  (Test)
  (Reassess)
  (Study)
  (Evaluate)

(3) *Feedback:*
  (Observations)
  (Discussions)
  (Demonstrations)
  (Reports)

The cycle of inquiry activates the sequence of the teaching act. Utilizing the concept of inquiry, the teacher does four things. She begins with her own criteria and develops a procedure. She gathers feedback about the results of the procedure's application. She utilizes this information to assess the procedure. Based on this assessment she

276   Inquiry

adjusts her criteria to the specific situation. This sequence of events shows the process of inquiry in operation.

The teacher has the responsibility to review this pattern of teaching continually. She must be able to ask of herself, "How do I permit questions to be asked?", "How do I take the pressure off the student so the student can move?", "What kind of example do I provide for the student to observe, pattern after or identify with in the learning situation?", "How do I work with other types of nursing service personnel?", "How do my colleagues and associates relate to me?" The teacher has the obligation to maintain responsible involvement with the nursing service and the nursing practice that is provided by the service agency. (Cross-application: concepts of leadership, team plan, group process)

The Learning Act—
        Student to self: "How can I learn what I need to learn?"
                    "How can I learn what I want to learn?"

The learning act involves these four dimensions:

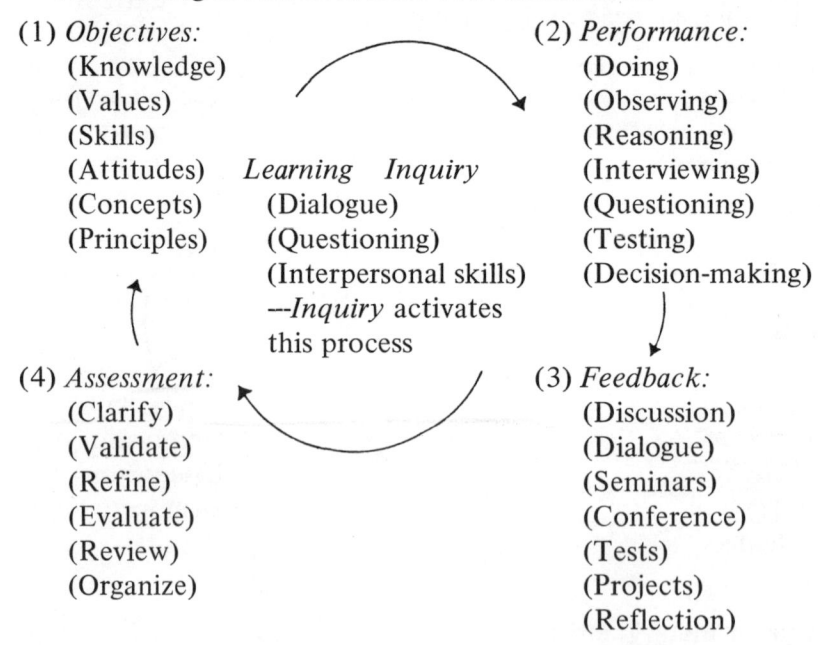

(1) *Objectives:*
   (Knowledge)
   (Values)
   (Skills)
   (Attitudes)   *Learning   Inquiry*
   (Concepts)   (Dialogue)
   (Principles)   (Questioning)
                  (Interpersonal skills)
                  —*Inquiry* activates
                  this process

(2) *Performance:*
   (Doing)
   (Observing)
   (Reasoning)
   (Interviewing)
   (Questioning)
   (Testing)
   (Decision-making)

(4) *Assessment:*
   (Clarify)
   (Validate)
   (Refine)
   (Evaluate)
   (Review)
   (Organize)

(3) *Feedback:*
   (Discussion)
   (Dialogue)
   (Seminars)
   (Conference)
   (Tests)
   (Projects)
   (Reflection)

The cycle of inquiry activates the sequence of the learning act. The learning act involves four dimensions that are counterparts of the teaching act. The student utilizes the concept of inquiry to perform in accordance with her own objectives, to gather feedback about her performance, to utilize this feedback to assess her performance, and to change her objectives according to the assessment that she makes in a specific situation. This is the process of inquiry on the part of the learner.

These two conceptual patterns, the teaching act and the learning act, merge to become a design of four interrelated and interdependent dimensions. The teaching-learning process requires that this sequence become a joint venture, a cooperative relationship between student and teacher. Cooperation depends upon effective communication which encourages the kind of relationship essential for the achievement of new levels of understanding. The concept of inquiry activates the continuum through which learning becomes change for both the student and the teacher. (Cross-application: concepts of group process, leadership, communication)

INQUIRY AS A CORE THEME

When today's college students arrive on the campus, they display a wide range of knowledge, active curiosity, eagerness to learn and a sincere confidence in their own abilities. They are aware of issues of cultural and social import and are becoming involved in social action and change. They possess active intellectual energy that is seeking expression through the specific academic curriculum in nursing. These students anticipate guidance and direction and expect education to affect their emotional outlooks and attitudes as well as their intellect.

Independent study is the procedure used herein to develop the concept of inquiry as one kind of intellectual tool that can be integrated throughout the basic curriculum.

The student must enter into creative scholarship at the earliest possible level of the nursing program. Independent study that requires the least complex process of inquiry is initiated through the use of specific reading assignments. This is a fundamental learning technic; but the timing, quality and pattern of completion of structured and unstructured assignments permit appraisal of student progress in independent study. The encouragement of independent study in the total learning experience emphasizes the interest, initiative, and responsibility which the student integrates into her own individual patterns of work: effective, reflective, physical or intellectual, in part or in total. (Cross-application: concepts of acceptance, leadership, autonomy)

A second approach to independent study as a learning procedure is the project or investigation that is undertaken by the individual student independently. Students need to comprehend how knowledge comes into being and how scholars arrive at their conclusions. To facilitate this kind of understanding the student should be given the opportunity to study and investigate a problem or a point of concern in an area of her own choice. A student who wants to study in an area outside the field of nursing should be free to do so. The problems that the students investigate need not be creative in the sense that new and unique outcomes will be produced, but they need to be creative in the student's terms. Whatever form the independent study project takes—an annotated bibliography, development of a set of activity procedures, a study of a problem in nursing practice, or a longer research effort—it must be more than an exercise of rote, repetition or regurgitation of what is or has been done. This project must be designed to assist the student, through logical reasoning and insight, to reach an understanding of how answers are found or why a problem persists. It takes time and patience on the part of the teacher to assist the student in the planning of a project, to guide the student progressively and then to evaluate the results of this independent creativity. For the student, the development of the project requires time and considerable intellectual energy along with imagination and enthusiasm. This form of the concept of inquiry motivates learning in a unique way. In conducting the independent study project, the student will be able to learn, understand and use experimental methodology consciously, sequentially and precisely. The process of inquiring as a disciplined intellectual approach can develop into a habit of mind for both the student and the teacher. The student can derive satisfaction from self-directed creative achievement and the teacher can share this satisfaction. (Cross-application: concepts of communication skills, self-esteem)

RECOMMENDATION

Research: The character of research that is recommended will involve and invoke the highly complex levels and patterns of the concept of inquiry. A searching study of nursing education as it now exists is mandatory. The short range goals of such a research should be to devise some new, creative ways to deal with the problems and issues that confront and confound collegiate nursing education. The long range objectives for this investigation should provide guidelines for the future. A forward look should include the design for a truly experimental program in an autonomous school of nursing in a college or university community that has never had such a school. Nursing education endeavors to provide two things for the individual student—a general liberal education and a more intensive education in nursing. The notion persists that perhaps the planners of a new truly experimental program in nursing would do well to review the conceptual pattern in operation at Antioch College, Yellow Springs, Ohio. This suggestion is on thin ice but it is possible that some useful ideas would be garnered from such an investigation since the fundamental premise at Antioch is essentially what nursing education endeavors to achieve for the individual student. To undertake such research, the thinking and resources of a range of experts would be required and the National Institute of Mental Health might be the logical structure to assume this leadership for nursing education.

CONCLUSION

John W. Gardner in the Annual Report of the Carnegie Corporation for 1962, wrote:

> ... if we indoctrinate the young person in an elaborate set of fixed beliefs, we are ensuring his early obsolescence. The alternative is to develop skills, attitudes, habits of mind, and the kinds of knowledge and understanding that will be the instruments of continuous change and growth on the part of the young person. Then we will have fashioned a system that provides for its own continuous renewal.[6]

A curriculum design that implements the concept of inquiry throughout the program provides for the development of aggressive learning which is an essential element in any effort to bring about change. The depth and breadth of the implementation of the concept of inquiry within nursing curricula could emerge as a focus of differentiation between the kinds of nursing programs.

It has been said that nursing responds to change but does not create its own change. The cycle of inquiry can evolve into a cycle of change ... a process of creativity that can deal with the here and now and still search for new horizons.

> ".... The imagination needs to be cultivated and developed to assure success in life. A man will never construct anything he cannot conceive."[7]

REFERENCES

1. Whewell, W.: The Philosophy of the Inductive Sciences. 2:16. 1847.
2. Webster's Collegiate Dictionary. p. 434. Springfield, Mass., G. & C. Merriam, 1956.
3. Parker, J. C., and Rubin, L. J.: Process as Content. p. 2. Chicago, Rand McNally, 1966.
4. Ryan, W.: Preventive services in the social context: Power, pathology, and prevention. *In* Bloom, B. L., and Buck, D. P. (eds.): Preventive Services in Mental Health Programs. p. 50. WICHE, Boulder, Colorado, 1967.
5. Rogers, C.: Personal thoughts on teaching and learning. Improving College and University Teaching, 6, 1:4-5.
6. Gardner, J. W.: Renewal in Societies and Men. New York, Annual Report of the Carnegie Foundation, 1962.
7. Stanford, L.: Stanford Today. p. 1. Stanford, California, March, 1962.

BIBLIOGRAPHY

Abercrombie, M. L.: The Anatomy of Judgment. New York, Basic Books, 1960.

Ammons, M. P.: Educational objectives: The relation between the process used in their development and their quality. Educational Horizons, Vol. 40, No. 2, Winter, 1961-62.

Anastasi, A.: Differential Psychology. New York, Macmillan, 1958.

Atkinson, J. W.: Motivational determinants of risk-taking behavior. Psychol. Rev., Vol. 64, 1957.

Bloom, B. S.: Taxonomy of Educational Objectives. New York, David McKay, 1956 and 1964.

Bruner, J. S.: The Process of Education. Cambridge, Mass., Harvard University Press, 1960.

Burton, G.: The instructor-counselor. J. Nurs. Educ., Vol. 1, No. 4, 1962.

Davis, F.: The Nursing Profession. New York, John Wiley & Sons, 1966.

Dixon, J. P.: Community dynamics and nursing education. Nurs. Outlook, 9, 10:627-629, October, 1961.

Gage, N. L.: Handbook of Research on Teaching. Chicago, Rand McNally, 1963.

Hargreaves, A. G.: The group culture and nursing practice. Am. J. Nurs., 67, 9:1840-1846, September, 1967.

Henderson, A., and Hall, D.: Antioch College: Its Design for Liberal Education. New York, Harper & Brothers, 1946.

Hilgard, E. R.: Teaching Machines and Creativity. Stanford Today, Series I, No. 6, September, 1963.

———: Theories of Learning. 2 ed. New York, Appleton-Century-Crofts, 1956.

Hunt, J. McV.: How children develop intellectually. Children, Vol. 2, No. 3, May/June, 1964.

Hyman, R.: The Nature of Psychological Inquiry. Englewood Cliffs, N.J., Prentice-Hall, 1964.

Jourard, S.: The Transparent Self. Princeton, Van Nostrand, 1964.

Larrabee, H. A.: Reliable Knowledge. Rev. New York, Houghton Mifflin, 1964.

Major, D.: Keys to a philosophy of teaching. Nurs. Outlook, 10, 8:506-510, August, 1962.

Office of Strategic Services: Assessment of Men. New York, Rinehart, 1948.

Rokeach, M.: Open and Closed Mind. New York, Basic Books, 1960.

Taba, H.: Curriculum Development. New York, Harcourt, Brace & World, 1962.

Team Teaching, A Special Issue. School & Society, Vol. 21, No. 2234, December 14, 1963.

Toward More Effective Teaching in WCHEN Schools. WICHE/WCHEN, Boulder, Colorado, 1964.

Toynbee, A. J.: Change and Habit. New York, Oxford University Press, 1966.

White, R. W.: Lives in Progress. New York, Holt, Rinehart & Winston, 1952.

15

Development of Awareness of Self for the Professional Nursing Student

Perquilla Callaghan

The nurse is exposed to a wide range of conditions in the physical, social, cultural and psychological aspects of human experience. Examples of these are physical disfigurement; problems of adjustment from birth through old age; the inevitability of death; attitudes of indifference and apathy toward health; neglect of health measures; dissension or disruption within families.

She must learn to cope with a myriad of reactions, such as denial, grief, aggressiveness and anger. She is confronted with a wide range of emotional states, such as apathy, hostility and depression, which may vary from mild to extreme.

Giving nursing care includes being involved in activities considered to be of a private nature by both the recipient and the nurse. Such activities include physical exposure for certain procedures, the revelation of certain information which in other circumstances may be kept private, the disclosure of very personal thoughts and feelings—kinds of activities the patient or client would not usually share with others.

In the course of practice, the nurse will react as a person as well as a provider of services. Though she may possess special knowledge and skills, these are not sufficient to enable her to give optimum nursing care unless she is able to look at herself and her responses in the nursing setting. Awareness and acceptance of various facets of herself can promote understanding and acceptance of others and is essential to her effectiveness.

Students come to the professional nursing program with a wide range of personal experience and development. They vary in their abilities to cope with problems presented in nursing. The nursing student, as a person, will react according to many factors derived from her personality and experience: her ideas, beliefs, feelings, predominant concerns, expectations and self-concept. Such actions as observing the patient's reactions, focusing on the patient's concerns, offering a nonthreatening environment and providing a consistent, safe relationship are essential in providing optimum patient care. Such actions as avoidance, withdrawal, expression of shock or displeasure in unpleasant situations, imposing one's own ideas, opinions and expectations upon the patient, and taking action primarily for one's own gain, may have an adverse effect in the performance of nursing services.

Although there is general agreement that awareness of self is an essential ingredient in developing nursing competence, nursing authorities lack consensus with regard to the *kind* of awareness which is desirable and the way in which the professional nursing student might be helped to achieve it. Ambiguity in the use of the term "self" may be one of the reasons for this lack of agreement.

The term "self" has been used in various ways in psychologic and psychiatric literature. Hall and Lindzey distinguish between two quite different uses of the term and state that it would be better to have separate terms for each meaning.[1]

One use, "self as process," refers to a group of psychological processes which control behavior and adjustment and include such mental activities as thinking, remembering and perceiving. It involves what the individual experiences, the meaning he gives to these experiences, and how he reacts.

Coleman writes more specifically about these psychological processes. He states that the individual builds a frame of reference (which must be accurate and realistic for him to function effectively) about the things he knows—about himself, other people, events, objects and ideas. In addition, the individual seeks or avoids things according to the meaning he attaches to them. As an active and responsible agent, the individual perceives a situation, "... processing all the information received from inner and outer sources—evaluating its significance, integrating it with previous knowledge, deciding what course of behavior it dictates; and pursuing a course of action...."[2] Factors involved in these processes may be in or out of awareness.

Developing awareness of oneself as an individual who carries out these processes involves identification and description of certain information—data an individual gets from inner and outer sources; his body of knowledge; the meaning which he attaches to it; what he plans to do; and what he actually does about it. In essence, awareness of oneself in this sense is focused on such questions as: What is (or was) going on within me? What is going on outside me? What do I know about all this? What does this mean? What am I going to do? What am I doing?

Another use of the term "self," as discussed by Hall and Lindzey, refers to what an individual thinks of himself, which ". . . denotes the person's attitudes, feelings, perceptions, and evaluations of himself as an object."[3] The meaning in this sense is referred to as "self as object."

Coleman states that "self as object" refers to one's self-image. He described this image as comprising three areas—self-ideal, self-evaluation and self-identity.

An individual's self-ideal encompasses his aspirations for growth and accomplishment and includes his assumptions of what is desirable and what he should be able to achieve or become. A sense of identity involves the individual's ideas of what he is really like. Part of the individual's sense of identity is derived from the different roles which he plays. The roles may be integrated into a master role, which contributes to the individual's stable sense of identity. On the other hand, an individual may show certain characteristics, abilities, attitudes and feelings in one role and not demonstrate these in another. A sense of worth and adequacy (or unworthiness and inadequacy) evolves from a person's experiences, beginning with appraisals from others in early relationships.[4]

Development of awareness of self in this sense would involve a compilation of many thoughts and feelings one has about himself. Awareness of "self as object" focuses on such questions as: Who am I? What am I like? What do I think about myself? How do I feel about myself? How do I value myself? What would I like to be? What do I want for myself? In this respect each individual is the only person who has access to the many thoughts and feelings he holds about himself.

Awareness of aspects of "self" using both meanings, "self as process" and "self as object," is important in the performance of nursing services. The nurse needs to be able to describe what she is experiencing or what she has experienced, what meaning she gives to these experiences and how she reacts (aspects of "self as process"). She also needs to know how she assesses herself as a person and in the professional role—as a provider of service (aspects of "self as object").

Following is a schema for use by the nursing student to develop awareness of herself. The specific goals are to help the student to identify, describe and compare data about herself and external events and to reach logical conclusions based on the comparison of these data. These goals may be approached in a systematic, developmental sequence. The steps of the proposed sequential schema are:

A. Self as Process—Collection and Comparison of Data.
    Step 1 Collection of data about self including:
        a. Data from inner sources about "internal events"—thoughts, feelings, expectations, wishes or wants, needs.
        b. Data regarding own actions.
        c. Data describing external events and their situational context.
    Step 2 Identification of similarities and differences in the data collected as they occur in similar and in different situational contexts.
    Step 3 Identification of compatibilities and incongruities in the data collected.
B. Self as Object—Collection and Comparison of Data.
C. Collection of Information from Others—Comparison with Data Previously Identified.

A basic assumption is that, using this schema, development of awareness of self should begin with self-identified and classified data and only later include collection of data about the self from others. That is, it is essential that the nursing student first gather, organize and compare her own data rather than be the passive recipient of statements or interpretations from others. If the student were to rely repeatedly upon such comments by others, she would be less likely to develop the ability to collect, examine and question data about herself. In nursing situations, a student might be given an appraisal of her performance so that she might effect an immediate behavior change or for other reasons. However, for the student's learning to be developmental, the student must be involved in the learning process and be an active participant in gathering and comparing data.

The student is the only person who has access to data from sources inside herself—her thoughts, feelings, needs, expectations, wishes. Other persons can observe, identify and describe her actions and verbal statements, but beyond this they can only make inferences as to their subjective origin. The manner in which the student identifies these data may not be consistent with inferences others may make about her, based on their observations.

Each individual has some degree of awareness of self, although of course complete awareness of self is never achieved. The usefulness of the nurse's self-awareness depends upon its extent, its accuracy and (because the self is both constant and changing) her predisposition to continue exploring facets of herself. The schema has two basic purposes: (1) to help the nursing student obtain a *beginning* awareness of self, using the term "beginning" to refer to basic or fundamental requisites which are believed to be essential, and (2) to provide a foundation for the student which will prepare her to develop further awareness of herself and which will promote within her predisposition to make continuous inquiry about herself. The limits of the schema can be stated by pointing out that it does not include exploring the appropriateness of a course of action, making general interpretations, or evaluating significance of the data and determining causation or possible motivating factors involved. Development of further awareness of self in nursing would include these areas.

A. Self as Process—Collection and Comparison of Data
   Step 1 Collection of data about self

"Internal events" may be categorized into thoughts, feelings, expectations, wishes, and needs, which are concomitants of every experience. Students vary in their ability to identify and describe data about their own "internal events." Frequently they make only a partial inventory of their internal events and have not learned to search for additional information in each of these categories. Also, the ability to distinguish between categories may be lacking. Though they talk freely about thoughts, feelings, wishes and needs, their statements frequently indicate an interchangeable use of these terms.

One student related the following account of her interaction with a patient.

As I left the room I had an odd feeling that he reminded me of someone—his reactions as well as physical appearance (way in which his eyes and mouth drooped, etc.). I realized that this feeling I was getting from him was quite

288 Development of Awareness of Self

similar to the one I got from Mrs. C., my first patient who had been in the hospital with the same symptoms.

As the morning progressed, this feeling of mine became quite pronounced and as we were conversing on a common subject—traveling—I realized that I was actually getting bored and rather tired. I found it hard to continue on the subject. After a while I realized I was looking out the window quite often, whether to keep myself from looking at him and becoming bored by the expressions he presented, or whether it was merely that I was distracted—I don't know. . . . I felt that the whole conversation was one way—I was asking too many questions.

The student's statements about her internal events are general, sketchy and ambiguous. The student did not discriminate between thoughts and feelings nor distinguish different kinds of feelings from one another. She uses the words "felt" and "feeling" to refer to a unique perception and an opinion. She acknowledges getting bored (an emotional reaction) and tired (a physical state).

Repeated opportunities to identify, describe and elaborate on "feelings" can enable students to distinguish between feelings and other internal events, as well as between different kinds of feelings, and to gather information about the duration and intensity of their feelings. This also applies to the category of "thoughts," which can be subclassified into various kinds such as: ideas based on fact; beliefs or opinions based on values; and tentative hypotheses, each of which have different functions in the cognitive process.

Another example of subclassifications which should be made within each category of internal events is illustrated by the following account:

Another thing that was interesting in caring for Miss M. was that the doctor had written "encourage patient to take part in group activities," so I expected myself to encourage her to do this, and I expected her to want to do things in groups. When she didn't want to do these things, I felt at several different times that I could only do so much to encourage her, so why not face it—if she doesn't want to, her feelings require respect, not the attitude of "you're not doing what the doctor wants." It could be easy to assume that it was my not doing a good job when she wouldn't want to do things, so I would feel inadequate, but it also must be necessary to take into consideration that the patient wouldn't want to do what we asked of her because of the nature of her problem.

This account illustrates various kinds of expectations. The student writes of expectations of herself and of the patient, and alludes to what she thinks the doctor expects of her.

Collection of data about "self as process" should include not only internal events, but the individual's perception of his own actions and the external environment in which they occur. One method of learning to collect these data is by the student's identifying her "internal events," her actions and perceptions of the environment in a situational context. Systematic collection of all the above kinds of data may be facilitated by the use of a series of questions designed to extend the student's inquiry and bring out additional information. The purposes of the questions are two-fold: to help the student think further about what has occurred or what is occurring within her, and, through this redirection, to help her learn to extend her exploration and make continuous inquiry about various facets of herself.

The following illustration provides examples of questions which might be used. In some instances, only a few questions may suffice. Discretion is necessary to determine the amount of exploration which can be profitably pursued at any given time. Development of awareness of various facets of self requires a period of time and many opportunities to make repeated explorations about oneself.

Student's account	Sample questions
As I left the room I had an odd feeling	What happened before this? What was the feeling? Describe it. What other name might you call it?
that he reminded me of someone—his reactions as well as physical appearance (way in which his eyes and mouth drooped, etc.).	What were his reactions? Anything else about his physical appearance?
I realized that this feeling I was getting from him	Who had the feeling? What was it? Describe it in another way. What else can you tell about it? In what way did you get the feeling?
was quite similar to the one I got from Mrs. C., my first patient who had been in the hospital with the same symptoms . . .	Tell about Mrs. C. What were her symptoms? What else can you say about her? What symptoms were the same as your first patient's? What things about her were different?

As the morning progressed,	What happened? What were you doing? What was the patient doing? What were you thinking? What were you expecting?
this feeling of mine became quite pronounced and	In what way did it become pronounced? What can you say about the degree of intensity? Anything else you can say about the feeling? What other feelings did you have at this time? What were you thinking?
as we were conversing on a common subject—	What was said? Who said it? How was it said? What did you do? What else was happening?
traveling—I realized I was actually getting bored and rather tired.	Elaborate about getting bored. In what way were you tired? What was happening when you realized this? What else were you feeling? What else were you thinking? What expectations did you have of the patient? What expectations did you have of yourself?
I found it hard to continue on the subject.	What did you do? What had you been doing before? In what way was it hard? What were you thinking?
After a while I realized I was looking out the window quite often, whether to keep	What else were you doing? What was the patient doing? What were you thinking? What were you feeling? What did you think about yourself sitting there looking out the window? What did you expect of yourself?
myself from looking at him and becoming bored by the expressions he presented	What did he do? What were his expressions? What did you think about them? How did you feel about them? What were your expectations of the patient?

or whether it was merely that I was distracted—I don't know.	In what way might you have been distracted? What else was going on? What were you thinking about? What did you want to do? What did you think you ought to do?
I felt the whole conversation was one way—I was asking too many questions.	Elaborate about this. What kinds of statements are you making? In what category would they belong? What questions were you asking? What happened?

The repeated use of such questions for purposes of refocusing and obtaining further information can help the student learn to search more systematically and diligently for the variety of thoughts, feelings, expectations, wishes and needs which may exist simultaneously. This exploration can contribute to the student's appreciation that "internal events" belong uniquely to her and can decrease the tendency to attribute these to others. Retrospect not only will help the student to identify more fully what she has experienced, but also will tend to heighten awareness of what she is actually experiencing at the time.

Step 2 Identification of similarities and differences in the data collected

The student may be helped to use the data systematically by identifying similarities and differences in her internal events and actions as they occur in similar or different situational contexts. For example, one student noted that she had a consistant reaction to similar situational contexts:

When I entered the patient's room I was apprehensive, as I am when entering the room of any patient I have not met before.

The systematic identification of similarities of her own internal events and actions in various situational contexts provides the student with an opportunity to identify some of her recurring basic reactions, patterns or themes which remain stable to some degree. Similarly, the identification of differences in her own internal events and actions provides the student with an opportunity to explore these differences and examine the situational contexts in which they occur.

292 *Development of Awareness of Self*

In the following account a student noted differences in her own feelings and actions in two situations, both involving patient observation:

I found from this experience that it is not as easy (for me) as I thought it would be to observe the patient outside the hospital. I thought it would be easier than in the hospital setting. I found that since this is outside the hospital it is a more relaxed atmosphere. I became more relaxed and most likely not as observant as in the hospital setting. Also, I found myself at times meeting my own needs (although I was not aware at the time) rather than the patient's needs. The fact that the patient became more relaxed (in speech and actions) I'm sure influenced my relaxation. And in this relaxation I tended to become less observant. I think that I could come to be more aware of meeting the patient's needs before mine if I were in more situations like this.

She notes two variables (the nursing setting and the patient's behavior) and reaches a conclusion that these variables influenced her feelings and actions. However, the reader will note that statements about what actually happened are missing. It is not uncommon for nursing students to reach conclusions about themselves based on inadequate and sometimes inaccurate data. If the student were to go back and fill in the missing data, as outlined in Step 1, she might or might not come to the same conclusions.

A student might be helped to make these comparisons more systematically and objectively by use of the method presented above. The following illustration demonstrates how the student might be helped to search for and identify the data and note the similarities and difference in her internal events and actions before she reached conclusions.

Student's account

I found from this experience that it is not as easy (for me) as I thought it would be to observe the patient outside the hospital.

I thought it would be easier than in the hospital setting.

Sample questions

(This is the conclusion which the student has reached about her performance.)

What about observing the patient outside the hospital did you think would be easier than in the hospital setting? What were your expectations of yourself in the hospital setting? What were your expectations of yourself outside the hospital?

Development of Awareness of Self 293

I found that since this is outside the hospital it is a more relaxed atmosphere.	What about the atmosphere seemed more relaxed to you? In what way was this evident? What else can you say about what was going on?
I became more relaxed	In what way did you become more relaxed? What else did you do? What were you thinking? What were you feeling?
and most likely not as observant as in the hospital setting.	What did you observe in the hospital setting? How did you make these observations? What did you observe outside the hospital? How did you make these observations? What observations did you make in the hospital setting which you did not make on the outside? What observations did you make outside the hospital setting that you did not make inside? What else can you say about your observations?
Also, I found myself at times meeting my own needs (although I was not aware at the time) rather than the patient's needs.	What were your own needs? How did you meet them? When did you become aware you were meeting your own needs? What was happening at that time? What were the patient's needs? Which of the patient's needs did you not meet? What are your expectations of yourself in meeting the patient's needs?
The fact that the patient became more relaxed	In what ways did the patient become more relaxed? Describe the patient's speech and actions. What did the patient say? How did he say it? What else can you say about the patient?

(in speech and actions) I'm sure influenced my relaxation.

And in this relaxation I tended to become less observant.

How did you feel before you noted that the patient was more relaxed? What was happening at the time you became more relaxed?

What did you do? What were you thinking? What were you feeling? What were your expectations of yourself? What were your expectations of the patient? What were your expectations of yourself and the patient in the hospital setting? In what way were you less observant? When did you become aware of this thought?

Compare your
   thoughts
   feelings
   expectations of yourself
   expectations of the patient
   needs
   own actions
   patient's actions
in the hospital setting and outside the hospital setting. What conclusions can you reach by making these comparisons?

I think that I could come to be more aware of meeting the patient's needs before mine if I were in more situations like this.

(Student's prediction of own future behavior under similar circumstances.)

Most of the questions are similar to those used in Step 1. Step 2 illustrates the importance of the student gathering sufficient data before she attempts to make comparisons or reach conclusions.

    Step 3 Identification of compatibilities and incongruities in the data collected

Further use of the data collected by the student in promoting awareness of self would be the identification of compatibilities or inconsistencies of her internal events with her actions and with reality.

One student noted inconsistency between what she thought and what she did:

Helping oneself is very important in the hospital setting. I get the urge to do everything for the patient, when actually the patient can do and should do a lot for his self care. My actions impede his progress and the staff's objectives. I am working on this factor.

The student states a belief about patient care and notes that this is not compatible with what she has the "urge" to do and with the outcome of her actions. She implies that she is attempting to change her behavior.

Festinger writes that the individual strives for consistency within himself—for harmony between what he thinks, believes, and does. However, the occurrence of inconsistencies or incongruities is common and almost inevitable. Festinger has coined the term "cognitive dissonance" to refer to the existence of non-fitting relations among cognitions, using "cognition" to mean any idea or belief about oneself, one's behavior and the environment.[5]

The first basic hypothesis of the theory of cognitive dissonance is: "The existence of dissonance, being psychologically uncomfortable, will motivate the person to try to reduce the dissonance and achieve consonance."[6]

Festinger writes further that pressures to reduce the dissonance and achieve consonance result in certain activities, including behavior changes, changes of cognition and exposure to new information and opinions.[7] In the student's account given above, her statement "I am working on this factor" illustrates an attempt of reduction of dissonance through behavior change.

Festinger also states that the most important determinant of cognitive content is reality, for when cognitive elements deviate from reality, ". . . *the reality which impinges on a person will exert pressures in the direction of bringing the appropriate cognitive elements into correspondence with that reality.*"[8] (author's italics)

In the following account, the student notes an inconsistency between her own thinking and reality.

I was assigned to Mr. F. The thought made me kind of nervous. I wondered what would be the patient's reactions to me—and my reactions to him on a more personal basis. It was a simple case of personality conflict. I had fostered a dislike for the very boisterous, overly he-man, intrusive type of personality. Previously I had sometimes dodged Mr. F., purposely telling myself that he didn't really like me. But after weighing these feelings I concluded that this was a projection, for I had no grounds at all for such a feeling. Mr. F. reacted to me as affirmatively as many others.

The student stated that she had dodged Mr. F., thinking that the patient didn't like her, but she noted that the patient reacted in a way that was not consistent with this thought (cognitive element inconsistent with reality). At this point the student was able to reach the conclusion that the dislike was coming from herself (change of cognitive element to correspond with reality).

Festinger's second basic hypothesis is:

When dissonance is present, in addition to trying to reduce it, the person will actively avoid situations and information which would likely increase the dissonance.9

The following excerpts from a student's account of her interaction with a patient and his wife illustrate this:

As I thought over the interaction with the patient, I felt that I should concentrate more on listening rather than getting my ideas in when he was talking. I think that if I concentrate on listening more and talking less, he will have a chance to say what he wants, using his own words rather than agreeing with my comments. I was quite satisfied with the way this visit went—I feel we got to know each other fairly well, and I hope the next time we visit he will feel as free to talk to me as he did at the close of the interaction.

The following incidents were related by the same student in subsequent interaction with the patient and his wife.

Student: Well, how are you?
Patient: If everything goes well, I can go home next Thursday. They plan to take out the stitches on Wednesday. (Explanatory note: the patient had not had the operation yet.)
S.: That's not too bad, is it?
P.: Well . . .
Patient's wife: It's not as long as last time is it?
P.: I think so. It was about 8 days; yeah, this is about seven days. (To student) Where will you go when you finish your assignment here?

(Patient's wife and student were talking alone.)
P's. wife: He's kind of worried about the operation.
S.: That's quite normal. Everyone is somewhat concerned when he is going to have surgery.
P's. wife: The doctor said it would be about an hour. He'll go up about 9 a.m.
S.: Uh huh. Yes, an hour sounds about right. (Here I think I should have explained to her about the recovery room—that he would be in there for a while afterward—but I was thinking at the time with a spinal he wouldn't go to the recovery room.)
P's. wife: It'll be only about an hour, so he should be okay. (She was definitely concerned and wanted reassurance—and perhaps when she expressed that he was concerned she was really meaning that *she* was concerned.)

The student wrote these remarks about the incidents:

I didn't get the feeling that they were dreading it (the operation), except for Mr. K. and the anesthetic. I think that it was convenient that the prep nurse came in and I had a chance to talk with Mrs. K. She had a lot of things on her mind and I think that by talking to someone other than her husband or a close friend, she was able to say some things which she might not otherwise have been able to verbalize.

The student did not give any indication that the incidents she related were additional examples illustrating her comment that she should concentrate on listening more and talking less, allowing the patient a chance to say what he wants. Though the student did not avoid reporting these situations, she did not see their pertinence to her former comments, which would have highlighted the dissonance or inconsistency between what she thought she ought to do and what she actually did.

It is not uncommon for students to lack awareness of incongruities (or dissonances) about themselves in situations. These incongruities can be made more obvious through questions focusing on the data bearing the incongruities. Following the above account, the student could be questioned regarding her expectations of herself and her assessment of what happened. For example:

You have said that you believe you should concentrate more on listening than getting your own ideas across to the patient. How do you think it went when you were talking with the patient and his wife about his stitches? How do you think this went when you were talking with the patient's wife?

The above questions do not reveal the discrepancy, but by their refocus give the student the opportunity to discover it. The student still may not note the inconsistency. If this occurs, questions focusing on the student's statements and what actually happened (the inconsistent data) would be appropriate. Examples of such questions are:

You have said that you believe you should concentrate more on listening than getting your own ideas across to the patient. What did you do when the patient said, "They plan to take out the stitches on Wednesday?"

or:

You have said that if you concentrate on listening more and talking less, the patient will have a chance to say what he wants, using his own words rather than agreeing with your comments. When the patient said, "They plan to take out the stitches on Wednesday," you replied, "That's not too bad, is it?" Do you think this statement is consistent with what you thought you should do? What did happen in response to your statement?

B. Self as Object—Collection and Comparison of Data

The development of awareness of "self as object" can be promoted in a way similar to that outlined above—through the collection of data and identification of compatibilities or incongruities in the data. Students might be asked a series of questions which would help them explore various ideas and attitudes which they have about their self-identity, self-evaluation and self-ideal. Such questions might be focused on a particular role. For example:

As a nursing student . . . . .
   (or as a professional person . . . ; as a member of a family . . . ; as a person . . .)
   What am I like? What characteristics do I have? What do I think about myself?
   How do I feel about myself? How do I value what I am doing?
   What do I want to be? What is important for me to accomplish?

A comparison of data from each of these questions would enable the student to identify the harmony and consistency (or lack of it) in her comments about herself.

In the following account a student makes comments about her past performance, self-evaluation and self-ideal as a nursing student:

Though I know I have improved over last semester I am not satisfied with my work. I feel I am capable of doing better work. I should be able to offer my patients complete nursing care to the fullest extent of my knowledge. This is impossible to attain when I feel I am not working to my full potential.

Ideally, the individual develops aspirations and goals which are compatible with his abilities, interests and opportunities. However, when his aspirations have little relationship to how he presently views himself, feelings of frustration and failure can result. In addition, feelings of worth and adequacy are more closely related to one's ideas about himself than one's actual achievement.[10] The student's comments indicate both frustration and a lack of satisfaction with her performance in the nursing role.

If the student were to be more explicit about her aspirations and goals, she would then be able to determine if her goals are reasonably attainable—within a specified time span. A more inclusive description of what she thinks she is really like in the student role might afford her the opportunity to recognize that she has met some of her goals in various ways.

An accurate appraisal of one's capabilities and limitations is important to the integration and harmony of one's own self-identity, self-evaluation and self-ideal. Limitations and inabilities do not necessarily incapacitate an individual or reduce his worth as a human being.[11]

   C. Collection of Information from Others—Comparison with Data Previously Identified

In this phase of the schema the student may be encouraged to explore a variety of sources which might provide further data about herself. In addition to seeking observations, ideas and opinions from others, she might review a video tape or tape recording of a situation in which she participated. Comparisons of feedback with the student's original data may show areas of validation or lack of it and stimulate the student to extend her inquiry.

REFERENCES

1. Hall, C. S., and Lindzey, G.: Theories of Personality. p. 468. New York, John Wiley & Sons, 1957.
2. Coleman, J. C.: Personality Dynamics and Effective Behavior. pp. 66-67. Chicago, Scott, Foresman & Co., 1960.
3. Hall, C. S., and Lindzey, G., *loc. cit.*
4. Coleman, J. C., *op. cit.,* pp. 63-66.
5. Festinger, L.: A Theory of Cognitive Dissonance. pp. 1-9. Evanston, Ill., Row, Peterson & Co., 1957.
6. *Ibid.,* p. 3.
7. *Ibid.,* p. 31.
8. *Ibid.,* p. 11.
9. *Ibid.,* p. 3.
10. Coleman, J. C., *op. cit.,* pp. 65-66.
11. *Ibid.,* p. 297.

BIBLIOGRAPHY

Bermosk, L. S., and Mordan, M. J.: Interviewing in Nursing. New York, Macmillan, 1964.

Coleman, J. C.: Personality Dynamics and Effective Behavior. Chicago, Scott, Foresman & Co., 1960.

Festinger, L.: A Theory of Cognitive Dissonance. Evanston, Ill., Row, Peterson & Co., 1957.

Hall, C. S., and Lindzey, G.: Theories of Personality. New York, John Wiley & Sons, 1957.

Jersild, A. T.: In Search of Self. New York, Teachers College, Columbia University, 1952.

Jourard, S. M.: Personal Adjustment. 2 ed. New York, Macmillan, 1963.

Moustakas, C. E.: True experience and the self. *In* Moustakas, C. (ed.): The Self. pp. 3-14. New York, Harper & Brothers, 1956.

Murray, J. B.: Self-knowledge and the nursing interview. Nurs. Forum, 2:69-78, 1963.

Peplau, H. E.: Process and concept of learning. *In* Burd, S. F., and Marshall, M. A. (eds.): Some Clinical Approaches to Psychiatric Nursing. pp. 333-336. New York, Macmillan, 1963.

Symonds, P. M.: The Ego and the Self. New York, Appleton-Century-Crofts, 1951.

Taba, H., and Hills, J. L.: Teacher Handbook for Contra Costa Social Studies Grades 1-6. Hayward, California, Rapid Printers & Lithographers, 1965.

Travelbee, J.: Interpersonal Aspects of Nursing. Philadelphia, F. A. Davis, 1966.

16

The Process of Role Change

Lucile L. Love

In nursing, as in all other creative aspects of life, the process is dynamic and presents ceaseless and often bewildering changes. Although the nursing profession is armed with a rich and varied backlog of knowledge and experience, its future is unpredictable. Nurses must necessarily adjust to situations for which no precedents have been established, no rules exist, and no laws have been written. This process of change outmodes many old and established practices and renders the present merely a period of transition. In the search for an understanding of successful ways of adjusting to the process of role change in nursing, examples can be found in the general approach to role theory.

The general idea of "role"—as the term is used by social psychologists—is borrowed from the drama. However, when the actors in a play portray a character, their performance is determined by the script, instructions from the director, the performances of fellow actors, and the reactions of the audience. In real life, each individual occupies a position, but his role performance in this position is determined by social norms, demands, and rules; by the role performance of others in their own positions; by those who observe and react to the performance; by the individual's particular capabilities and personality; and by role models. The social "script" may be as constrictive as that of a play, but frequently it does allow more options: the "director" is often present in real life as a supervisor, teacher, parent, or coach; the "audience" in real life consists of all those who observe the position member's behavior; the position member's "performance in life," as in the play, is attributable to his familiarity with the "part," his personality and personal history in general, and, more significantly, to the "script" which others have defined. In essence, performance of a role results from the social prescriptions and behavior of others, and individual variations that occur are expressed within the framework created by these factors.[1]

Although role theory is a relatively new concept, its intent is to provide understanding, prediction, and control of the particular phenomena involved in its domain of study. In real life, these phenomena are observable in behavior during genuine, on-going social situations.[2]

The concept of role theory has become more and more important because it provides a framework for a study of the ways in which a society or subculture (in this particular instance the nursing profession) transmits to the novice the group prescriptions for the behavior patterns appropriate to positions or status recognized and accepted within the structure of the society.[3]

The process by which culture and its norms are transmitted is known as socialization. Through this process the individual acquires attitudes, values, discipline, aspirations and ambitions; assumes new and different roles; and learns the skills required in these roles. Socialization is a dynamic process which has a beginning but no end.[4]

Because the process of role development is an orderly one, and can be structured, the concept of role change is an especially useful tool in the socialization process of the nursing student. To facilitate this role change, both teacher and learner can benefit from such knowledge, since it is mainly through daily interpersonal relationships that a person's behavior is learned. A knowledge of role theory and the process of role development is helpful in the teaching-learning process because it enables both teacher and learner to: (1) understand how and what is influencing their behavior; (2) evaluate their relationships with others (e.g., patients); and, (3) learn on a reciprocal basis the nature of role conflicts, role confusion, and other indications of dissensus.

The disciplines of psychology, sociology and anthropology have made contributions to the concept of role theory, but social psychology has contributed most toward its actual development. This mixture may account for the impression of disorder and lack of systematization in the theory.

At the present time, the language of role theory still lacks clarity: one term may refer to more than one concept, while even the technical meaning is not always exact. For this reason, the following terms have been assigned stated definitions throughout this paper:

Role: A constellation of behaviors that emerge out of an interaction between self and others, that constitute a meaningful unit and are a consistent expression of the sentiments, values and/or goals that govern or provide direction for that interaction.[5]

Status: A position in a particular social pattern or hierarchy.[6]

Position: Often called status, referring to a place occupied at a given time.[7]

Role Conception: The actor's understanding of the norms appropriate to a particular circumstance. Role conception varies with: (1) social class differences; (2) differences in occupational specialization; (3) regional or subcultural differences, and (4) different positions occupied by the actor.[8]

Role Congruency: A situation in which the incumbent perceives that the same or highly similar expectations are held for him.[9]

Role Conflict: A situation in which the incumbent of a focal position perceives that he is confronted with incompatible expectations.[10]

Role Model: A person playing a role whose organization of attitudes, behaviors, and values are considered a standard of excellence to be imitated.[11,12]

Role Play: An experimental procedure; a method of learning to perform roles more adequately (e.g., social interaction).[13]

Role Taking: Imaginatively assuming the position and point of view of another.[14]

Role Validation: Role performance about which there is agreement and which is based on principles that can withstand criticism or objection.[15,16]

Role Consensus: Role performance about which there is agreement based on the degree of similarity on given behaviors. There may be consensus of behaviors within such specific areas as prescription, evaluation, description or sanction of the role, according to which is being analyzed.[17]

Role Dissensus: Dissent or disagreement of the role performance (behaviors). This may take two forms: (1) polarized, in which there is no agreement, or (2) nonpolarized, in which all possible areas are in about equal disagreement (e.g., prescription, description, evaluation, or sanction). Sometimes called "role conflict" or "norm conflict."[18]

Role Rejection: Refusal to play a role or to accede to a role.[19,20]

Role Failure: Role performance in which the overt behavior was not carried out or prescribed emotions were not experienced.[21]

Role Ambivalence: Conflicting feelings about the role play.[22]

Role Confusion: Role performance in which the actor becomes disorganized, bewildered, embarrassed or chaotic in the social interaction.[23]

Role Repertoire: The entire range of roles employable by the participant—which may range from zero to a wide variety of alternative behaviors.[24]

Referent Groups: The group, real or imagined, whose standpoint is being used as a frame of reference by the actor.[25]

Social Forces: The community or national norms which offer a system of rewards or punishment (e.g., the law, social structure, social movements. etc.).[26]

Interpenetration: Penetration of each other (i.e., ego and alter).[27]

Ego: The self.[28]

Alter: The other.[29]

Roles define mutual, reciprocal, or complementary relationships, and indicate the position of the self (ego) and the other person or group (alter) in such relationships. A variety of roles (role repertoire) is known to and employed by most people, and these roles act as guides to action in both social and occupational situations.

Roles become defined in the course of group activities and interactions. The definition and the role responses that they call for are part of the learning patterns of group members; they become, in other words, part of the tradition, and are then passed on to new members of the group.[30]

All societies devote a great deal of time and energy to training the younger members of the group to interact in various situations. However, roles differ greatly: some are ritualistic and inflexible while others have broad limits. Roles in nursing run the gamut, and the socialization of the student to the projected professional status and roles in nursing is extremely complex and challenging.

The process of role theory can be analyzed. Roles can be anticipated; they can be evaluated either before or after any given interaction. There are logical, systematic steps which are operative in the socialization process (role change). The steps involved in the process of role change are presented graphically in the accompanying paradigm (see Fig. 16-1)

What is the socialization process? The stages of socialization of the student are role prescription, role taking, role playing, internalization, and evaluation (role validation). Because roles are constantly changing, the process is a continuous and open-ended one, proceeding from level to level in an inverse pyramidal structure.[31] For example, a person wishes to become a nurse, at which time a wide base of nursing roles are prescribed: the student interacts with her peers, instructors, and other members of the profession by role playing

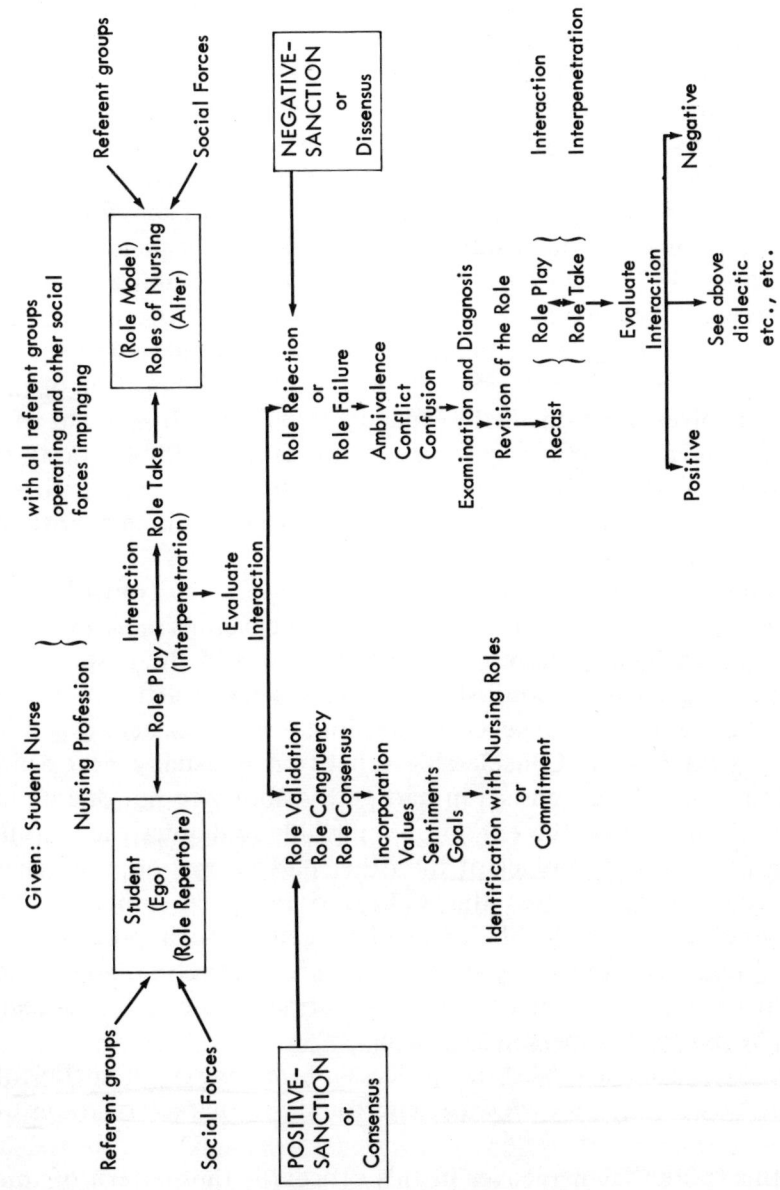

DIALECTIC OF PERSONAL GROWTH IN ADULT SOCIALIZATION

Fig. 16-1.

(ego) and role taking (alter). She validates her role with each and all of the groups whose behavior and attitudes impinge on the professionalization process. At each step of this process she either internalizes (i.e., incorporates or identifies) certain aspects of the prescribed role, or she does not. What has been internalized becomes a part of her repertoire of roles and is a value to which she becomes committed. The pyramid begins to grow as the process is repeated. Since there is a body of formal and informal knowledge and skills to be acquired, and role conception is necessary, this process will be repeated many times before acquisition of the desired behavior.

How does the capacity for role playing and role taking develop? Role playing is dependent on many things other than the acquisition of a body of knowledge. Equally important is the development of self-awareness. Self-concept consists of more than delineation of the body; it involves the individual's capacity to see himself as a part of a social system—a system recognizing a set of claims and obligations. It is control over one's conduct, and the ability to locate himself within the interpersonal and cultural matrices into which he is cast, both as an actor and a recipient of acts.[32]

In today's subtle and complex society, learning to control one's conduct and to interact in the prescribed role develops more gradually and is considerably more difficult than it was in the past, and is often characterized by confusion between what is attributable to oneself (ego) and those aspects of the situation which belong to the outside world (alter). Considerable repetition is usually necessary. Successful role taking consists in part of the ability to put oneself in the role of another to the extent of being able to deduce the accompanying feelings and motives of the other person or group. In other words, role taking involves the ability to recognize other human beings as objects capable of independent action, to appreciate the range of responses they may display in a given situation, and to be prepared to respond to an affirmative situation. These processes constitute the dialectic of personal growth.

Learning a role involves the process of moving with sufficient freedom between one's own experiences and the characterizations of others.

Another potential maneuver in this process is the pattern of role play—role take—evaluate—recast. This may be necessary when alter either refuses to assume his role or does not understand it. One example might be the case of a young student who assumes the role of nurse with a 45-year-old male patient who assumes, at the outset, the role of father. In time, the patient may be persuaded to accept the patient role instead of the father role, although the operation may have to be repeated many times before the desired role is achieved. Most often in role taking and recasting, alter responds to intentions. However, when role taking, it is well to evaluate ego simultaneously to make certain that there is no discrepancy between overt behavior and inner disposition in both actors.[33]

Since roles define mutual relationships, they indicate the identity of ego and alter. Difficulties in learning roles occur when students are exposed to: (1) contradictions, (2) too many constraints, (3) excessive flexibility, or when roles switch too rapidly.[34] For example, too many constraints interfere when the instructor allows the student little or no ego judgment in a situation and perceives role primarily as specific function. Contradiction occurs when role consensus is low or absent; excessive flexibility provides no guidelines by which the student may orient ego. Set limits are a necessary component in the socialization process. Furthermore, when the learner is introduced to a new role there should be sufficient time allowed for the experiential learning of the new role before being presented with another. And, of course, as a role is learned and internalized, commitment to that role increases. At the same time, new roles are more readily learned and the roles in the inverted pyramid grow and are simultaneously reinforced.

Initially, students may be ambivalent about their roles. They start out being somebody (in this particular instance, the nurse), for an hour or so, and then step out of the nursing role. They may then revert to a variety of previously learned social roles. Being unable to remain in the present or live up to the prescribed role of nurse, they relinquish what they held of the role at a given moment. At this point the student and instructor may find it necessary to trace the dialectic of personal growth repeatedly in order to pinpoint the problem involved, in order that possible solutions to the ambivalence may be identified and implemented.[35] The nursing profession and—more specifically—the nurse instructor, expect that the student will be socialized into the nursing role. But at the same time, both may place obstacles in the path prescribed (e.g., constraints, contradictions, excessive flexibility, too rapid switching of roles), and they may fail to explore the dialectic of personal growth as a process of negotiating solutions to the problems created.[36] In such a situation long and delicate negotiations between the actors may be required.

In order to accomplish the socializing process of the nursing student with the least possible confusion to the learner, the profession's own collective values, sentiments, and goals must be consensually validated in order to erase or minimize the conflicting messages that we as professionals and role models present. The school of nursing is, of course, only one part of the total institutional complex which makes up professional nursing, but it is the agency primarily responsible for the transmission of the "culture" of nursing.

A few examples may explain how the framework of role theory and role change enhances the understanding of the socialization process of the individual.

While administering medications to a patient, a student discovered that an error had been made repeatedly by the staff nurses. She reported her discovery to the head nurse, who thanked her for observing and reporting the error. The student was, however, bewildered because the head nurse's concern was about the possibility of a suit, not the patient's welfare, and the records were changed to hide the errors. The student's behavior was given positive sanction, but she experienced conflict over concealment of the errors. This behavior was not congruent with the standards of excellence expected of the role model, and consequently the role model was rejected.

Examples of role conflict and failure may be found in situations where roles are not clearly prescribed, described or sanctioned.

One student was assigned the role of team leader, and was required to make the assignment for the team and discuss it with the head nurse. The student herself assigned all the medications and treatments, and the role model (the head nurse) gave no information or direction to the student. By mid-morning the student became aware that she had spent so much time performing tasks that she could not function as team leader. The student felt acutely uncomfortable because she could not make nursing rounds to give assistance or guidance to the team members. Both role model and student had allowed impossible and conflicting expectations to be established.

Positive sanction can be demonstrated by the experience of another student who was acting as team leader.

One of the team members, also a student, was caring for an 85-year-old woman and had taken an excessive amount of time giving her morning care. As a result the patient was virtually exhausted. The nursing instructor arrived and told the team member to get the patient up in a wheelchair. However, the team leader assessed the patient's immediate need for rest and explained why the patient should remain in bed. The team leader's evaluation of the situation was approved and accepted, and the team leader's role was thus validated in all four areas of prescription, description, evaluation and sanction.

In summary, the socialization process in the nursing profession begins with "givens": (1) the person who wishes to become a nurse, and (2) the nursing profession with all the attendant referent groups and other social forces which have impinged on them to this (given) moment in time. The novice enters a school of nursing where nursing roles are prescribed. In the dialectic of personal growth, roles are tried on by role taking and role playing with the referent groups of the student and the profession, the patient and other work groups on the team. As the student interacts with these individuals or groups, she is influenced—and influences—in her role performance. To the degree that there is interpenetration, socialization into nursing roles occurs. An evaluation of the interaction can confirm the extent of socialization.

A discussion of the evaluation process is another essay; in this paper it may be sufficient to say that the process serves to confirm or deny the extent to which a person is socialized, and those aspects of a role or roles that have been rejected by the learner. In socialization the student receives positive sanctions and there is role consensus with the profession. Within this framework there are role validation and role congruency, which the learner incorporates into her repertoire of roles as values, sentiments, and goals. To the extent that this process occurs, the learner then identifies with nursing roles and commitment occurs. In subsequent role performances this is reinforced.

Evaluation of the interaction may reveal that there are usually certain roles or aspects of certain roles that for one reason or another are rejected. Negative sanctions have, of course, the opposite effect of positive sanctions, at least to the extent that there may be dissensus in the role performance. As in most situations where there are expectations in opposition to each other or goals which have not or cannot be achieved, there is resultant ambivalence, conflict, and confusion. As these rejected aspects of nursing roles are explored and closely examined the problem may be pinpointed, a diagnosis made, and a new or revised role prescription made in an attempt to remedy the situation. The learner is then recast in the new role, and following interaction the evaluation process is again employed in order to assess the degree to which the revised or newly-prescribed role has been effective in the socialization process of the learner into nursing roles. This process is repeated over and over throughout life, and has been termed the dialectic of personal growth.

REFERENCES

1. Biddle, B. J., and Thomas, E. J.: The nature and history of role theory. *In* Role Theory: Concepts and Research. pp. 3-4. New York, John Wiley & Sons, 1966.
2. *Ibid.*, p. 17.
3. Moment, D., and Zaleznik, A.: Role Development and Interpersonal Competence. p. 15. Boston, Division of Research, Harvard Business School, 1963.
4. Folta, J., and Deck, E. S.: The venture: Sociological concepts. *In* A Sociological Framework for Patient Care. p. 13. New York, John Wiley & Sons, 1966.
5. Turner, R. H., as quoted by Hadley, B. J.: The dynamic interactionist concept of role. J. Nurs. Educ., 6, 2:5-6, April, 1967.
6. Linton, R.: Status and role. *In* Borgatta, E. F., and Meyer, H. J. (eds.): Sociological Theory: Present Day Sociology from the Past. p. 174. New York, Alfred A. Knopf, 1964.
7. *Ibid.*
8. Haas, J. E.: Role Conception and Group Consensus. Bureau of Business Research Monograph No. 117. pp. 3-4. Columbus, Bureau of Business Research, College of Commerce and Administration, The Ohio State University, 1964.
9. Gross, N., *et al.:* Explorations in Role Analysis. p. 248. New York, John Wiley & Sons, 1958.
10. *Ibid.*
11. Linton, R.: Status and Role. *In* Coser, L. A., and Rosenberg, B. (eds.): Sociological Readings. p. 359. New York, Macmillan, 1964.
12. Webster's New World Dictionary. p. 945. New York, World Publishing, 1958.
13. Biddle, B. J., and Thomas, E. J., quoting Jacob L. Moreno, *op. cit.*, p. 7.
14. *Ibid.*, p. 6.
15. *Ibid.*, pp. 6, 33.
16. Webster's New World Dictionary, *op. cit.*, p. 1608.
17. Biddle, B. J., and Thomas, E. J., *op. cit.*, p. 33.
18. *Ibid.*, pp. 33, 34.
19. *Ibid.*, p. 6.
20. Webster's New World Dictionary, *op. cit.*, p. 1226.
21. *Ibid.*, p. 521.

22. *Ibid.,* p. 46.
23. *Ibid.,* p. 308.
24. Biddle, B. J., and Thomas, E. J., *op. cit.,* p. 59.
25. *Ibid.,* pp. 47-49.
26. *Ibid.,* pp. 311-318, 325-326.
27. Webster's New World Dictionary, *op. cit.,* p. 746.
28. Biddle, B. J., and Thomas, E. J., *op. cit.,* pp. 10-24.
29. *Ibid.,*
30. Lindesmith, A. R., and Strauss, A. L. (eds.): Social Psychology. p. 375. New York, Dryden Press, 1957.
31. Merton, R. K., Broom, L., and Cottrell, L. S., Jr. (eds.): Sociology Today. p. 35. New York, Torchbooks, Harper & Row, 1959.
32. Shibutani, T.: Society and Personality. pp. 504-505. Englewood Cliffs, N.J., Prentice-Hall, 1961.
33. *Ibid.,* p. 506.
34. Jourard, S. M.: The Transparent Self. pp. 111-113. New York, Rheinhold Books, Van Nostrand, 1964.
35. Ruesch, J.: Therapeutic Communication. p. 431. New York, W. W. Norton & Co., 1961.
36. Shibutani, T., *op. cit.,* p. 519.

BIBLIOGRAPHY

Biddle, B. J., and Thomas, E. J.: The nature and history of role theory. *In* Role Theory: Concepts and Research. New York, John Wiley & Sons, 1966.

Borgatta, E. F., and Meyer, H. J.: Sociological Theory: Present-Day Sociology From the Past. New York, Alfred A. Knopf, 1961.

Coser, L. A., and Rosenberg, B. (eds.): Sociological Theory: A Book of Readings. 2 ed. New York, Macmillan, 1964.

Davis, K., and Scott, W. G.: Readings in Human Relations. 2 ed. New York, McGraw-Hill, 1964.

Elliott, M. A., and Merrill, F. E.: Social Disorganization. 4 ed. New York, Harper & Row, 1961.

Erikson, E. H.: Childhood and Society. Rev. New York, W. W. Norton & Co., 1968.

Gross, N., Mason, W. S., and McEachern, A. W.: Explorations in Role Analysis. New York, John Wiley & Sons, 1958.

Folta, J., and Deck, E. S.: The venture: Sociological concepts. *In* A Sociological Framework for Patient Care. New York, John Wiley & Sons, 1966.

Haas, J. E.: Role Conception and Group Consensus. Bureau of Business Research Monograph Number 117. Columbus, Bureau of Business Research, College of Commerce and Administration, The Ohio State University, 1964.

Hadley, M. J.: The dynamic interactionist concept of role. J. Nurs. Educ., 6, 2:5-10, 24-25, April, 1967.

Holmes, M. J., and Werner, J. A.: Psychiatric Nursing in a Therapeutic Community. New York, Macmillan, 1966.

Jerslid, A. T.: When Teachers Face Themselves. New York, Teachers' College Press, Columbia University, 1955.

Jourard, S. M.: The Transparent Self. New York, Rheinhold Books, Van Nostrand, 1964.

La Piere, R. T., and Farnsworth, P. R.: Social Psychology. 3 ed. New York, McGraw-Hill, 1949.

Lindesmith, A. R., and Strauss, A. L.: Social Psychology. ed. 2. New York, Dryden Press, 1957.

Linton, R.: The Cultural Background of Personality. New York, Appleton-Century-Crofts, 1945.

Mead, G. H.: George Herbert Mead on Social Psychology. Chicago, The University of Chicago Press, 1964.

Merton, R. K., Broom, L., and Cottrell, L. S. (eds.): Sociology Today. New York, Torchbooks, Harper & Row, 1959.

Milton, O., and Walker, R. G.: Behavior Disorders—Perspectives and Trends. 2 ed. Philadelphia, J. B. Lippincott, 1969.

Moment, D., and Zaleznik, A.: Role Development and Interpersonal Competence. Boston, Division of Research, Harvard Business School, 1963.

Munroe, R. L.: Schools of Psychoanalytic Thought. New York, Holt, Rinehart & Winston, 1955.

Parsons, T.: Essays in Sociological Theory. Rev. New York, The Free Press of Glencoe, 1954.

Parsons, T., Shils, E., Naegele, K. D., and Pitts, J. R.: Theories of Society: Foundations of Modern Sociological Theory. New York, The Free Press of Glencoe, 1961.

Ruesch, J.: Therapeutic Communication. New York, W. W. Norton & Co., 1961.

Rose, A. M.: Sociology—The Study of Human Relations. New York, Alfred A. Knopf, 1956.

Shibutani, T.: Society and Personality. Englewood Cliffs, N.J., Prentice-Hall, 1961.

Skipper, J. K., Jr., and Leonard, R. C.: Social Interaction and Patient Care. Philadelphia, J. B. Lippincott, 1965.

Taves, M. J., Corwin, R. C., and Haas, J. E.: Role Conception and Vocational Success. Bureau of Business Research Monograph No. 112. Columbus, Bureau of Business Research, College of Commerce and Administration, The Ohio State University, 1963.

Webster's New World Dictionary. New York, World Publishing, 1958.

17

Stigma

Betty Blackwell

In this article, I will present material from the literature on stigma (particularly that of Erving Goffman and Beatrice A. Wright), comment on relevant nursing literature, and suggest some implications for nursing education and intervention.

According to Goffman, a person is stigmatized when there is a difference between an expectation based on a value judgment of what that person or anyone with a similar social identity should be, and what he actually presents to other persons. Inherent in the assignment of stigma is a judgment that the social worth of the person is less than was anticipated. If his stigmatizing aspect is visually obvious or his personal history is available, he is termed "discredited." If his disability is not obtrusive, either by sensory or cognitive means, he is defined as "discreditable."

For instance, the Skid Row alcholic is discredited; the middle class alcoholic who continues to meet his role obligations is discreditable. The student who is caught cheating is discredited; the successful cheater is discreditable. The teen-age unwed mother who maintains her primary and secondary group relationships and continues her pregnancy to term is discredited; the teen-age unwed mother who interrupts the pregnancy before it becomes visible or who severs primary and secondary relationships prior to delivery is discreditable.

Goffman declares that the major assumption made in the response of normal persons to the stigmatized is that the stigmatized person is not human. On this assumption, normals develop a stigma theory to explain the stigmatized's inferiority and to account for his danger to the social structure. This process permits one to use words with negative emotional connotations such as "bastard," "cripple," and so

317

on. Gradually, a mythology evolves which imputes a "wide range of imperfections on the basis of the original one, and . . . some desirable but undesired attributes, often of a supernatural cast, such as 'sixth sense' or 'understanding'."[1]

This phenomenon is called expectation discrepancy by Beatrice Wright. She lists the following conditions underlying it: spread, position of the subject, requirements of mourning, wish for improvement, and blurring of perception owing to anxiety.[2]

Wright states that reconciling the discrepancies in expectation "may be accomplished by such cognitive changes as *expectation revision, altering the apparent reality* and *anormalizing the person.*"[3] In the last manuever, anormalizing the person, the laws that apply to normal persons are transcended.

> Anormalization that reconciles a discrepancy in which expectations are lower than the apparent reality leads to sanctification, but where the expectations surpass the apparent reality, anormalization leads to vilification.[4]

Wright, like Goffman, concedes that every human being experiences increased tension in situations that are perceptually unclear, unstructured or ambiguous. Both writers also hypothesize that the frequency of such encounters is greater for the disabled person, and that any of his social interactions may carry undertones of ambiguity or unanticipated behavioral response.

In discussing spread, Wright emphasizes the significance of physique in determining one's own and other's expectations regarding character and personality. Physique is seen as the central feature in the assessment of an individual. Deviations from normal, especially when the viewer considers physical perfection important—and few Americans are not imbued with the cult of youth, health and beauty—may cause the viewer to impute to the disabled a sensitivity to the needs of others. This sensitivity is presumed to arise out of suffering; a vocational capability is assumed to grow out of a handicap. Intelligence, or the lack of it, stems from a typical physical behavior, and so on. In short, the viewer may attribute all the disabled person's intrapersonal difficulties to his disability.

The disabled person's acceptance of such imputations may make him uncertain, in recurring social situations, as to whether he is being treated in a stereotyped fashion. His acceptance also may put into play all the dynamics of the self-fulfilling prophecy.

In addition to the features of this mythology that Goffman specified, I believe that others develop, such as the extreme beliefs about the inherent rights and value of the individual regardless of his social contribution. For example, many in our society favor the maintenance of physical life after present or future social life has ceased. It is better to be alive, some hold, even though stigmatized or socially dead.

This mythology places the stigmatized person in the position of expecting to be treated like anyone else of his social position although at the same time he recognizes that such expectations may not be realistic because of his disability. Goffman says that the disabled person in the presence of normal people may feel as if his privacy were being invaded—"a kind of nakedness experienced most acutely perhaps when children simply stare at him."[5] He joins other not-quite-people, such as policemen and children, in being considered approachable by strangers. He is asked personal questions about his conditions. Goffman states that this is considered proper providing the questioning is "sympathetic to the plight of persons of his kind."[6]

Goffman describes two categories of persons who significantly affect not only the stigmatized individual but public opinion about him. These classifications are the *own* and the *wise*. The *own* are sufferers from the same affliction. The *wise* are nonsufferers who have become or are considered knowledgeable and understanding of the sufferer's plight. Goffman distinguishes between two types of the *wise*. The first of these are persons such as doctors, nurses, social workers, police, bartenders, and so on with whom the individual relates because of his condition. For the purposes of this paper, I suggest these be called the *professional wise*. Goffman's second type includes those who participate in a primary group relationship with the individual. These I shall call the *intimate wise*.

Wright's description of the *inside* position corresponds to Goffman's *wise* and *own*. The *outside* position is maintained by strangers.

Goffman stresses that the main task for both the normal and the discredited in a mixed interaction is the management of tension. In the interactions between the discreditable and the normal, the principal task is the control of information about the defect.

These points are of prime importance to this paper and will be discussed at length under implications for nursing the discredited and the discreditable.

Wright summarizes the effects of being disabled—discredited—this way:

> [The disabled] "rarely has the kind of group sanction and personal valuation that endorse behavior reflecting the disability. Rather, the typical advice is to appear as much like a nondisabled person as possible, and his adjustment is often measured in terms of his skill as an actor. Even where there is a high degree of acceptance of the disability, there is a resistance against behavior that unnecessarily spotlights the handicap."[7]

After describing the trying psychological states of shame, self-pity, and inferiority, their effects on the disabled person, and the tendency to hide or weaken one's identification with a devalued group, Wright notes that "the vigilance required for covering up leads to strain, not only physically but also in interpersonal relations, for one must maintain a certain distance in order to fend off the frightening topic of the disability."[8]

Discussing the acting that the disabled must do in attempting to emulate the able-bodied person, she says that:

> Even should the person with a disability achieve or surpass the standards of normal performance, this by no means guarantees a success experience, for as long as he views his disability as a stigma, he can have only the feeling that at best he is an imperfect facsimile of a nondisabled person.[9]

Internalizing culturally derived standards of behavior, even about such matters as the proper way to walk or talk, can produce feelings of shame and guilt—shame at being inferior and guilt for violating a moral code. "Thus, the means of extricating oneself from more shame becomes the means of submerging oneself further."[10]

The desire to escape identification with a devalued group leads to avoidance of that group. This avoidance protects the disabled from reminders of his implicit membership in that group. Furthermore, avoidance removes the threat of discovery "for by the mere fact of contiguity he fears that likeness will be exposed; he may also sense that a person like himself will see through his mask."[11] However, avoidance of the group may be accompanied by guilt feelings.

One obstacle that the disabled faces in establishing understanding human relationships is the pretense by both participants that the disability does not exist. This pretense leads to "the feeling that the person with a disability is only seemingly accepted, i.e., that he is not really accepted at all."[12]

Wright describes the technics used by the disabled to manage the curiosity of others. These methods are:

> 1. attacking the offender with either biting sarcasm or dramatic prevarication
> 2. excluding the disability from the situation by an ostrich reaction or by redirecting the course of the interaction
> 3. minimizing the disability and preserving the relationship by good-natured levity and superficial discourse.[13]

I believe that the individual who is disabled (discredited) has problems in both the psychological and social spheres. His central activity is to manage tension in social interactions. Also, no matter what the disability is, I see similarities in both the psychosocial problems and the activities required to attenuate them. The activity required when discreditability is involved, on the other hand, is the management of information. With both the discredited and the discreditable, the nurse may be one of the *wise*.

A survey of recent nursing literature discloses a rather standard approach to the nursing care of the disabled. The usual paper is either a personal case history by a disabled author or an attempt by a knowing nurse author to communicate the status of the disabled, his response to attitudes and feelings expressed by others, and suggestions about how to treat him. Most of the literature deals with individuals in a specific disease category such as the blind, the cerebral palsied, those with muscular dystrophy, and so forth.

Generalizations applying to the conclusions and recommendations of all articles reviewed are: (1) that nurses interact with the discredited in the same manner as does the general society; (2) that the discredited are worthwhile, thinking, feeling beings who should be treated like anyone else except that one should do specified things for them; and (3) that the nurse who has common sense, empathy, and so forth will intuitively behave in a helpful manner.

Wershow departs somewhat from this uniform approach by suggesting that norms for the abnormal should be established when one is caring for the patient (and the family of the patient) who has muscular dystrophy.[14]

IMPLICATIONS FOR NURSING THE DISCREDITED

Two aspects of nursing practice relate to the individual who is discredited. The first is how the nurse assists the patient to manage tension during nurse-patient interactions. The second is how the nurse helps him manage tension with others.

In nurse-patient situations, both parties ordinarily will anticipate that the disability is a topic of mutual concern. Depending upon such variables as length of time discredited and previous experience with nurses, the patient may expect that the nurse knows the medical implications of his condition, is willing to assist him in regaining the best health possible, sympathizes with his suffering, and knows about others who have his condition.

Tension management in nurse-patient interactions has been discussed at length in the nursing literature. In "Reassurance," Gregg described fully the rationale, technics, and anticipated outcomes of nursing practice with such an objective.[15] (Also see Chapter *4*, "Shame" and Chapter 7, "Humor."

The second nursing aspect, helping the patient manage tension with others, has been less explored but is critically important. If one regards many of the teaching and rehabilitative tasks of nurses as assisting the patient to manage tension with others, it follows that the nurse aids him to develop a cirlce of *own* and *intimate wise* with whom he can experience support and decreased tension. This process is illustrated by the following examples:

1. When the family of an individual who is paraplegic is taught how to assist in his care, the primary objective is the prevention of complications. Secondary objectives include an adjustment in the family's values regarding paraplegics and acceptance of the individual as essentially unchanged in his humanness and therefore deserving of continued love.

2. When the patient who has had a laryngectomy is told about the Lost Chords, one objective is to assist him to learn techniques for speaking. Another is to provide him with a ready made group of *own* from whom he can learn technics of managing tension and with whom he can relax.

3. When the family of a mentally retarded child or of an alcoholic is referred to voluntary agencies, one objective is to provide the family with a source of information on technics for helping their

relative. An equally important objective is the provision of an audience and a climate for the expression of feelings, the family situation, and possible outcomes without shame. Further application of this frame of reference reveals that the intent of some nursing practices is to change the individual's status from discredited to discreditable. For example:
   a. After a patient has had a leg amputated, the primary objective of teaching and rehabilitation is to restore mobility. A secondary objective is to provide a lifelike prosthesis and thereby enable the patient to share information about his disability only with those whom he chooses.
   b. For the patient with a colostomy, the primary objectives of the nurse are maintenance of nutrition, elimination, and skin integrity. Of equal importance are measures that permit the patient to maintain his privacy.
   c. When a woman has had a mastectomy, the teaching related to a prosthesis is done solely to permit her to control the information about her disfigurement.

IMPLICATIONS FOR NURSING THE DISCREDITABLE

Despite the wide publicity given the ills suffered by today's prominent figures, the value of a person in this culture usually depreciates when information about his lack of health is available to coparticipants in an interaction. The individual is held increasingly responsible for becoming sick, probably because of modern medical knowledge and mass communication concerning preventive measures.

In this society, in which more and more information that previously was private now becomes a matter of public record, where such a word as "repersonalization" is coined and a movement of concern develops, it appears that the professional nurse must make a philosophical decision about the issue of privacy.

If the nurse believes that the patient has a right to control the spread of information about his health status, then she must devise technics and skills to help him prepare for this task.

Two factors that make the nurse a potential discreditor of individuals with whom she works are the growing emphasis on community participation and the need for adequate information to plan personalized nursing care plans. For example, certain types of behavior, life styles, and socioeconomic ills once were considered outside the purview of nursing. Now these are regarded, with an attendant increase in degree of involvement, as legitimate nursing concerns. There is increasing expectation that nurses understand and work with the so-called culturally deprived.

When hospitals had one routine for all patients—time for bathing, for eating, for visiting—there was less reason for the nurse to secure information which might discredit the patient. With the present trend to personalize care, the nurse often obtains such information. She needs personal information if she is to personalize care. The hospital patient may be asked for minute data regarding his sleeping, elimination, dietary, and exercise habits. Answering such questions may make him feel that he is discrediting himself.

Besides facing requests for information that is potentially discrediting, the patient encounters an army of personnel. He cannot be certain which workers have access to the information; but if he knows anything about the team approach in health practice, he can be sure that the information he supplies will have wide dissemination.

Four conclusions for nursing practice are that (1) the nurse must be able to justify the seeking of information, for both short and long term goals, (2) she must anticipate receiving some inaccurate information if the patient is cognizant of cultural mores, (3) she is responsible to the patient for controlling the spread of the information, and (4) she is responsible to the patient for assisting him to learn methods for managing information.

While the first three conclusions are important, I should like to concentrate on the fourth because it states a nursing responsibility that has been less emphasized in the past and promises to be one that can help determine nursing action.

The three examples of nursing and medical actions associated with helping the patient control information about his health status cited also demonstrated how the patient's status was changed from discredited to discreditable. A logical next step is the discussion of measures to assist the individual to control information about his discreditability.

In a Utopian world, alterations from the norm in health status undoubtedly would not be labelled stigmata. Since we are far from Utopia, it would seem logical to help the patient develop technics for protecting himself from attacks on his self-image. There should be no encouragement to the patient to deny his illness, but rather to identify those aspects of his behavior which cause him to snarl up his relationships with others.

Examples from everyday practice that illustrate this sort of help include the following:

1. Teaching the blind to "look at" the person speaking to them eases the tension of the interaction and at times prevents awareness that the blind person cannot see.

2. Suggesting that the ex-patient who has been hospitalized for mental illness supply this information only when asked protects him from stigmatization.

3. Diet teaching for the individual with diabetes not only assists in the maintenance of his health, but also permits him to control the spread of information about his illness.

4. Instruction in caring for the newborn not only safeguards the infant's health, but also helps the mother achieve the status of a good parent.

In each of these examples, the management of tension or information has been a fortuitous occurrence. Conscious application of the concept would enhance the total nursing care plan.

All of us have worries about our possible behavior in untried situations which we wish to control. Within the context of the nurse-patient interactional system, there are several factors that limit the patient's ability to control information about himself. Among these constraints are the stress ordinarily connected with health-illness matters, cultural expectations in terms of the sick role, and the health institution as a social system.

Applying the concept of stigma to some relatively simple yet often stressful situations provides new insights for nursing practice. For example:

1. When an adult is waiting to be immunized or to give blood, one concern is about pain. Another and perhaps the major concern is whether his behavior will meet adult norms. If he should cry or faint, he fears he may discredit himself.

2. The person awaiting general anesthesia worries about pain, outcome of the procedure and death. An equally important concern is of unintended disclosure of information, including unruly behavior.

3. When an individual knows but does not practice dental hygiene, he fears that a dental examination may provide information that will discredit him.

Active participation in the treatment program is a major responsibility of the sick person in this society. Examples are numerous and obvious of individuals who must provide discrediting data in order to enter the sick role: the person with diabetes who does not follow his treatment regimen, the individual who attempts suicide, the alcoholic who drinks, the person with emphysema who smokes, and many others.

IMPLICATIONS FOR NURSING EDUCATION

There are three principal implications in the concept of stigma for nursing education. The first implication relates to the special burdens borne by the stigmatized in a society which many contemporary authorities call alienated. The concept of alienation is presented in most nursing curricula. So, too, the concept of stigma should be a common thread throughout the nursing major because nurses are in daily contact with most persons whom this society defines as inferior—the mentally and physically disabled, minority group members, and lower socioeconomic group members.

Utilization of this concept, if one accepts Goffman's conclusions, could lead to a categorical presentation of content and thus decrease the discussion of typical patient and public responses to a specific disease entity. An understanding of stigma could make students more sensitive in planning care for individual patients.

The second implication is that nurse educators should consider the education of the nursing student as the preparation of the professionally *wise*. Although the nurse may become one of the *wise* with many and varied groups, it is doubtful if at present she is. Notable exceptions may be nurses in some rehabilitation, psychiatric or special care units. Possibly education to be one of the *wise* with many persons is not a feasible objective of an undergraduate program.

Integrating the stigma concept into nursing education dramatizes what seems to have been a latent purpose of clinical experience. Like the family of the discredited patient, the student nurse must achieve a drastic revision in values. This revision involves not one individual with a particular stigma, but large numbers of people with a multitude of conditions devaluated by the larger society. Nursing educators, perhaps intentionally, have tried to hasten this change in students' value systems by diversifying patient assignments and by emphasizing patients' strengths instead of weaknesses.

The third implication relates to the student nurse as discreditable. Applying the concept of stigma raises troubling questions. Do some stresses the student encounters arise from expectations that she is a fully accredited practitioner, at least a safe one? It seems apparent that the student, the instructor, and the patient collaborate to prevent the fact that she is not fully accredited from spoiling the student-patient interaction. What is the effect of the "as if" performances when a patient and student cooperate to keep the instructor from learning that the student's performance has been less than satisfactory? And how much stress does the student experience when the information that all have been trying to hide finally obtrudes and the student is discredited?

REFERENCES

1. Goffman, E.: Stigma: Notes on the Management of Spoiled Identity. p. 5. Englewood Cliffs, N.J., Prentice-Hall, 1963.
2. Wright, B.: Physical Disability—A Psychological Approach. p. 72. New York, Harper & Row, 1960.
3. Wright, B., *op. cit.,* p. 73.
4. Wright, B., *op. cit.,* p. 77.
5. Goffman, E., *op. cit.,* p. 16.
6. Goffman, E., *op. cit.,* p. 16.
7. Wright, B., *op. cit.,* p. 19.
8. Wright, B., *op. cit.,* p. 24.
9. Wright, B., *op. cit.,* p. 25.
10. Wright, B., *op. cit.,* p. 27.
11. Wright, B., *op. cit.,* p. 40.
12. Wright, B., *op. cit.,* p. 211.
13. Wright, B., *op. cit.,* pp. 212-216.
14. Wershow, H. J.: Muscular dystrophy: A positive approach to care. Nurs. Outlook, *14,* 1:49-53, January, 1966.
15. Gregg, D.: Reassurance. Am. J. Nurs., *55,* 2:171-174, February, 1955.

BIBLIOGRAPHY

Goffman, E.: Stigma: Notes on the Management of Spoiled Identity. Englewood Cliffs, N.J., Prentice-Hall, 1963.

Gregg, D.: Reassurance. Am. J. Nurs., *55,* 2:171-174, February, 1955.

Jackson, G. D.: How blind are nurses to the needs of the visually handicapped. Nurs. Outlook, *13,* 9:34, September, 1965.

MacGregor, F. M., *et al.:* Facial Deformities and Plastic Surgery: A Psychosocial Study. Springfield, Ill., Charles C Thomas, 1953.

Stoll, K.: A patient's humiliation. Am. J. Nurs., *65,* 10:95, October, 1965.

Wershow, H. J.: Muscular dystrophy: A positive approach to care. Nurs. Outlook, *14,* 1:49, January, 1966.

Wolanin, M. O.: They called the patient repulsive. Am. J. Nurs., *64,* 6:72, June, 1964.

Wright, B. A.: Physical Disability-A Psychological Approach. New York, Harper & Row, 1960.

18

Relationship Control

Mary R. Lawrence

In recent years, in nursing education and practice, increasing emphasis has been placed on the nature of the relationships the nurse has with the patient. Many books and articles have been published and numerous papers presented all stating in effect that in order to meet the patient's needs, the nurse must know how to conduct effective interactions; that in order to improve these contacts, she must have sufficient understanding of human behavior in general and specifically of the patient and of herself.

The literature also indicates that nurses are working toward the improvement of relationships to reinforce the therapeutic process. However, in the process of discussing these interactions with many nurses I have been impressed with the frequency of the comments, "The patient was controlling me and the relationship," "I *felt* I was controlling the relationships," and "I was *in* control." These statements had different meanings to me, yet each raised the same question: Is it important who controls? Apparently, in some situations it is and for that reason we need to deal directly with the concept of control and its ramifications.

The definitions of relationship and control will be made at this point in relation to context. A relationship will be considered the interaction of one or more individuals with another. The persons involved communicate; or at any rate, the action or behavior of each person affects the other. Control is not as easily defined unless its meaning is limited; for our purposes, we will consider control simply as one person exercising influence over the other.

While accepting this definition of control, one should at least be aware of the many other ways in which the word can be viewed, and is employed. Some dictionaries list as many as 15 categories. However, it is generally considered the act or fact of exercising power or authority; dominating or regulating; censuring or calling to account; curbing or holding from action, to list a few. The synonyms for control include: restrain, rule, direct, overpower, and command. This list also encompasses: check, subdue, govern and test. Exposure to control from the above lists can stimulate resistance, anger, fear, submission or acceptance in subsequent experiences depending on the outcome of each contact. Consequently, control can be received as positive or negative, that is, considered good or bad.

Man has increased and refined his ability to exercise control over other men's thoughts and actions, and this power has raised many fears of abuse. Will sophisticated methods of control be used to violate the ethics of a profession, infringe on the freedom of man, or impose the values of one on another? We shudder when we hear of brainwashing, prediction, constriction and manipulation. On the other hand, can we ignore the benefits derived as man endeavors to understand, predict, influence and control human behavior—his own and that of others? Is it not possible to exercise control relationships in nursing constructively for the benefit of the patient and recognize when they are not being used properly?

Dr. William Schutz has developed what he calls a three-dimensional theory of interpersonal behavior in an attempt to understand the behavior of individuals and groups. He states that each individual has a personal need for control. He defines this behavior as the "need to establish and maintain a satisfactory relation with people with respect to control and power." This satisfactory relation includes: "(1) a psychologically comfortable relation with people somewhere on a dimension ranging from controlling all the behavior of other people to not controlling any behavior of others and (2) a psychologically comfortable relation with people with respect to eliciting behavior from them somewhere on a dimension ranging from always being controlled by them to never being controlled by them."[1]

Macgregor and others who have analyzed nursing interactions feel that if the nurse of the future is to give effective care and obtain personal satisfaction, she must be able to work effectively with her super-ordinates, her peers, and her subordinates.[2] Yet it is generally assumed that nursing is practiced within a power hierarchy and it is here that care is given to patients. The hospital combines many lines of authority, from the administrator, the trustees, and the medical staff to the nursing staff. According to Wilson, the nursing staff operates as the day-to-day decision-makers who fix the hospital's image.[3] Yet nurses are the ones who take the orders issued all the way down the line. They are responsible for patient safety and care as set forth by the administrators of the hospital, and for therapeutic intervention as expected by each physician. The two lines of authority meeting at the patient's bedside can create problems for the staff as well as for the patient. The administrators want consistency and efficiency, the physician wants his orders carried out, and the patient wants care and cure.

Nurses are aware of this situation, but what about the patient? Ida Jean Orlando states "It is apparent that all kinds of things happen to patients. Many of their experiences are satisfying; others help them and still others distress them. Experiences which are satisfying and helpful to the patient presuppose that his care was at least adequate. However, in assuming the responsibility for optimum care, the nurse must understand how the patient's experiences may interfere with his sense of adequacy or well-being."[4]

Margaret Newman reported in Nursing Forum her results in attempting to determine the most common and urgent needs of hospitalized patients. She found, as did others before her, that these needs are emotional in nature. She was able to categorize them under identity, control, safety and comfort. The problems concerning control were especially interesting because patients were able to be rather specific about their feelings. These problems were: (1) lack of information regarding treatment or routine, (2) feelings of helplessness due to lack of control over matters pertaining to self, (3) manipulative behavior, (4) fear of loss of (self) control.[5]

When one considers the concept of control, he should be aware of it in a teaching-learning situation. Students will be having experiences in clinical areas which are part of a controlled institution—the hospital—and under the supervision of an instructor, who by the nature of her role must exercise some control over the student's behavior. The staff on the wards cannot be excluded since they are the representatives of the administration, plus the fact that they as individuals have the same basic human needs as the patients, administrators, physicians, other hospital workers, and the man on the street.

Because not all of nursing is practiced in the hospital, it is important to consider the nurse and patient in the community. In the community clinic or agency there are controls which affect all who are exposed to their facilities, patients and nurses alike. Lines of control may not be as rigid, but they are present. In the patient's home, even though the nurse goes in as a member of a helping profession, she is a guest and subject to the controls of that environment.

Usually the student nurse is in the late adolescent years with all the desires of youth to be of direct help to fellow humans. She has a great deal of enthusiasm, idealism and curiosity. These qualities and the true commitment to nursing can be guided and enhanced if individuals in nursing education and nursing service are aware of the influence they exert over her. Many graduate nurses today are highly skilled and dependable in giving physical care to patients; however, contemporary nursing literature makes the point that the interpersonal relationships between nurse and patient can affect the outcome of a patient's problem more than the routine technical procedures. It is important that both students and graduates understand and accept the responsibility for their own actions, including their management of interpersonal situations, which should be based on reliable observations and sound decisions derived from tested knowledge. The performance of the graduate assumes greater importance as she becomes the role model for the student.

Some individuals are more naturally skilled than others in the management of interpersonal relationships. However, intuition alone is never sufficient for consistently dealing with interpersonal problems in nursing. The educative process is essential. Some basic concepts important to effective relationships, such as theories of human growth, development, behavior and personality and of the individual in his social context must be learned. Exposure to experiences promoting the development of insights which are dependent upon theoretical knowledge must be supplied. Appreciation of the many facets of an individual or an institution can influence behavior and aid in the development of self-awareness which is basic to a therapeutic relationship. The educative process involves control on the part of both educator and student. That controlled relationships are a part of everyday living in the classroom, hospital or community is obvious. However, the reactions to these interactions will be based on the needs and the judgment of the persons involved.

It is a fact that we cannot live without controls of some kind; they are essential. As citizens of a nation that developed out of rebellion against too much control, we continue to object (quite overtly to-

Relationship Control 335

day) to any semblance of control which we can label arbitrary, unjust or unnecessary. Yet it is generally accepted that some type of control must be exercised in all of human relationships. Can one recognize this paradox and use it in a positive and therapeutic way? We must at least try, because someone has to be ready to exercise (or relinquish) control in a therapeutic interaction; control that is perfectly compatible with a democratic attitude and is not tyrannically exercised or submissively received.

The following clinical incidents will be used to demonstrate control relationships as they reinforce the feelings voiced by nurses in their comments, "The patient was controlling me and the situation," "I *felt* I was controlling the relationship," and "I was *in* control."

"The patient was controlling me and the situation."

1. Miss S. was to give Mr. A. his morning bath; when she told him so he shouted at her, "No, you will not. I can take my own bath when I want to, I don't want to be bothered. You get out of here, I'm tired of all this fooling around." Miss S. left the room and reported, "I tried to explain, but he just kept on yelling at me to get out."

2. Mr. P. was 2 days post-op and wanted to bathe and shave in the bathroom. The student said he was not strong enough and she would do it for him. The student left the room to get the bath equipment. On her return, the patient was in the middle of the room on his way to the bathroom. He said, "I can do it, leave me alone." He went into the bathroom and shut the door.

3. The student reported to her teacher that she was not able to talk to Miss K. about anything with meaning. The patient chatters all the time about insignificant things, and won't talk about herself or her condition. When her condition is mentioned she cries, "I don't know what to do."

4. While the student nurse was making a home visit, the patient continued to watch TV, and only nodded occasionally while the nurse was talking. Finally the student gave up and left.

5. There were many complaints from the night staff that Mr. L. was "uncooperative and always wants his own way." He kept his TV on after hours, he said, because he was not used to going to bed that early and he couldn't sleep anyway, even if he tried.

The previous incidents demonstrate that the patient's actions influenced the nurse to the extent that she was not able to follow through on her predetermined plan of care. This was managed by the use of different kinds of behavior. Mr. A. in incident no. 1 shouted to show his anger and hostility. He said he was "tired of being bothered." Because the nurse did not realize that Mr. A. had had a series of tests that morning, she became his target. There had been nothing he could do about the tests, but the nurse presented a situation that he could at least attempt to control by rejecting her care and ordering her to leave.

In incident no. 2, the patient actually separated himself from the nurse by going into the bathroom and shutting the door. Miss K., in the next nursing situation, was able to avoid the topics she feared, and the nurse felt were important, by introducing distractions. The fourth and fifth incidents showed the patients controlling the relationships by ignoring the nurse and hospital policy.

"I *felt* I was controlling the relationship."

6. Miss S., student nurse in Public Health, made a home visit. On several occasions during the visit, the patient mentioned that she was concerned about her husband. Each time the student continued with her teaching plan for the mother and her baby.

7. Mrs. R., student nurse, was to give nursing care to a patient who was several days post-op and who was ambulating. The student told the patient that she was going to give her a bath. The patient stated that she could take her own bath, but the nurse said, "Today you are my patient and I will bathe you."

8. The nurse was giving a liquid medication to a four-year-old girl who was resisting, crying and spitting the medication from her mouth. The child twisted her head sideways, back and forth, and gave the nurse a difficult time. Finally the nurse held the child's hands above her head, and another nurse assisted in holding the child down while the child's mouth was squeezed open and the medication poured in. Between coughing and crying, the medication was swallowed.

9. Mr. Q., with a long-standing permanent colostomy, was scheduled for daily irrigations, when previously his irrigations had been done every other day at home. The latter method had been effective over a long period of time, according to the patient, and he refused the irrigation. He expressed himself with a great deal of hostility. The team leader stated, "He will have his irrigation. It is the rule of the hospital and while he is here, he will do as he is told."

10. Mr. Z. was due for a treatment, but the doctor had not yet arrived. Mr. Z. put his light on several times within a 20-minute period to ask if the doctor had arrived. The nurse told Mr. Z. quite firmly that he would know when the doctor arrived and not to put his light on again as she did not have time to answer it.

When considering the incidents just presented, it is important to note that some of the kinds of behavior exhibited by the nurses in controlling the relationship were similar to those used by the patients. For instance, in situation no. 6, Miss S. gave no evidence of listening to her patient and in no. 7, Mrs. R. heard the patient, but ignored her comments and proceeded with her plan.

Incident no. 8 is an example of physical force, which is viewed by many as the least acceptable method of handling a situation though at times there may be no alternative. There is the necessity to recognize when there is an immediate need for medication and when there is time enough to try different methods of administration. The age of the child is important in determining the most reasonable method to use.

The team leader in no. 9 invoked hospital rules as a reason for not giving consideration to the patient's request. And in incident no. 10, the lack of time became the reason. The patient's need for relief from anxiety went unrecognized. In these last two incidents, the nurses' remarks were delivered with a great deal of hostility.

In the preceding incidents, the means used to control the actions of others were force, negativism, refusal and hostility, silence, avoidance, withdrawal, insignificant chatter, yelling, crying and the imposition of rules from those in authority. Awareness that these methods are being utilized is not always present. But nurses must recognize them for what they are; otherwise effective patient care is in jeopardy. It is possible to handle most of the situations already listed in a more therapeutic manner. In so doing the nurse can manage the interaction by first analyzing the facts and then deciding when it may be advantageous to the situation to yield control and to what extent.

"I was *in* control."

In incident no. 1, Miss S. returned to the patient's bedside after conferring with the team leader and looking at the patient's chart. She began by saying, "Mr. A., you have had quite an uncomfortable morning...." She followed by encouraging him to tell about the tests and offering him the choice of having his bath or resting awhile first. Because she gave some consideration to his feelings and did not attempt to force him into a bath, he was able to elect to go ahead with the care necessary. The nurse did not feel that the patient was attacking her personally. She was concerned about him as the patient and not with the danger of his attempting to control the situation; consequently, she was able to influence his behavior and carry out her plan for care.

The same approach could have been used in the second incident. Some consideration to the patient's desire to bathe and shave in the bathroom might have helped. Was it possible for him to do this in stages, or do one in the bathroom and the other in the bed, or use a wheelchair? On the other hand, would the patient be up to going to the bathroom? If not, the nurse would have to make sure the care was taken in bed or at the bedside, and that the patient was given a rational explanation. In either instance, she remains in control of the situation.

Incidents 7 and 9 can be considered here also. If the patient is capable of giving himself care, should the nurse allow him this opportunity to exercise some control? She still remains in control unless the hospital rules are especially rigid, or unless she has an overwhelming desire to do it herself.

The patient (in incident no. 3), who doesn't talk about herself or her condition, is not unusual, and so the nurse must consider her own motives. Is it the patient's or the nurse's needs that are to be met? If it is the patient's needs, then the nurse must work at developing a relationship of trust with the patient so that feelings can be expressed, or else attempt to find someone in whom the patient can confide.

Hospital policy or lack of time (such as in incidents 9 and 10) can be legitimate reasons for determining the kind of care a patient receives. However, they should not be used to impose unnecessary controls over the patient's behavior so that the nurse can ignore her responsibility of giving effective care to the patient.

Is the patient who is chattering and crying to avoid talking about her problems (no. 3) so different in her behavior from the nurse who continues with her teaching plan and doesn't allow the patient to express her concerns? (no. 6)

The forms of behavior used to control a relationship can be recognized, but it should be realized that these are also reactions to the feelings of being controlled. For instance, incident no. 1 can be used again to demonstrate this. Mr. A. felt controlled because of the doctor's orders and hospital routine; he reacted with angry behavior in an attempt to regain control. Miss S. could have retaliated with anger in order to maintain control. Or she could have left the room and avoided the patient, and as a result both would have felt angry, rejected and helpless. Instead, she was aware of a nontherapeutic atmosphere and made inquiries to obtain more information that would help in determining his needs. The result was an effective relationship in which she allowed the patient some control, and yet she remained *in* control by influencing his behavior in a positive way.

Some very common everyday nursing situations have been used to demonstrate the effectiveness of relationship control. Consideration of this concept can provide a framework for action and for the teaching of other concepts.

Relationship control is essential to the maintenance of a therapeutic interaction. As the nurse becomes increasingly astute in recognizing when she moves to and from the position of controller and controllee, she tends to become more adept in maintaining this relationship. In reality she remains in full control of the overall relationship between nurse and patient.

REFERENCES

1. Schutz, W. C.: FIRO: A Three-Dimensional Theory of Interpersonal Behavior, p. 18, New York, Holt, Rinehart & Winston, 1958.
2. Macgregor, F. C.: Social Science in Nursing: Applications for the Improvement of Patient Care. p. 15. New York, Russell Sage Foundation, 1960.
3. Wilson, R. N.: The social structure of a general hospital. *In* Skipper, J. K., Jr., and Leonard, R. C. (eds.): Social Interaction and Patient Care. pp. 233-244. Philadelphia, J. B. Lippincott, 1965.
4. Orlando, I. J.: The Dynamic Nurse-Patient Relationship: Function, Process and Principles. p. 5. New York, G. P. Putnam's Sons, 1961.
5. Newman, M. A.: Identifying and meeting patients' needs in short-span nurse-patient relationships. Nurs. Forum, 5, 1:79, 1966.

BIBLIOGRAPHY

Abdellah, F. G., *et al.:* Patient-Centered Approaches to Nursing. New York, Macmillan, 1960.

Abramovits, A. B., and Burnham, E.: Self Understanding in Professional Education. Madison, Wisconsin State Board of Health, 1965.

Erikson, E. H.: Insight and Responsibility: Lectures on the Ethical Psychoanalytic Insight. New York, W. W. Norton & Co., 1964.

Glasser, W.: Reality Therapy: A New Approach to Psychiatry. New York, Harper & Row, 1965.

Hassenplug, L. W.: Editorial. J. Nurs. Educ., *3,* 3:2-3, August, 1964.

Hays, S. I., and Anderson, H. C.: Are nurses meeting patient's needs? Am. J. Nurs., *63,* 12:96-99, 1963.

Jourard, S. M.: The Transparent Self. Princeton, Van Nostrand, 1964.

Macgregor, F. C.: Social Science in Nursing: Applications for the Improvement of Patient Care. New York, Russell Sage Foundation, 1960.

Newman, M. A.: Identifying and meeting patient's needs in short-span nurse-patient relationships. Nurs. Forum, *5,* 1:76-86, 1966.

Orlando, I. J.: The Dynamic Nurse-Patient Relationship: Function, Process and Principles. New York, G. P. Putnam's Sons, 1961.

Peplau, H. E.: Interpersonal Relations in Nursing. New York, G. P. Putnam's Sons, 1952.

Schutz, W. C.: FIRO: A Three-Dimensional Theory of Interpersonal Behavior. New York, Holt, Rinehart & Winston, 1958.

Skipper, J. K., Jr., and Leonard, R. C.: Social Interaction and Patient Care. Philadelphia, J. B. Lippincott, 1965.

Sullivan, H. S.: The Interpersonal Theory of Psychiatry. New York, W. W. Norton & Co., 1953.

Thibaut, J. W., and Kelley, H. H.: The Social Psychology of Groups. New York, John Wiley & Sons, 1959.

Ulrich, R., *et al.:* Control of Human Behavior. Chicago, Scott, Foresman & Co., 1966.